Breaking Free from Depression

Pathways to Wellness

Jesse H. Wright, MD, PhD

Laura W. McCray, MD

THE GUILFORD PRESS
New York   London

© 2012 The Guilford Press
A Division of Guilford Publications, Inc.
72 Spring Street, New York, NY 10012
www.guilford.com

Library of Congress Cataloging-in-Publication Data

Wright, Jesse H.
    Breaking free from depression : pathways to wellness / Jesse H. Wright and Laura W. McCray.
        p.   cm. — (The guilford self-help workbook series)
    Includes bibliographical references and index.
    ISBN 978-1-60623-919-3 (pbk.)
    1. Depression, Mental—Popular works.   2. Self-care, Health—Popular works.
I. McCray, Laura W.   II. Title.
    RC537.W743 2012
    616.85′27—dc23
                                                                2011024716

Dr. Jesse H. Wright may receive compensation from Empower Interactive and Mindstreet, publishers of software for computer-assisted therapy of depression described in this book.

To our family members,
who have given us so much loving support:

Marion Wright
Susanne Wright
Ian and Jesse McCray
Andrew, Stacy, Ada, and Harriet Wright

Contents

Preface

One of the great challenges of depression is that it can rob you of the very powers you need to put it behind you. When you need energy to tackle the problem, you may find yourself exhausted. Just when you need a solid dose of self-confidence, you may be riddled with self-doubt. And when you need hope that things will improve, you may feel that a cloud of gloom has been cast over your dreams for the future. We've seen so many people struggle with this problem. But fortunately, we've also seen them emerge from the darkness of depression. Their joy in gaining power over depression has enlivened us and galvanized our work over many years. Their recoveries have inspired this book.

If you've been living with depression for years, you may very well have tried valiantly to follow the path of a single treatment that, statistically speaking, works for many people but turns out not to work very well for you. Perhaps you then turned to a second and even a third treatment but still feel beaten down by depressive symptoms. Why does feeling better have to be so hard?

The answer begins with the fact that, when it comes to depression, one "size" definitely does *not* fit all. Research has found that there are many possible causes of depression, and thus a single form of treatment may not work for everyone—or it might not work by itself. The good news is that the discovery of this diversity of causes has revealed many effective ways to treat depression. The six paths to recovery described in this book are all evidence based, meaning that a substantial body of research, along with clinical experience such as ours, has documented their benefits. Even better, many of these methods incorporate actions you can take yourself to reduce symptoms.

In our work as a psychiatrist and family physician, we've found that developing a multifaceted plan that includes some practical and effective self-help strategies can smooth the road to recovery. Therefore our goal in this book is to make the six paths—*thoughts-action, biology, relationships, lifestyle, spirituality,* and *mindfulness*—as accessible and easy to use as they can be. Each path is based on a different way of understanding depression and overcoming it. Our worksheets, tips, and concise descriptions of the six paths are designed to walk you through all of the key options, allowing you to select the ideas that appeal to you—the choices that you believe could give you the most help. You can keep it simple and draw methods from just one path or a small number of paths. Or you can gradually build a multilayered plan that taps into resources from many of the paths. Whatever itinerary you choose, this book is intended to help you overcome the road-blocks that have prevented you from achieving wellness in the past.

One of those obstacles might be that you've heroically tried over and over to just "snap out of it." We know that doesn't work. As we tell all of our patients, depression is a medical illness. Having the illness is not your fault, and neither is the fact that the road to recovery can be difficult to map. But just like other complex medical problems, such as diabetes and heart disease, depression deserves to be understood fully and treated effectively. This principle is at the heart of how we treat our patients, and this book reflects the diverse clinical experiences we have had with trying to unravel the enigma of depression for them in both psychiatric and family medicine settings. As a psychiatrist who is a professor and director of the Depression Center at the University of Louisville, one of us (JHW) has geared his clinical and research efforts toward improving the treatment of depression for more than 30 years. The other (LWM) is a family physician who teaches and has a clinical practice at the University of Vermont. She also completed a master's degree program and research fellowship at the University of Pennsylvania that focused on treatment of depression in primary care practice.

Year after year, we have seen women and men recover from depression by adopting a combination of well-researched treatments such as cognitive-behavior therapy and other proven psychotherapies; antidepressant medications; lifestyle modifications such as simple shifts in eating, sleeping, and activity habits; and other health-promoting practices that increase overall well-being and even help people regain a sense of meaning in life. This abundance of methods can offer you and many others facing the same challenges a hope-filled future.

Because your experience of depression is unique, and you deserve to have a plan for wellness that *does* fit you, this book starts by helping you understand some basics about the diagnosis of depression in general and then about your depression in particular. Next we give a "satellite view" of the six paths so you can start to get a sense of the direction you'd like to take. You can then explore all the paths in more depth or pick the one you'd like to get started on first and then try other paths as needed. The final chapter will help you pull all the elements of your plan together, troubleshoot obstacles to success, and design strategies for staying well.

If you are receiving professional treatment, we encourage you to take this book with you to appointments and to ask your doctor or therapist to weave the self-help exercises, tip lists, and other suggested activities into your therapy. We've developed the book to help facilitate effective professional treatment. If you do not have a doctor or therapist, you can use the book to learn more about effective therapies and to build skills for coping with depression.

To our knowledge, we are the only father–daughter team to write a self-help book for depression. As you might expect, the opportunity to work together on a book that can help with a problem that affects so many people but can respond so well to treatment is something we treasure greatly. We hope that reading and using this book will empower you as much as writing it has moved us. And we wish you great success on your path to wellness.

Authors' Note

To help explain strategies for overcoming depression, we describe many examples of people who have received treatment for this problem. Although we draw these examples from our work as a practicing psychiatrist (JHW) and family physician (LWM), we use composites of our clinical experiences. Names, genders, ages, personal backgrounds, and details of treatment have been modified so that none of our patients can be identified. However, we use the convention of writing about people as if we have actually treated them, to improve the flow and appeal of the text. To avoid repeated use of the phrase "he or she" (or exclusive use of either "he" or "she"), we alternate use of personal pronouns when describing clinical examples.

This book is not intended as a substitute for treatment with a doctor or professional therapist but is offered only as a self-help guide to understanding and coping with depression. The depression questionnaire introduced in Chapter 1 and used throughout the book should not be used as a method of diagnosing depression or assessing suicide risk. Readers who suffer from significant depression should see a health care professional for diagnosis and treatment. Persons who have suicidal thoughts or plans should seek help immediately.

Acknowledgments

Chris Benton and Kitty Moore, our editor and publisher at The Guilford Press, were wonderfully encouraging partners and always gave "spot-on" advice. We wish that every author could have the pleasure of working with these two talented and affirming people. We also want to thank Carol Wahl and Heather Jones, who provided much needed assistance in preparing the manuscript, and Ann Schaap, Deborah Dobiecz, and Leslie Pancratz, librarians at Norton Healthcare in Louisville, who helped us find key scientific articles about the treatments described in the paths to wellness. A special note of appreciation goes to Tom Peterson, Chair of the Department of Family Medicine at the University of Vermont, and Allan Tasman, Chair of the Department of Psychiatry and Behavioral Sciences at the University of Louisville, who supported our work on this book.

Several experts in different treatment approaches kindly agreed to read chapters and give us feedback. We deeply appreciate the assistance of Giovanni Fava, MD, who advised us on developing the chapter on well-being in the thoughts–action path; Michael E. Thase, MD, who assisted with the biology path; John Markowitz, MD, who gave excellent suggestions on the relationship path; Ryan Wetzler, PsyD, who made recommendations for the section on sleep for the lifestyle path; Kris Small, PhD, and Allan Josephson, MD, who gave thoughtful recommendations on the spiritual path; Paul Salmon, PhD, who provided guidance on the mindfulness path; and Mary Hosey, LCSW, who helped review the overall concept for the book. The contributions of all of these colleagues and friends gave us important support in our efforts to produce a book that gives accurate and up-to-date information on how to overcome depression.

1
Getting Started

Chapter Highlights

▸ Going on the offense against depression

▸ Diagnosing depression

▸ Measuring depression and charting your progress

If you have experienced depression, you know how much it hurts. You've suffered from low moods and difficulty enjoying life. Probably there have been strings of days filled with worries and many nights of troubled sleep. You may even have passed through some especially difficult times when it seemed like your problems were too much to bear.

Perhaps you have already had some success in your battle against depression. Or maybe you are still struggling to learn how to get symptoms under control. Wherever you are in your path to recovery, you're probably searching for answers on how to beat this disease and keep your life headed in a positive direction.

We wrote this workbook to help people find the answers that work best for them and develop practical and effective recovery plans. For most people, these plans will include getting professional help. But as practicing doctors we know that our patients who spend time outside treatment sessions learning about depression and taking actions to combat this disease often have better results.

Because you have decided to read this book, you may be like so many of our patients who want to do more than simply take a pill for depression. Even if an antidepressant is a cornerstone of your treatment, you will want to know more about how it works, how to manage side effects if they occur, and which medications to consider if the current prescription isn't fully effective. And if you are like most people with depression, you will have personal stresses, self-doubts, relationship issues, physical illnesses, or a variety of other concerns that may play a role in the depression. Addressing these types of problems can be an important part of the recovery process.

This book will help you learn about the best treatments available today and how to put them into action. The starting point for our work together is to lay out an overall strategy for overcoming depression.

Going on the Offense against Depression

Depression can sap energy and motivation, make it harder to accomplish tasks, and lead to a sense of defeat and demoralization. People who have had depression for a while often feel that they are only playing defense—just hanging on in the face of a sea of problems. When we see people with depression in our medical practices for the first time, we try our best to appeal to their fighting spirit, to somehow get them back on offense.

There are three key actions that you can take to break out of depression and regain control of your life.

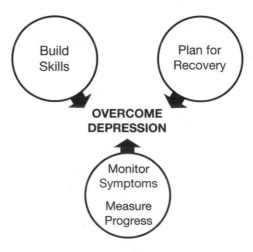

Action 1: Build Skills

Our patients who recover from depression often acquire a number of useful depression-fighting skills along the way. You may already have some of these skills and are putting them into action. However, for most people there is usually room to add to and sharpen their tools for getting depression under control.

If you wanted to build your skills in a sport, a hobby, or an area of work performance, you would need to practice. You would build your competence gradually as you learned the basics and then gained more and more experience. The same process holds true for becoming skilled in managing depression.

Sometimes when people who are depressed first hear about the prospect of learning skills to manage the disease they have thoughts such as: "It will be too much work ... I don't have the energy to do anything ... I'd rather just take a pill." Are you having any similar thoughts about the difficulty of building your abilities to combat this disease? If so, the negative and pessimistic thinking style of depression may be clouding your vision.

You may be having trouble seeing that you do have the capacity to grow your strengths and learn new ways of moving from depression to wellness. Later in the book (in Chapter 4, "Fighting Negative Thinking") we'll help you learn how to recognize and change the depressive thinking that may be standing in the way of your recovery.

The process of building skills does not have to be too hard. You can target a few things that you want to learn the most or think may have the biggest payoff, and you can take it at your own pace. Or, if you are feeling very positive about getting involved in the learning process and are excited to get to work, you can stake out a more ambitious agenda. Either way, we believe that you have the potential for gaining valuable skills that can help you on your path to wellness.

Some of the depression-fighting skills that we teach in this book are listed in the first exercise. You can use the checklist to get a preliminary picture of what you might like to accomplish.

We have included a number of learning exercises in this book that we hope will be interesting, stimulating, and helpful in building your skills for overcoming depression. You may want to go through the book in sequence, taking each chapter in turn. Or you may decide you want to focus only on certain topics such as "Getting the Most from Antidepressants" (Chapter 8) or "Restoring Energy and Enjoying Life" (Chapter 5). In Chapter 3, we will help you take an inventory of your interests and potentials and then plot a course for effective change.

Action 2: Plan for Recovery

Treatment for depression works, but many people are not getting the full benefit of the useful therapies that are available. One of the most startling statistics we have seen is that only 20% of people in the United States who have depression are receiving adequate treatment for it. Could you be one of those people who are missing out on therapy methods that could offer answers?

QUICK TIPS   To give yourself the best possible chance of recovery from depression:

- Choose at least one treatment approach that has been scientifically proven to be effective.

- Give treatment a full opportunity to work.

- Consider developing a comprehensive plan that is tailored to your needs, strengths, and interests.

You may be thinking, "How can I know which treatments are effective and which may be the best for me?" In Chapter 3, we outline the most important approaches to depression and explain the concept of "evidence-based" therapy—relying on scientifically tested interventions for the core of your treatment program. In later chapters, we also suggest guidelines for giving treatment a full opportunity to work. For example, you will

Overcoming Depression: A Skills Checklist

Skill	I already have some of this skill	I want to build this skill
Find and effectively work with a doctor and/or therapist		
Identify medical illnesses and drugs for physical problems that can cause depression		
Change negative, worrisome, or self-defeating thoughts		
Get better organized and complete tasks		
Increase energy and stimulate interest in life		
Have healthy self-esteem		
Enhance feelings of well-being		
Understand medication options for depression		
Minimize and manage side effects of antidepressants		
Deal effectively with relationship issues that may be affecting depression		
Improve sleep, diet, exercise, or other habits		
Find a deeper sense of meaning or purpose		
Spend less time worrying and being stressed; spend more time being aware and appreciating the good things in life		
Troubleshoot problems in reaching full recovery		
Prevent depression from returning		

learn about the optimal dose and duration for treatment with antidepressants and what to do if the first medication doesn't give you full relief.

Sometimes the path to recovery from depression can follow a single track. One possibility is that people can have a superb response to the first medication they try; the antidepressant seems to do the trick, and nothing more is needed. Other people may choose to focus exclusively on psychotherapy (talk therapy) and find this method relieves depression for them. Still others may opt for alternative, nontraditional approaches and have success. Yet for most people a more comprehensive plan for recovery may lead to the best outcome.

We have several reasons for recommending that you look at more than one option for building your plan for recovery from depression.

1. Although people with depression usually have similar symptoms, everyone has a unique blend of personal history, current concerns, strengths, and preferences. Instead of a "one size fits all" approach, many people with depression, and their doctors and therapists, prefer an individualized, multifaceted plan.
2. Research has shown that there can be a wide variety of contributors to depression, such as genetics, medical illnesses, psychological influences, and social stresses. And there is scientific evidence that diverse treatment approaches can be effective.
3. More than 30 years of studies on medication and psychotherapy for depression have found that combining the two treatments can provide a greater overall treatment benefit than receiving medication or psychotherapy alone.

To give an example of how a comprehensive recovery plan might be developed, we'll introduce you to Kate, a woman who had been struggling with depression but eventually had success in overcoming this problem.

Kate's Story

Kate's depression had been dragging on for more than 6 months. It seemed to have been triggered by a relationship breakup that rocked her self-esteem and drained her energy and motivation. As so often happens with depression, she gradually pulled away from many of the activities and relationships that used to give her enjoyment and a sense of purpose. It was as if the depression were driving her into a shell.

Kate was still able to go to work, but when she came home she spent much of her time alone, staring at the TV or doing "mindless" tasks. After Kate had made repeated excuses for avoiding social activities, many of her friends either called her only infrequently or had stopped calling her altogether. As the gloom of depression intensified, Kate began to think of herself as a "failure" and a "loser."

Prior to becoming depressed, Kate had led a fairly healthy lifestyle. She took yoga classes, rode a bicycle two or three times a week, or went to the gym to do aerobic exercise. She sang in a choir and attended church services regularly. Now, however, the only activity she enjoyed outside of work was having dinner with her family on Sunday evenings. Kate had tried dating again about 3 months ago, but the relationship foundered. Now she had decided that she was "better off alone."

When Kate first consulted one of us for treatment of depression, she mentioned that she had tried an antidepressant for about 4 weeks, but it didn't seem to help. She had also had three counseling sessions with an employee assistance professional. However, Kate had not yet had the opportunity to benefit fully from therapies that have been proven scientifically, and there appeared to be several promising opportunities for helping her overcome depression.

There were other encouraging signs that suggested a good outcome was likely. Kate was very interested in learning how to control her symptoms. She had many strengths to use in the fight against depression, as we describe in the next section of the chapter. And she appeared much more hopeful after we worked together to sketch out some plans to help get her life back on track.

If you have read other books on depression or have been coached on depression by a doctor or therapist, you may be starting to get some ideas about what Kate might need to do to get better. Even if you're just starting to learn about depression, you may be thinking of options for helping Kate. Is an antidepressant the only answer? Or are other possibilities coming to mind? If Kate was starting to develop a comprehensive plan to fight depression, what might she consider including in the plan? As you work through this book, we hope you'll get lots of good ideas for tackling depression. If you're in Kate's position, we hope you'll be able to collaborate effectively with your doctor or therapist to find solutions that lead to recovery.

The treatment plan that Kate developed included several different strategies. We briefly outline the plan here. Later in the book, you will learn more about how to organize multifaceted plans for overcoming depression.

Kate's Plan

1. *Identify and use personal strengths.* As happens so frequently with depression, all Kate had been able to see was her problems and her frailties. She had been downplaying or ignoring many personal strengths, such as her musical interest and talents, excellent work performance, an ability to be a good friend, a sense of humor, and a variety of interests in activities such as cooking, bicycling, and gardening. Part of her plan was to recognize and tap her personal strengths as she fought depression.
2. *Give medication another try.* After learning more about the possible benefits and risks of antidepressant therapy, Kate decided to become more aggressive in using medication to fight depression. Although the first medication that we chose didn't lead to a full recovery, she stuck with treatment and within 10 weeks was able to find a medication plan that worked well.
3. *Start cognitive-behavior therapy (CBT).* This form of psychotherapy has specialized methods for depression and has been shown to be effective in more than 300 randomized research studies (in which the study participants receive a treatment as opposed to a placebo or a control therapy). CBT targets negative thinking in depression (for example, low self-esteem, unproductive self-talk, hopelessness) and behaviors that make the depression worse (for example, inactivity, isolation,

helplessness, procrastination)—problems that Kate had been experiencing over the past few months. The methods are usually easy to understand and often can be learned fairly rapidly. CBT also encourages use of self-help to amplify the benefits of treatment. Because CBT is such a powerful approach to depression, we draw heavily from its methods in this workbook (see, for example, Chapter 4, "Fighting Negative Thinking," and Chapter 5, "Restoring Energy and Enjoying Life").

4. *Gradually resume exercise and other healthy activities.* Exercise has been shown to be an effective treatment for depression, and it obviously has many other health benefits as well. Kate's participation in CBT helped her re-engage in exercise and also gave her tools for rekindling interest in things that could give her a sense of meaning and pleasure. Resuming stimulating activities, especially ones that involve increased contact with people, is often a key element of successful recovery plans.

If you want to develop your own comprehensive plan, you can explore the possibilities by talking with a doctor, a therapist, a spiritual counselor, or someone else who has experience in helping people. And you can use this book to learn about different strategies for coping with depression. Your plan does not have to be complex, but it should have several good prospects for how to fight symptoms. In Chapter 3 we will help you recognize your best opportunities for change.

Take a moment now to do another self-help exercise. Use the worksheet on page 8 to record some of the treatments or strategies that you may have tried for depression. Then do a bit of brainstorming about some methods that you think might help. As you read through this book, you'll be able to investigate whether these ideas are worth pursuing.

Action 3: Monitor Symptoms and Measure Progress

Research has shown that using rating scales to measure symptoms helps both patients and doctors stay on course toward reaching goals. Also, studies of the effectiveness of efforts to change behavior, such as sticking with an exercise plan or a diet, have solidly supported the value of self-monitoring or logging (keeping a written record). One example of the value of monitoring and measuring is the program at the gym where one of us works out on a regular basis. This gym uses a computerized recording system that keeps track of all of the exercise done on both aerobic and strength training machines and gives regular feedback to users on their progress. Seeing these reports strengthens motivation and provides guidance for taking positive steps to move forward.

FAST FACT Scientific studies have found that efforts to measure and monitor depression enhance treatment.

Checklist of Ways to Fight Depression

Instructions: A partial list of commonly used strategies for fighting depression is provided in this worksheet. Place check marks in the columns to indicate whether you have tried this approach, whether it has helped, and whether it may have potential to help. Please remember that things you tried in the past may not have been given a full opportunity to work. For example, maybe you had some counseling sessions that weren't useful, but a different therapist or a more specific therapy for depression could lead to a breakthrough.

Method or Strategy	I've Tried It	It Has Helped	It Hasn't Helped	It May Have Potential to Help
Using antidepressants or other medication for depression				
Obtaining counseling or psychotherapy				
Exercising or making other lifestyle changes				
Light therapy				
Looking for a medical illness or medication that could cause depression				
Meditating				
Reading a self-help book				
Tapping spiritual resources				
Working to draw strength from and/or improve relationships				

There are three core opportunities to use measuring and monitoring techniques to strengthen treatment plans for depression.

QUICK The three ways that you can use measuring and monitoring in your plan for fight-
TIPS   ing depression are:

- Use rating scales or questionnaires to help define the problem.
- Use rating scales to monitor progress.
- Write out and review self-help exercises.

---

1. *Use rating scales or questionnaires to help define the problem.* Do I have depression? What type of depression is it? How severe are the symptoms? Your doctor will ask questions to help define the problem because it is very important to know the diagnosis before suggesting a treatment plan. An example of the importance of making an accurate diagnosis is that a common type of mood disorder called "major depression" often responds very well to antidepressant medication. But antidepressants may be of little value for less severe forms of depression.

Some doctors use rating scales routinely, but research has shown that doctors don't employ these valuable tools as often as they might. In the next section of this chapter, you will be able to use a rating scale to give you a better idea of what your symptoms mean.

CAUTION When you use rating scales, keep in mind that self-rating scales can't take the place of an assessment by a health care professional. But you can learn a lot from completing a rating scale, and you can share the results with your doctor or therapist.

2. *Use rating scales to monitor progress.* We suggest that you use the depression rating scale on page 15 to check your progress in getting over depression. You could take the depression test every week or every other week to see how you're coming along. We use this depression test routinely in our clinical practices and find that it provides very valuable information. Of course, it's always heartening to see people recovering from depression. The positive feedback from seeing declining rating scale scores helps all of us feel good. But even when progress isn't all that patient and practitioner desire, we can take stock of the results, consider the alternatives, and adjust the plan to put the person back on a path to wellness.

3. *Write out and review self-help exercises.* Throughout this book, we recommend self-help exercises that will help you build skills. Some of these exercises will work best if you do them more than once. For example, if you're learning to reduce negative thinking, a tool called a "Thought Change Record" (described in Chapter 4) can be used multiple times to identify and modify depressing thoughts or worries. People who use this form usually get better at spotting and changing negative thoughts if they practice doing it regularly.

Many of the self-help exercises from this book can be downloaded from The Guilford

Press website (*www.guilford.com/breakingfreeforms*). You can print them out or copy them from the book.

QUICK TIP   We strongly recommend that you take the time to monitor your progress with the rating scale in this book and that you fill in the exercise forms and review what you wrote. These efforts can have a big payoff in gaining skills for overcoming depression.

Diagnosing Depression

Now that we have outlined the actions you can take to "go on the offense" against depression, it's time to start putting these strategies to work. In this last section, we'll help you learn to sort out the different types of depression and measure and monitor symptoms.

Types of Depression

The American Psychiatric Association has developed specific criteria for diagnosing the different forms of depression. The full criteria are published in the fourth edition of the *Diagnostic and Statistical Manual* of the American Psychiatric Association. An abbreviated form of the criteria is provided here so that you can start to think about what kind of depression you might have.

Major Depressive Disorder

Major depression is the most common form of depression that responds to antidepressants and/or psychotherapy.

FAST FACTS
- About 17% of people in the United States will suffer from major depression during their lifetime.
- In any given year 7 to 8% will have a depressive episode.
- The annual cost of depression in the United States is about $87 billion for lost productivity and treatment.

CRITERIA FOR DIAGNOSING MAJOR DEPRESSION

The diagnosis is made when a person has *five* of the following symptoms nearly every day for at least 2 weeks and one of the first two symptoms is present*:

*Reprinted with permission from the *Diagnostic and Statistical Manual of Mental Disorders, Fourth Edition, Text Revision.* Copyright 2000 by the American Psychiatric Association.

1. Depressed mood
2. Loss of interest or decreased ability to experience pleasure
3. Low energy or excessive fatigue
4. Insomnia or sleeping too much
5. Decreased appetite and/or weight loss; or increased appetite and/or weight gain
6. Low self-esteem or guilt feelings
7. Decreased ability to concentrate
8. Getting agitated or being slowed down
9. Thoughts of suicide or wishing you were dead

CAUTION
- If you are having significant thoughts of suicide, contact a health care professional immediately.
- Depression increases the risk of suicide, but getting help saves lives.
- Professional help is always needed when suicidal thoughts are present.

Dysthymic Disorder

Dysthymic disorder is a chronic lower-grade depression that is present all the time for at least 2 years. People with this condition have a depressed mood most of the day, more days than not, and they have at least two other symptoms of depression. Often people who have dysthymic disorder go on to develop major depression later in their lives.

Minor Depression

The term "minor depression" is used in the American Psychiatric Association diagnostic system, but we think that using the term "minor" can downplay the extent of the problem. Any depression can cause significant suffering. This diagnosis is made when depressive symptoms have lasted for at least 2 weeks but the full criteria for major depression (five depressive symptoms) haven't been met. One of the differences between minor depression and dysthymic disorder is that dysthymic disorder lasts a very long time (more than 2 years without relief). Many of the people with depression who are treated by primary-care doctors may have minor depression. Thus there is some concern that antidepressants can be prescribed to people who won't benefit from them. We discuss the usefulness of antidepressants for the different types and severity levels of depression in more detail in Chapter 8.

FAST FACTS
- Research studies have shown that antidepressants can be very helpful for many people with major depression.
- But antidepressants may work no better than a placebo (sugar pill) for "minor depression" or other milder forms of depression.

Bipolar Disorder

Bipolar disorder is characterized by mood swings in both the depressed and manic directions. When a person with bipolar disorder is depressed, the symptoms are just like those of major depression. During manic or hypomanic (a less extreme upswing) periods, the symptoms are usually the opposite of depression—feeling too good, having too much energy, and being overactive.

FAST About 4% of people in the United States develop bipolar disorder in their life-
FACT time.

People with bipolar disorder can have many different patterns of mood swings. For some, depressive spells far outnumber the times they develop mania or hypomania. Others mostly experience manic symptoms and very rarely become depressed. Sometimes the mood swings occur many years apart, and people feel completely normal between episodes. However, others may have "rapid cycling" in which they switch from depression to mania or hypomania very frequently.

FAST The definition of "rapid cycling" is four or more episodes a year, but people with
FACT this form of bipolar disorder can have mood swings as often as several times a
day.

Because this workbook is focused on the treatment of depression, we don't include detailed treatment recommendations or self-help strategies designed explicitly for bipolar disorder. However, some of the exercises may be useful for people who are in the depressed phase of this condition. There are several excellent books that can help people with bipolar disorder. We particularly recommend *The Bipolar Disorder Survival Guide* by David Miklowitz and *The Bipolar Workbook* by Monica Ramirez Basco (see the Resources at the back of the book).

We include bipolar disorder in our discussion about making a diagnosis because it is very important that you recognize this condition if it is the source of your depression.

FAST • Studies have found that about 60% of people with bipolar disorder are either
FACTS undiagnosed, misdiagnosed, or not receiving appropriate treatment for this disease.

• The most common misdiagnosis is major depression.

Bipolar disorder can be treated effectively, but it is an illness with very strong biological roots that almost always requires a mood-stabilizing medication. Treatment with an antidepressant alone (without a specific mood-stabilizing drug) is not ideal treatment. In fact, there is concern that use of antidepressants alone can worsen the course of the disease in some people with bipolar disorder. So if you truly have bipolar disorder, it is best to recognize the condition and use the kinds of treatments that can help solve your problem.

DIAGNOSIS OF BIPOLAR DISORDER

The diagnosis of bipolar disorder is made when a person has a history of at least one episode of mania or hypomania (a less intense upswing). If mania has occurred, the diagnosis is bipolar disorder type I. If the severity of the upswing(s) has only reached the level of hypomania and the person has a previous history of a depressive episode, the diagnosis is bipolar disorder type II.

Some of the common symptoms of mania are*:

- Abnormally elevated, expansive, or irritable mood.
- Inflated self-esteem or grandiose thinking.
- Reduced need for sleep.
- Talking more rapidly than usual.
- Distinct increases in activity levels or agitation.
- Getting involved in activities likely to have a bad outcome, such as buying binges or sexual indiscretions.

Symptoms of *mania* need to last at least a week and cause marked impairment (such as causing yourself financial disasters, getting little or no sleep for three or more nights, and being significantly hyperactive) to make the diagnosis of bipolar disorder type I. The criteria for diagnosis of a *hypomanic* episode are about the same, but the symptoms only have to last 4 days and don't cause marked impairment. Instead of withdrawing your life savings to invest in a stranger's business venture, for example, you might find yourself spending more than usual and feeling more upbeat and energetic. But you don't drain your assets or get less than 75–80% of your normal sleep. If you think you may have symptoms of bipolar disorder, we recommend that you see a doctor for a full diagnostic assessment.

Measuring Depression and Charting Your Progress

As mentioned earlier, it's very helpful to your recovery to monitor your depression regularly, such as once a week or every other week. Why not start right now, with Exercise 1.3?

---

*Reprinted with permission from the *Diagnostic and Statistical Manual of Mental Disorders, Fourth Edition, Text Revision*. Copyright 2000 by the American Psychiatric Association.

The Patient Health Questionnaire–9

The Patient Health Questionnaire–9 (PHQ-9) was developed to help doctors and patients screen for depression and monitor the progress of treatment. This scale is easy to use and takes only a few minutes to complete. All of the nine core symptoms of major depression identified by the American Psychiatric Association are included in the scale. We suggest that you rate your symptoms of depression now using the PHQ-9 and that you use this scale repeatedly to check on how you are doing in your quest to overcome depression. Additional copies of the scale can be downloaded from *www.guilford.com/breakingfreeforms*.

How to Interpret PHQ-9 Scores

The total score on the PHQ-9 can be used to get a general idea of the severity of depression. After you add up the total score, you can use this table to see how your symptoms compare to others who have taken the PHQ-9.

Total score	Depression severity
1–4	Minimal depression
5–9	Mild depression
10–14	Moderate depression
15–19	Moderately severe depression
20–27	Severe depression

A diagnosis of any depressive disorder is suspected if:

1. There are <u>4</u> or more ratings of a severity of at least 2 (more than half the days).
2. One of these ratings is either item 1 or item 2.

A diagnosis of major depressive disorder is suspected if:

3. There are <u>5</u> or more ratings of a severity of at least 2 (more than half the days).
4. One of these ratings is either item 1 or item 2.

Tracking Progress with the PHQ-9

Kate's Record of PHQ-9 Scores

Kate took the PHQ-9 weekly for the 12 weeks after she started using her new treatment plan. As you can see from looking at the graph on page 16, she made good overall progress. It took a little while for the benefits to start showing, as might be expected in a person who had been depressed for a while. But the ultimate outcome was excellent.

Patient Health Questionnaire–9 (PHQ-9)

Name: _____ Date: _____

Over the *last 2 weeks*, how often have you been bothered by any of the following problems?

(*Circle a number or use "✓" to indicate your answer.*)

	Not at all	Several days	More than half the days	Nearly every day
1. Little interest or pleasure in doing things	0	1	2	3
2. Feeling down, depressed, or hopeless	0	1	2	3
3. Trouble falling or staying asleep or sleeping too much	0	1	2	3
4. Feeling tired or having little energy	0	1	2	3
5. Poor appetite or overeating	0	1	2	3
6. Feeling bad about yourself—or that you are a failure or have let yourself or your family down	0	1	2	3
7. Trouble concentrating on things, such as reading the newspaper or watching TV	0	1	2	3
8. Moving or speaking so slowly that other people could have noticed. Or the opposite—being so fidgety or restless that you have been moving around a lot more than usual	0	1	2	3
9. Thoughts that you would be better off dead or of hurting yourself in some way	0	1	2	3

Add columns: _____ + _____ + _____

Total: [   ]

The PHQ-9 is adapted from PRIME MD TODAY, developed by Drs. Robert L. Spitzer, Janet B. W. Williams, Kurt Kroenke, and colleagues, with an educational grant from Pfizer, Inc. Additional copies of this exercise can be downloaded from *www.guilford.com/breakingfreeforms*.

At about week 5, she experienced a temporary worsening of symptoms. She had some work stress at that time and had more problems with insomnia and self-critical thinking. However, she worked in CBT to promote sleep and increase her self-confidence. After 3 months, her depression was in total remission, and she was able to shift her focus in treatment toward ways of staying well.

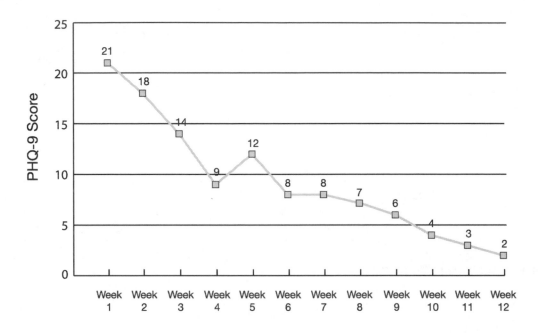

Your Record of PHQ-9 scores

You can use the chart in Exercise 1.4 to measure your success in overcoming depression. You can also construct your own graph on paper or on a computer.

Summary

Depression can sap your energy, undermine your self-esteem, disrupt your normal functioning, and make it hard to accomplish tasks. Fortunately, there are many powerful tools for reversing the downward spiral of depression. These can include scientifically tested psychotherapies, antidepressant medications, exercise and other lifestyle changes, drawing strength from relationships, tapping spiritual resources, mindfulness meditation, and other valuable approaches.

This book is designed to help you build skills for overcoming depression and to develop an effective plan for recovery. In this chapter, you identified some of the depression-fighting skills you may already have and some of the skills you may want to strengthen. You listed treatment strategies that you may be interested in using. And you learned about the value of making an accurate diagnosis and monitoring progress.

The next chapter is designed to help you recognize the influences of physical con-

My Depression Score Record

Date	PHQ-9 score	Comments/ideas/suggestions

ditions on depression. Because medical illnesses and prescription drugs can trigger or worsen depression, it is usually a good idea to consider physical health in your path to wellness. If you have had a recent evaluation by your medical doctor and are sure that you know about your physical status and any impact it might have on depression, you could skip ahead to Chapter 3. But if you have any questions about the association between general health and depression, we recommend you pause briefly to learn about this important link.

2

Medical Illness and Depression

> **Chapter Highlights**
>
> ▶ The medical illness–depression connection
>
> ▶ Learning from examples: Four common physical conditions associated with depression
>
> ▶ Am I taking any medications that could make me depressed?
>
> ▶ My plan for physical wellness

All of the symptoms of depression can be produced by medical illnesses or the drugs used to treat them. Even suicidal thinking can be stimulated by physical disorders or treatments. That's why a health care professional who evaluates you for depression will consider the possibility that a medical condition is causing or aggravating symptoms. So we recommend that you do "first things first"—find out whether a medical illness could be part of the problem before launching a full plan for overcoming depression.

The Medical Illness–Depression Connection

A very large number of medical problems have been reported to increase the risk for depression, worsen symptoms, or make it more difficult to achieve recovery. However, there are also very large numbers of people who have significant medical problems and are not depressed. Although having a medical illness doesn't necessarily load the dice against your recovering from depression, most doctors recommend that you try to recognize and treat physical illnesses and depression simultaneously. Improvements in physical health and optimal management of medications for medical problems can play a significant role in reducing symptoms of depression. And, in turn, relief of depression may have positive effects on physical health.

Take a look at this list of some of the more common medical conditions that have been associated with depression. Do you have any of these problems?

Medical Problems Associated with Depression

Adrenal gland deficiency or excess (rare conditions that affect production of the hormone cortisol)

Anemia

Cancer

Chronic fatigue syndrome

Chronic kidney disease

Chronic pain

Coronary artery disease

Diabetes

Fibromyalgia

Hyperthyroidism (excess thyroid hormone)

Hypothyroidism (thyroid hormone deficiency)

Irritable bowel syndrome

Multiple sclerosis

Parkinson's disease

Seizure disorder

Sleep apnea

Stroke

Vitamin deficiencies (possibly folate, vitamin D, and vitamin B_{12})

Some of the conditions on this list, such as Parkinson's disease, seizure disorder, chronic pain, and stroke, have obvious symptoms. But other problems have subtle symptoms that may appear at first to be much like depression—low energy, lack of interest, poor sleep, difficulty concentrating, changes in appetite and weight. So how do you know whether your depressive symptoms are being influenced by a medical condition that has yet to be diagnosed? Or how can you sort out the relative contributions of medical illnesses you know you have and the psychological parts of depression?

The only definitive answer to these questions is to team with a physician to screen for medical illnesses and to develop a comprehensive treatment plan. But you can prepare to help your doctor figure out what's going on and how to treat your problems if you know what some typical interactions between medical illnesses and depression look like. In the following pages we describe four common medical problems—hypothyroidism, chronic pain, sleep apnea, and vitamin deficiencies—that can silently masquerade as depression or make depressive symptoms worse. With these examples in mind, you may be better prepared to collaborate with your doctor in making medical treatment a part of your plan for recovery from depression.

SCIENCE CORNER
- Studies have found high rates of depression in a wide variety of medical conditions.

- Approximately 20% of people with coronary heart disease (CHD) have depression.
  - People with depression and CHD have double the risk of dying in the year following a heart attack!
- Among people with diabetes:
  - Up to 30% will experience depression symptoms sometime in their life.
  - Depression is associated with diabetic complications such as neuropathy, kidney failure, and eye problems.

Learning from Examples: Four Common Physical Conditions Associated with Depression

We can't provide an exhaustive list of all of the symptoms that might be signs of medical illnesses, and therefore indicate the need for a checkup, or describe the key features of all the frequently occurring physical conditions that have been linked to depression. We can, however, give you a few tips on how you might work with your doctor to spot and manage these four problems that can drag you down for long periods of time.

Hypothyroidism

The thyroid is a hormone gland located in your neck, just below your adam's apple, that produces thyroid hormone. This hormone is responsible mainly for energy level, metabolic rate (how fast or slow we move and how efficiently we burn calories), and healthy skin, hair, and nails. Low levels of thyroid hormone (hypothyroidism) can be caused by several disorders but are most often seen in autoimmune destruction of the thyroid (thyroiditis) and are more common in women who are older or who are in the postpartum period (just after childbirth). At any one time, up to 2% of people will have hypothyroidism.

Because the thyroid is responsible for energy level, low levels of thyroid hormone can make people feel slow, sluggish, tired, and depressed. Use the symptom checklist in Exercise 2.1 to see if hypothyroidism might be contributing to your depression.

A simple blood test, ordered by your doctor, can be used to diagnose hypothyroidism. If the test shows low levels of thyroid hormone, a prescription replacement hormone (such as levothyroxine) will usually be needed to normalize metabolism and relieve symptoms. Although thyroid hormone therapy is usually quite safe, regular monitoring is required. Excess levels of thyroid hormone can cause dangerous heart rhythms or electrolyte imbalances.

Chronic Pain

A common medical problem that is usually quite obvious but may be vexing to both patients and doctors, is chronic pain. People can feel down because of the pain itself or

EXERCISE 2.1   Symptom Checklist for Hypothyroidism: Are Low Thyroid Levels Contributing to Your Depression?

Instructions: Check off any symptom that you're experiencing on a regular basis. If you checked 3 or more items, consult your doctor to discuss whether you may need thyroid screening. Keep in mind that some of the symptoms below may overlap with depression or other medical illnesses.

Symptom	I have this symptom
Extreme fatigue	
Inability to tolerate cold (very sensitive to cold temperatures)	
Dry skin, hair, or nails	
Slow mental processing (takes a long time to complete mental tasks)	
Weight gain	
Constipation	
Heavy menstrual periods	

From *Breaking Free from Depression*. Copyright 2012 by The Guilford Press.

functional limitations related to the pain (such as having to give up a job or favorite activities). A study by Drs. Ohayon and Schatzberg at Stanford University found that pain and depression can be tied together very closely. The authors discovered that pain was worse when people had poor sleep, fatigue, or stress.

People with coexisting depression and pain are more likely to miss work, be bedbound, or report that the pain interferes with their daily activities. Depression can make the pain worse, and in turn pain often makes depression worse. If you have both pain and depression, try Exercise 2.2 to see if you can detect an association between your pain level and your mood.

Does the exercise reveal a connection between your "bad" pain days and your mood? Can you think of ways to break the vicious cycle between pain and depression? Would it be targeting the pain, the depression, or perhaps both? Regarding the issue of pain control, we encourage you to talk with your doctor to explore different medication options, physical therapy, referrals for interventional therapies, or even alternative therapies (such as acupuncture).

EXERCISE 2.2	**Pain and Depression**

Instructions: Over the next week, log your average level of pain and mood for each day. See whether there is a connection between your pain level and depression. You can use a 0–10 scale for depression, or use the PHQ-9 from Chapter 1 to rate your depression.

Day of the week	**Rate your level of pain** (0 = no pain, 10 = worst pain)	**Rate your level of depression** (0 = no depression, 10 = worst depression), or insert your daily PHQ-9 score (see Chapter 1, page 19)
Monday		
Tuesday		
Wednesday		
Thursday		
Friday		
Saturday		
Sunday		

People with pain and depression can benefit from both medication and nonmedication treatments for the depression component of the problem. Several studies suggest that treating depression may improve pain. One specific antidepressant medication, duloxetine (Cymbalta), has been found to be effective in treating pain associated with diabetic neuropathy (a painful condition affecting the feet in people with long-standing diabetes), fibromyalgia, and chronic musculoskeletal pain.

Cognitive-behavior therapy (CBT) has also been shown to improve pain symptoms and mood in people with chronic pain syndromes. The benefits of CBT on mood seem to be long-lasting too. So if you are living with chronic pain, try using some of the powerful CBT techniques from Chapters 4, 5, and 6. As an example, let's look at the experience of Trisha, who suffers from chronic pain from a back injury.

Trisha

Trisha is a 46-year-old mother of two who has been living with pain from back problems for 10 years. Although she can go work as a teacher, she feels pain daily, especially in her low back and down into her right leg. Most days, Trisha's pain is bearable, but when she has a flare-up, she feels like she can't get out of bed and often calls in sick. Lately, Trisha has been feeling down about her chronic pain and has noticed that she is losing her motivation and interest in doing things she normally enjoys, such as playing Ping-Pong with her teenage kids or taking walks with the dog. Trisha hasn't been sleeping well due to both the pain and her mood, finding herself thinking at night, "If only the pain would go away, I could have a normal life."

When Trisha went to see Dr. McCray, they talked about medication options, such as increasing her pain medications (gabapentin and ibuprofen), but Trisha wanted to try some nonmedication treatments for the pain and depression first.

For the pain, Trisha had had some success in the past doing low-impact exercise. So she worked out a safe exercise plan with Dr. McCray and got a referral for physical therapy. She was also happy to hear that exercise was a reasonable treatment option for depression (see Chapter 11). The idea of CBT was new to Trisha. At first she thought that CBT couldn't help because her pain was "real" and "beyond my control." Dr. McCray explained that although Trisha's pain was quite real, and was produced by disc and arthritic problems in her back, there was room to learn coping strategies from CBT, such as interrupting the volleys of negative thoughts that just made her pain and depression worse (explained in Chapter 4). The action plan they developed proved helpful in reducing symptoms of depression and assisting Trisha in managing her pain, but additional steps were eventually needed to move her closer to recovery. You'll learn more about Trisha's treatment later in the chapter.

Sleep Apnea

Although there has been increased awareness about sleep apnea, this problem typically goes unrecognized for months or years before it is discovered and treated effectively. People with sleep apnea have many periods during sleep in which they pause in breathing. Typically, they also snore loudly and sleep very restlessly. During the day, they may suffer from excessive drowsiness, concentration problems, morning headaches, and other symptoms related to getting poor sleep and not having enough oxygen when they stop breathing. Continuous positive airway pressure (CPAP) and several other treatments can be very useful for sleep apnea.

Approximately 7% of people in the United States have sleep apnea, and many of these people also experience depression. A study by Dr. Daniel Schwartz and associates found that 40 out of 41 people with sleep apnea and depression who were treated with CPAP had substantial decreases in self-ratings of depression. So screening for sleep apnea could pay big dividends—not only in treating the basic medical condition but in relieving depressive symptoms as well. Do Exercise 2.3 to get an idea of whether you might be experiencing sleep apnea.

EXERCISE 2.3　　　**Quiz: Is Sleep Apnea Contributing to Your Depression?**

Instructions: Circle "yes" or "no" to answer the following questions. If you answer "yes" to items 1 and 2 or to 3 or more questions, consult your doctor to discuss whether you may need testing for sleep apnea. Keep in mind that some of the symptoms below may overlap with depression or other medical illnesses.

Question	Answer
1. Do you have excessive daytime drowsiness?	Yes/No
2. Do others tell you that you snore loudly?	Yes/No
3. Do you awaken feeling unrefreshed?	Yes/No
4. Do you have difficulties with concentration or memory?	Yes/No
5. Do you have problems with low energy or excessive fatigue?	Yes/No
6. Do you have headaches in the morning?	Yes/No
7. Do others tell you that you are a restless sleeper?	Yes/No

Vitamin Deficiencies

There is no solid evidence that taking vitamins will help reduce depression in people who *do not* have vitamin deficiencies, so we don't recommend routine vitamin supplements for everybody with depression. Yet when actual deficiencies are present, vitamins can make an important contribution to recovery. The three vitamins that have been studied most in the treatment of depression are folate, vitamin D, and vitamin B_{12}. To identify a vitamin deficiency, you will need to be evaluated by your doctor and have blood tests.

SCIENCE CORNER
- A study reported by Drs. America and Milling in the *Journal of Behavioral Medicine* found that daily supplements with multivitamins or B-complex vitamins were <u>not</u> effective in helping relieve depressive symptoms in people who did not have a documented deficiency of these vitamins.
- In contrast to the findings in non-vitamin-deficient individuals, some research studies have supported the usefulness of supplements for those who have low levels of certain vitamins.

Folate

One of the B vitamins, folate, has been studied the most extensively for possible connections with depression. This vitamin influences the production of the neurotransmitters involved in depression and has been used as a booster for antidepressants in people who have folate deficiencies. A review of research on folate supplements conducted by Drs. Fava and Mischoulon at Harvard University noted that several forms of folate are available, including methylfolate, folic acid, and folinic acid. Their review found evidence for the usefulness of folate augmentation of antidepressants for residual symptoms of depression. However, a review by Dr. Gelenberg in *Biological Therapies in Psychiatry* concluded that more research was needed before folate supplements could be recommended as a routine strategy for treatment-resistant depression. Authors of both of these reviews commented that methylfolate may be better tolerated than other forms of folate.

Vitamin D

There has been increasing interest in the role of vitamin D in depression. A review of studies of the association between vitamin D and depression that was conducted by Dr. Bertone-Johnson at the University of Massachusetts concluded that research had produced inconsistent results. Yet a large study conducted in Norway discovered a significant relationship between low vitamin D levels and depression and a positive effect of vitamin D supplements on improving the symptoms of depression. Also, a study of depressed women with low vitamin D levels that was conducted at Washington State University found depression scores fell substantially when vitamin D supplements were given. Although routine use of Vitamin D for depression is not recommended, it may be a good idea to check for a deficiency in this vitamin if other therapies don't seem to be working or if you are stuck in depression.

Vitamin B_{12}

Deficiencies of vitamin B_{12} can cause a medical condition called *pernicious anemia* that can be associated with many physical and emotional symptoms such as weakness, depression, and mania. Vitamin B_{12} deficiencies are diagnosed by doctors with blood tests and other diagnostic studies. Significant deficiencies in this vitamin usually need to be treated with injections of B_{12}.

"Could Medications Be Making Me Depressed?"

Are you taking medication for a chronic medical illness, such as high blood pressure, seizures, or chronic pain? If so, your medication could be causing some of your depression symptoms. Despite the proven health benefits of some medications, no medication is without potential side effects. We hope your doctor or pharmacist routinely counsels you about possible medication side effects whenever you begin a new prescription and monitors you closely for any possible long-term side effects. Take a look at the list of medications that can cause symptoms of depression (such as low mood, poor sleep, or loss of interest) in Exercise 2.4.

Remember, you should weigh the pros and cons of taking medication with your doctor before stopping any medication. Most medications on the list in the exercise have proven health benefits (for example, beta-blockers such as metoprolol have been shown to help prevent heart attacks in people with coronary artery disease). Also, many of these medications are only occasionally reported to cause depression. If you are depressed and are taking one of these medications, it is entirely possible that the medication is not the culprit. So, review your options with your doctor before making a choice about how to proceed.

My Plan for Physical Wellness

To pull together and organize your ideas for promoting physical health as part of your strategy for overcoming depression, it could help to write out a *Plan for Physical Wellness*. Typical interventions could include working with your doctor to deal with medical problems that need attention, revising a medication regimen, or instituting some of the positive lifestyle modifications (such as improving diet or exercising regularly) detailed in Chapter 11. Other methods described in this book such as CBT (Chapters 4, 5, and 6), well-being therapy (Chapter 7), and mindfulness (Chapter 13) can also be used to reduce stress and help you cope better with medical illnesses.

Let's do some work now on creating a *Plan for Physical Wellness*. We'll check in with Trisha first so you can follow her example.

Trisha

Trisha had been seeing Dr. McCray regularly and had already had a thorough medical evaluation. And she had already decided to get started with CBT for depression as well as a gradual increase in exercise. Both of these actions had seemed to help, but she still had some ongoing pain, and her ratings on the PHQ-9 scale were staying in the range of moderate depression (12–17). When she completed a Plan for Physical Wellness (see page 29), some additional ideas came to mind.

Trisha seemed to find some very good options for additional treatment that could help her overcome both pain and depression. Now it's your turn. As you complete Exercise 2.5, remember that you don't have to develop or implement a plan by yourself. Discuss your ideas with your doctor or other people who may be able to help. And you can take the actions at your own pace. Everything doesn't need to be done at once. The important thing is to recognize that depression and physical health are tied so closely together that it makes sense to consider your total health as you move forward to overcome depression.

Did you identify several actions that you might take? Most people would probably do the same, so don't worry. We don't want this exercise to feel overwhelming, and we don't expect you to tackle all these opportunities at the same time, especially if you're feeling

Medication Checklist

Instructions: Review the following list of medications that may cause symptoms of depression. Put a check mark by any medications you are currently taking and take this list to your doctor to discuss whether your medication might be contributing to depression. This list is not exhaustive, so be sure to examine your current medication list with your doctor.

Medications that may cause depression symptoms	Check here if taking
Beta blockers (such as metoprolol [Lopressor or Toprol XL], atenolol [Tenormin], or carvedilol [Coreg])—used for high blood pressure and cardiac conditions	
Calcium channel blockers (such as verapamil [Calan], diltiazem [Cardizem], and nifedipine [Procardia])—used for high blood pressure and cardiac conditions	
Anticonvulsants (such as gabapentin [Neurontin] or divalproex [Depakote])—used to treat seizures	
Narcotic medications (such as oxycodone or morphine)—used for pain	
Antianxiety medications (such as benzodiazepines like lorazepam [Ativan] or diazepam [Valium])	
Varenicline (Chantix)—used to help people stop smoking	
Oral steroids (prednisone)—used for steroid replacement therapy and to treat some chronic diseases	
Metoclopramide (Reglan)—used for gastrointestinal problems	
Interferon alpha—used for hepatitis B, C, and some cancers	
Isotretinoin (Accutane)—used for acne	
Bromocriptine (Parlodel)—used for muscle spasms and neurological disorders	
Acyclovir (Zovirax)—used to reduce relapse rate of herpes infections	

My Plan for Physical Wellness: Trisha's Example

Instructions: Review possible actions on this checklist. Circle any of the actions that you might want to take within the next 1 to 3 months. Then get specific. Write down the things you actually plan to do.

Possible actions	This action might improve my health	I've already done this	Actions I plan to take/comments
See a doctor for a medical evaluation if I have not done so within the last year.		X	
Get screening tests for hypothyroidism, anemia, or (sleep apnea.)	X	X	The blood tests were all normal, but I'll take Dr. McCray's suggestion to get evaluated for sleep apnea. My sleep is poor. I never feel rested, and my partner tells me I snore at night.
Get checked for vitamin deficiencies.		X	
Get checked for other possible medical conditions that haven't been diagnosed.		X	
See doctor to reevaluate and improve management of chronic pain. Or use additional therapies for pain.	X	X	Make appointment with Dr. McCray to discuss alternative treatment options. Check insurance to see if it will pay for massage therapy for back pain.
Get help from doctor in more effective management of a chronic medical illness such as heart disease, diabetes, or a neurological condition.			
Receive more intensive treatment for depression (such as antidepressants or CBT) that could also help me cope with physical problems.	X	X	Keep going with CBT. It's helping, and I've had only 5 sessions. Take Dr. McCray's advice to try an antidepressant that may also help with pain.
Make lifestyle changes (such as increased exercise, improved diet, reduced use of alcohol or drugs).	X	X	Continue the walking program. Consider trying swimming or water aerobics exercises.

My Plan for Physical Wellness

Instructions: Review possible actions on this checklist. Circle any of the actions that you might want to take within the next 1 to 3 months. Then get specific. Write down the things you actually plan to do. You can ask your doctor for help in putting the plan into action.

Possible actions	This action might improve my health	I've already done this	Actions I plan to take/comments
See a doctor for a medical evaluation if I have not done so within the last year.			
Get screening tests for hypothyroidism, anemia, or sleep apnea.			
Get checked for vitamin deficiencies.			
Get checked for other possible medical conditions that haven't been diagnosed.			
See doctor to reevaluate and improve management of chronic pain. Or use additional therapies for pain.			
Get help from doctor in more effective management of a chronic medical illness such as heart disease, diabetes, or a neurological condition.			
Receive more intensive treatment for depression (such as antidepressants or CBT) that could also help me cope with physical problems.			
Make lifestyle changes (such as increased exercise, improved diet, reduced use of alcohol or drugs).			

depressed. It might help to break it down into small, achievable steps. You can also come back to this exercise after you have worked on some of the other chapters and are feeling better. As you follow your own path to recovery, you may find that you want to modify your plan for physical wellness; additional copies of this worksheet can be downloaded from *www.guilford.com/breakingfreeforms*.

Summary

This chapter on medical illness appears very early in this book because we think it's especially important to find possible physical contributions to depression before proceeding with treatment. Although a medical illness or a drug for a physical illness is rarely the sole cause of depression, sometimes a condition such as hypothyroidism can play a major role in producing depressive symptoms. And for many people, physical problems are part of the multistemmed path that has led to depression. If you have or think you might have a medical condition that is contributing to depression, take the time to get the help you need. Doing so will put you in a better position to benefit from the methods detailed in the rest of this book.

3

Paths to Depression: Paths to Wellness

> **Chapter Highlights**
> ◗ The thoughts–action path
> ◗ The biology path
> ◗ The relationship path
> ◗ The lifestyle path
> ◗ The spiritual path
> ◗ The mindfulness path

One of the most fascinating facts about depression is that there can be so many different paths that lead toward the illness and so many paths that can be taken to wellness. Fortunately, you do not just have to choose one path out of depression. You can combine ideas and methods from more than one perspective on depression to craft a plan that works best for you. In this chapter, we explain the major approaches to fighting depression and help you decide which paths you may want to emphasize in your journey to recovery.

The Thoughts–Action Path

The thoughts–action path is based on the principles of cognitive-behavior therapy (CBT)—the most widely used psychotherapy designed specifically for depression.

| DEFINITION | Cognitive-behavior therapy (CBT) is a treatment for depression that focuses on changing negative thinking and altering behaviors. |

To get a quick idea of how CBT works, let's do an exercise. Imagine for a moment that you are trying to help Kate, the woman with depression whom you met in Chapter 1. Do you remember that Kate dropped out of lots of her usual activities after she became depressed?

When Kate considers breaking out of the rut of spending time alone, staring at the TV, she often has thoughts that just drag her further down. Your goal in Exercise 3.1 is to generate some ideas that might help Kate start to make progress in the fight against depression.

Were you able to come up with some more realistic or helpful ways of thinking about the event? Examples of some of the thoughts that we might have tried to help Kate identify are: "I've been depressed, but I still can be a good friend. I'm not my usual self, but I'm not a total mess. It's an exaggeration to say that I'm a failure. I'm still doing well at work, and I have some interesting things to say. I would probably enjoy the movie and dinner. Going out with my friends would be good for me. It would be worth pushing myself to do this."

Whether you are getting treatment with CBT from a professional therapist or trying to learn CBT self-help methods on your own, you will be encouraged to "think about your thinking" so that you can recognize how your thought patterns may be inducing or worsening depression.

Of course, many people with depression have significant real-life problems, such as relationship strains or breakups, job losses, or physical illnesses. You may have had many negative experiences in your own life. We have certainly had our share of bad things happen. CBT doesn't minimize real problems, but it does try to help people avoid "adding insult to injury" and think in clear and objective ways about solving their problems.

FAST
FACTS

- The thoughts–action path is based on CBT—an effective treatment for depression.

- CBT teaches people how to recognize and change thinking patterns that may be promoting or worsening depression.

- When people face tough problems such as relationship breakups, unemployment, or other personal stresses, CBT helps to build problem-solving strategies.

Have you started to consider any of your own ways of thinking that could be part of depression? The checklist in Exercise 3.2 on page 35 could help you target some common thoughts that you might like to change.

Background Information: One of Kate's old friends from school called to ask her to join some other people they knew for some social activities on Saturday evening. The plan was to go to an early movie and then have dinner together. Here is what happened:

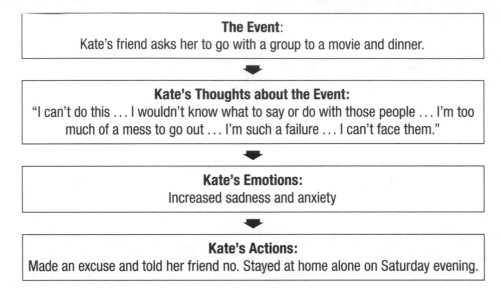

The Event:
Kate's friend asks her to go with a group to a movie and dinner.

Kate's Thoughts about the Event:
"I can't do this . . . I wouldn't know what to say or do with those people . . . I'm too much of a mess to go out . . . I'm such a failure . . . I can't face them."

Kate's Emotions:
Increased sadness and anxiety

Kate's Actions:
Made an excuse and told her friend no. Stayed at home alone on Saturday evening.

Be Kate's Helper: Are you thinking of some ways that Kate could have had a healthier response to the invitation? Did you spot the negative tone of Kate's thoughts? Depression often seems to cast a dark cloud on people's thinking. It can distort perceptions and make things seem worse than they actually are. If you knew that Kate actually was a good conversationalist, and it was likely that her friends didn't see her as a failure, what kinds of thoughts would you wish she could have? Try to rewrite Kate's thoughts so that a happier conclusion is reached.

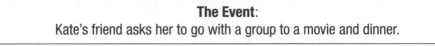

The Event:
Kate's friend asks her to go with a group to a movie and dinner.

Write down some positive yet realistic thoughts that would help Kate accept the invitation.

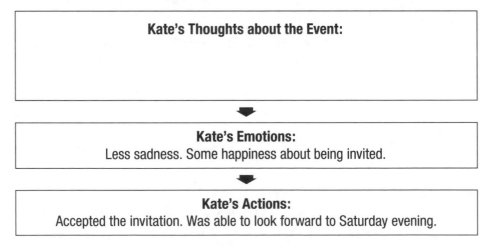

Kate's Thoughts about the Event:

Kate's Emotions:
Less sadness. Some happiness about being invited.

Kate's Actions:
Accepted the invitation. Was able to look forward to Saturday evening.

EXERCISE 3.2 | **A Checklist of Common Negative Thoughts in Depression**

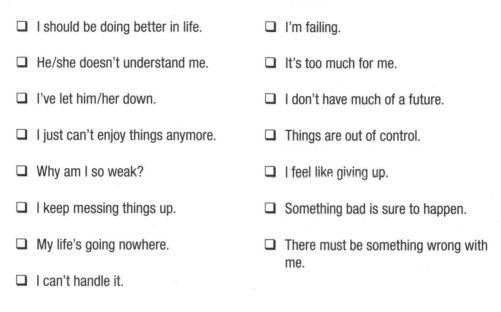

❏ I should be doing better in life.

❏ He/she doesn't understand me.

❏ I've let him/her down.

❏ I just can't enjoy things anymore.

❏ Why am I so weak?

❏ I keep messing things up.

❏ My life's going nowhere.

❏ I can't handle it.

❏ I'm failing.

❏ It's too much for me.

❏ I don't have much of a future.

❏ Things are out of control.

❏ I feel like giving up.

❏ Something bad is sure to happen.

❏ There must be something wrong with me.

The Link between Thoughts, Emotions, and Actions

The example we gave of Kate's response to the invitation illustrates a very common pattern in depression.

Events ◀▶ Thoughts ◀▶ Actions

1. *Events* (or memories of events) trigger *thoughts* that are negative, depressing, or anxiety provoking.
2. Distressing *thoughts* stir up unpleasant *emotions* such as sadness, anxiety, anger, or irritability.
3. Depressing thoughts and emotions lead to *actions* that can reinforce or deepen the depression.

FAST FACTS
- The relationship between thoughts and actions is a "two-way street."
- If you have negative thoughts, you may act in a self-defeating way.
- If your actions include behaviors such as giving up pleasurable activities, isolation, procrastination, and not treating yourself well, you may be likely to think less of yourself or to have other negative thoughts.

We often use the term "vicious cycle" to describe the negative, downward spiral that can occur in depression. Thoughts and actions feed on one another to drive people deeper into depression and to prevent them from getting better. However, CBT offers much hope for interrupting this cycle.

How Effective Is CBT?

Many research studies have shown that CBT reduces symptoms of depression, anxiety, and a large number of other problems. The following graph, adapted from the work of Drs. Steven Hollon and Edward Friedman and their associates, should provide encouragement about the prospects of getting help from CBT. It shows results of four of the large studies that looked at the effectiveness of three types of treatment for major depression: (1) CBT alone (2) antidepressants alone, and (3) combined CBT and antidepressants.

When researchers have examined results of all of the studies of combining CBT and medication, they have found that CBT and medication are each effective, but the two treatments together can be more powerful than either one alone.

Are There Any Negatives to Using CBT?

As you can see from looking at the graph below, CBT doesn't work for everyone. Like all other effective treatments for depression, the degree of response varies from person to person. Also, CBT may take more effort and time than treatment with an antidepressant. Another factor to consider is that psychotherapy may cost more than medication over the short term if your insurance pays most or all of your drug costs and you have to pay for therapy sessions yourself or have a significant copay. However, studies of the cost–benefit ratio of receiving different forms of treatment for depression have found solid support for the value of receiving CBT, both for acute treatment and for relapse prevention. An especially appealing feature of CBT is that it usually has very long-lasting effects—it teaches

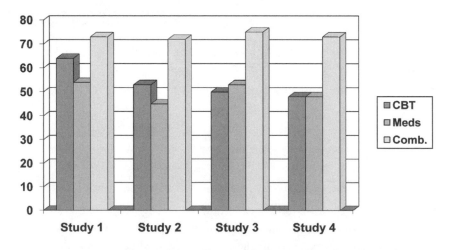

Response rates for CBT, antidepressants, and combined therapy.

coping skills and depression management techniques that can be used for a lifetime. In a way, CBT is a "gift that keeps on giving." Studies have shown that the longer-term outcome after stopping treatment is better for CBT than for medication.

Computer-Assisted CBT

Several computer programs have been developed to help people learn how to use CBT to overcome depression. These programs can be incorporated into professional treatment to enhance the therapy experience and to reduce the amount of time that people need to spend attending sessions with a clinician. Computer programs can also be used as self-help tools to build CBT skills. One program that has been tested in scientific studies and found to be useful is "Good Days Ahead" by Drs. Jesse Wright, Andrew Wright, and Aaron Beck. If you are interested in using a computer program as part of your way out of depression, you can check the websites listed in the Resources section of this book.

SCIENCE CORNER
- Research on computer-assisted CBT (CCBT) has found that people typically like working with these programs and find them helpful in reducing symptoms of depression and anxiety.
- A study conducted by Dr. Jesse Wright and associates found that people with depression had large decreases in depressive symptoms when treated with CCBT (a combination of brief visits with a clinician plus working with the "Good Days Ahead" program) and that the improvement was the same as in standard CBT (longer visits with a clinician but no use of the computer program). Also, the people who received CCBT had greater increases in knowledge about CBT than those who were treated with standard CBT.

Well-Being Therapy

Well-being therapy is a form of CBT developed by Dr. Giovanni Fava that focuses specifically on helping people develop positive life experiences. This therapy uses all of the methods of CBT plus exercises that show you how to find practical, everyday ways to promote feelings of well-being. Research studies have found that well-being therapy is effective for people with chronic depression and for those who have not had a full response to medication. In Chapter 7 we explain Dr. Fava's important contributions to CBT and show you how to put these useful methods into action.

How Does CBT Work?

If you receive CBT from a health care professional who is skilled in this approach, you will notice right away that teamwork is very important. You and your therapist will work together to identify how your thinking and your behavior are dragging you down. You will learn how to spot negatively biased thinking in depression and to develop a healthier thinking style. And you will build practical skills for improving energy, enjoying life, becoming more productive, and solving problems.

FAST FACTS

- Professional treatment for depression with CBT usually requires 8 to 20 sessions.

- Therapists typically recommend that you do "homework" with self-help exercises between sessions to solidify your learning and to put the therapy lessons to work in real-world situations.

- Some of the homework suggestions can include reading books such as this one to increase knowledge and strengthen skills.

Self-help is a very important part of CBT. Although we recommend professional treatment for people with significant depression, some studies have shown good results with self-help alone. Whether you have the opportunity to receive CBT from a trained therapist or you are trying to learn these strategies on your own, we have designed this book to provide some of the most powerful CBT methods for changing thoughts and actions.

EXERCISE 3.3   **My Interest in Using the Thoughts–Action Path**

Instructions: Place a mark on the ruler to indicate your interest in using the thoughts–action path to overcome depression.

| 0 | 1 | 2 | 3 | 4 | 5 | 6 | 7 | 8 | 9 | 10 |

None   Moderate   Maximum

The Biology Path

Biological treatments are used by millions of people to overcome depression and are becoming increasingly popular methods of treating this disease. Antidepressant use in the United States more than doubled in a recent 10-year period, and antidepressants are some of the most frequently prescribed drugs in medical practice.

Antidepressants are frequently a mainstay of treatment for more severe major depressions and for prevention of relapse. The scientific evidence solidly supports their use for these indications. However, their effectiveness for an acute episode of milder or "minor" depression has been questioned.

SCIENCE
CORNER

- The overall research findings on medication for major depression have been so strong that treatment guidelines published by leading professional organizations and universities recommend antidepressants as a top choice for treatment of this illness.
- However, there is some scientific evidence that antidepressants may not be superior to a placebo for milder or "minor" depression.

The biological pathways to depression are being unraveled by investigators working all around the globe. They are hunting for clues that will lead to a better understanding of the causes of depression and are working to develop improved treatments. We describe some basics of the biology of depression here. In Chapter 8 you'll be able to learn much more about how to benefit from biological treatments for depression.

The Genetics of Depression

If one of your parents or other close relatives has depression or bipolar disorder, your chances of developing depression are much higher than for people who have no family history of depression. The risk for major depression is about doubled if you have a parent with this problem, and the risk for bipolar disorder may be 10 times greater if you have a parent who has suffered from this type of mood disorder.

These findings have stimulated an intense research effort to try to identify specific genes that may be involved in producing the disorders. An important goal of these investigations is to uncover the details of how the genes influence the chemistry and/or the structure of the brain to induce depression. If the genetic mechanisms can be decoded, then new medications or other biological treatments could be designed to correct these abnormalities.

Although the promise of genetic studies hasn't been realized yet, there are many good leads. Investigators have found that it is unlikely that depression can be traced to one single gene. It is much more likely that a number of genes will be discovered that interact with the person's environment (for example, life stresses, medical illnesses, lifestyle, relationships) in the development of depression. An area of research that has been a special target for genetic studies is the function of the genes that control serotonin—a brain chemical that you will learn more about in the next section of this chapter.

Do you know your own family history of depression? Many of our patients tell us of people in their families who either have been diagnosed with depression or may have had this condition but never received professional treatment. If you have a family history of depression, you can use the next exercise to trace the pattern. You could share this chart with your doctor to help her better understand your depression.

EXERCISE 3.4	My Family History of Depression				

Relative	Treated for depression	Not treated for depression, but may have had this problem	Treated for bipolar disorder	Not treated for bipolar disorder, but may have had this problem	Treatments received, if known
Mother					
Father					
Maternal grandmother					
Maternal grandfather					
Paternal grandmother					
Paternal grandfather					
Maternal aunts or uncles					
Paternal aunts or uncles					
Cousins					
Children					

The Chemistry of Depression

Antidepressants and other biological treatments for mood disorders are thought to work, at least in part, by correcting imbalances of chemicals in the brain called neurotransmitters. These chemicals are responsible for connecting the billions of nerve cells (called neurons) in our brains. Without neurotransmitters, our brain cells could not send messages to one another—they would be like lone voices in the wilderness. Neurotransmitters are an essential part of an elaborate and effective communication system that allows us to think, feel emotions, make decisions, and perform all of the brain functions needed for life.

When people become depressed, they can have changes in their neurotransmitter functions that need to be returned to normal. The three main neurotransmitters that are culprits for causing depression are:

- Serotonin
- Norepinephrine
- Dopamine

Researchers have found that these neurotransmitters play an important role in functions that can become imbalanced in depression, such as mood, sleep, appetite, energy, and a sense of well-being.

Antidepressants can reverse abnormalities in neurotransmitters in several different ways, as shown in the diagram below.

Newer research is finding that antidepressants and other medications used to treat mood disorders (described in Chapter 8) can have positive influences on the brain beyond their impact on neurotransmitters. For example, these medications can reverse problems with function of the brain sites for depression described in the next section, and they can stimulate growth of certain brain cells.

FAST FACT Antidepressants work in multiple ways to correct the brain dysfunction that can occur in depression.

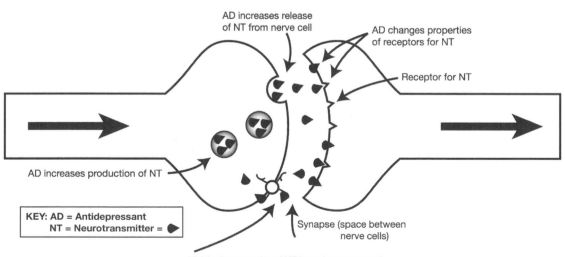

AD increases release of NT from nerve cell

AD changes properties of receptors for NT

Receptor for NT

AD increases production of NT

KEY: AD = Antidepressant
NT = Neurotransmitter =

Synapse (space between nerve cells)

AD blocks reuptake of NT back into nerve cell, thus increasing the amount of NT in synapse

The Anatomy of Depression

In the 1600s Robert Burton wrote what was to become a famous book about depression called *The Anatomy of Melancholy*. The term *melancholia* was used then (and sometimes still is) to describe depression because people with this condition suffer from a melancholic (sad) mood. Although the author made some very interesting observations about depression, he obviously did not have the tools of modern science to study the brain. Therefore he attributed the condition to a variety of possible causes such as "passions and perturbations of the mind, bad air, and distemperature of particular parts [of the body]."

An explosion of research in recent years has helped us understand what happens in the major centers of brain activity when people become depressed. Unlike the research on neurotransmitters, hormones, and other tiny molecules, studies of brain anatomy and physiology focus on some of the larger structures of the brain that are shown in the diagram below.

The anatomy of depression probably varies from individual to individual, so researchers doubt that one brain center will be found that will be abnormal in all people with depression. However, scientific studies have been adding to our knowledge of how certain biological treatments, and even psychological treatments, may work.

Some of the most important findings of research on the anatomy of depression are:

1. The *cortex* (outer layer) of the front of the brain becomes *underactive* in many people with depression. The cortex is the part of the brain responsible for our conscious thinking. If you have a depressing thought such as "It's hopeless," or an encouraging thought such as "I'll get better if I keep trying," these thoughts are generated in the cortex.

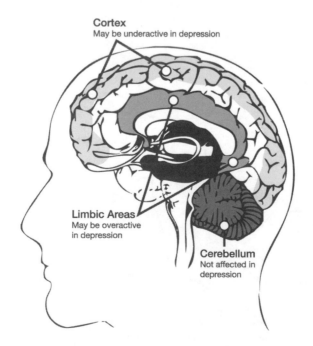

2. The *limbic* parts of the brain are located deep beneath the surface. The limbic areas are brain centers for emotions such as sadness, anxiety, anger, happiness, or joy. Some of the limbic portions of the brain are *overactive* in many people with depression.

3. Research has shown that antidepressant drugs work first by correcting abnormalities in the limbic or deeper parts of the brain.

4. Studies have found that CBT has biological effects on the brain. CBT works first by improving functioning in the front of the cortex. Thus CBT appears to work from the "top down," and medication appears to work from the "bottom up."

Biological Treatments for Depression

Most people who receive biological treatments for depression are prescribed antidepressants such as sertraline (Zoloft), escitalopram (Lexapro), fluoxetine (Prozac), or other medications that can correct chemical imbalances. Some of the other types of medication used for depression include mood stabilizers (such as lithium), atypical antipsychotic drugs (for example, quetiapine [Seroquel], aripiprazole [Abilify], and buspirone [Buspar]. These medications can be added when standard antidepressants aren't fully effective on their own or when other symptoms are present. Chapter 8 will help you learn about using these treatments to overcome depression and also will describe some other biological treatments, such as brain stimulation methods (electroconvulsive therapy and transcranial magnetic stimulation), that can be considered for very severe depression that doesn't respond to medication.

Although antidepressants are used frequently in current medical practice and help a great number of people, they do have potential downsides, such as the chance that they may not work to relieve symptoms, produce side effects, or lead to mild withdrawal symptoms when they are discontinued—problems that will be fully explained in Chapter 8. Also, some people prefer not to take medications when nondrug alternatives have been shown to be effective. You'll learn more about these options when we describe the other paths to wellness.

FAST
FACTS

- There are many biologically based tools that can be used to fight depression.
- Antidepressant medications are the most frequently used biological treatments.
- Other medications such as mood stabilizers, Abilify, or buspirone can be used to boost the effects of antidepressants.
- Brain stimulation methods are used infrequently, but they can help for very severe or refractory depression.

Now that you have learned some of the basics of taking the biology path, you can use the ruler in Exercise 3.5 to indicate how much you would like to use biological treatments in

| EXERCISE 3.5 | **My Interest in Using the Biology Path** |

Instructions: Place a mark on the ruler to indicate your interest in using the biology path to overcome depression.

```
 0     1       2      3      4      5      6      7      8      9     10
```

None   Moderate   Maximum

your plan for recovery. Because you will explore many other options for fighting depression in this book, the estimate can be revised later as you put together a comprehensive plan.

The Relationship Path

Relationships with family, friends, coworkers, and others can play a role in depression in three major ways:

1. *Relationship problems are triggers or causes of depression.* Part of Kate's path to depression was the sense of loss and rejection she felt after a breakup of a long-term relationship. Another "failure" just seemed to make things worse. These events reinforced her negative self-talk and decreased her motivation for forming new relationships.

Relationship difficulties don't have to be as dramatic as the ones Kate experienced to have an impact on depression. For some people, a subtle but steady erosion of a significant relationship can be a contributing cause. Or persistent criticism from a partner, parent, or other person can have a damaging effect. And for others chronic loneliness can be a factor. Research has shown that the fewer interpersonal relationships a person has, the more likely he is to experience depression.

2. *Depression causes relationships to suffer; and as relationships become strained or dwindle, the depression becomes worse.* When Kate became depressed, she didn't feel like being around other people. She pulled back from friends and others who could offer support or help her get involved in positive interests and activities. Her social isolation made her life even more depressing.

Depression can impair relationships in many ways. Because people with depression have lowered energy and interest, they can become less engaged in important relationships than when they are feeling well. If they have an understanding partner, parent, or friend, the changes may not have a negative influence on the relationship. However, there is a risk that depression can take a toll on relationships when others don't respond with empathy and caring.

3. *Relationships help in the recovery process.* Even though depression had caused Kate to back away from friends and family, she had some strong relationships that could be part of her recovery plan. When we described the thoughts–action path earlier in this chapter, we asked you to help Kate change her negative reaction to a friend's invitation for a social occasion. Kate had many other opportunities to recognize and take advantage of relationship strengths to fight depression. For example, she could ask her family to help her with plans to get more involved in social activities. Social supports have been found to play a very important role in coping with depression.

When people become depressed, they often turn inward. They can become so absorbed with the pain of the depression that they don't realize that good resources for fighting the depression can be found in their significant relationships. We'll help you troubleshoot relationship difficulties and tap relationship resources in Chapters 9 and 10.

Does Therapy Focused on Relationships Work to Relieve Depression?

In a word, yes. Many studies have shown that therapies directed at relationship problems are effective in treating depression. Although CBT most frequently uses an individual therapy format, the focus of interventions often is on the impact of relationship problems, and efforts to build and sustain healthy relationships are a very common element of treatment. When relationship problems are especially problematic, CBT can be done with couples and families.

Another form of talk therapy—interpersonal psychotherapy—is designed to help people deal with common relationship problems that may induce or aggravate depression. Interpersonal therapy (IPT) is much like CBT in being a practical method that teaches coping strategies. IPT is often used to help people (1) work through grief and loss, (2) improve troubled relationships, and (3) enhance relationship skills. Although it has been shown to be an effective treatment for major depression in several large research studies, IPT has not been studied as extensively as CBT, and many fewer therapists have been fully trained in IPT than in CBT.

We've tried to include some good tips and self-help exercises in this book for strengthening relationships in your fight against depression. The suggestions are drawn from both CBT and IPT. Let's begin in Exercise 3.6 with a brief inventory of relationship stresses or changes.

If you checked some of the items in the problems–opportunities inventory, there is probably a good chance that the relationship path could offer useful ways to battle depression.

The Lifestyle Path

Kate had stopped exercising and was having trouble with insomnia. She often stayed up late at night, had fitful sleep, and then was exhausted the next day. She was also giving

EXERCISE 3.6	**Relationship Problems and Opportunities**

Instructions: Place a check mark beside any problems or opportunities that you may have.

Problems

❑ I have had a relationship loss (for example, death, separation, break-up) that is still troubling me.

❑ I have pulled away from significant relationships.

❑ I am lonely.

❑ I tend to isolate myself.

❑ I have relationship conflicts.

❑ I am in a relationship with someone who criticizes me excessively.

❑ Depression makes it hard for me to maintain good relationships.

Opportunities

❑ I have family members who care about me.

❑ I have friends who care about me.

❑ I could reach out to family members in the fight against depression.

❑ I could reach out to friends in the fight against depression.

❑ I could work on coping better with grief or loss.

❑ I could work on improving one or more of my relationships.

❑ I could get professional therapy to help a troubled relationship.

From *Breaking Free from Depression.* Copyright 2012 by The Guilford Press.

EXERCISE 3.7	**My Interest in Using the Relationship Path**

Instructions: Place a mark on the ruler to indicate your interest in using the relationship path to overcome depression.

```
  0       1       2       3       4       5       6       7       8       9      10
```

None   Moderate   Maximum

From *Breaking Free from Depression.* Copyright 2012 by The Guilford Press.

little thought to purchasing or preparing healthy food. Kate knew that she had fallen into a habit pattern that was deepening her depression, but she couldn't figure out a way to change. It was like she was on a giant ship that was sailing in the wrong direction, and she couldn't turn it around.

In Chapter 11, we explain how to work toward healthier habits. For now, let's just sketch out some of the lifestyle patterns that you might think of changing.

Exercise

Many research investigations have provided solid evidence that exercise can be used to help depression. Yet many people are like Kate—they can't seem to get in gear to get walking or get to the gym. Scientific studies have suggested that exercise may work by increasing the neurotransmitters that we described in the biology path, or they may elevate levels of endorphins—brain chemicals associated with a feeling of well-being. Exercise can also enhance self-esteem, relax tension and anxiety, and improve general health and vigor. So there are many reasons to recommend exercise as part of a plan to fight depression.

FAST
FACTS

- Exercise is an "evidence-based" treatment for depression.
- One study found that exercise three times a week was as effective as an antidepressant medication.
- Exercise may work by increasing levels of neurotransmitters or endorphins.

Sleep Management

Sleep disruption is one of the core symptoms of depression, and methods to improve sleep can be an important part of the recovery process. CBT has been found to be an especially effective nondrug treatment for sleep problems. You can learn about CBT self-help methods for sleep in Chapter 11. But if sleeping problems persist, you can ask your doctor for advice. Some antidepressants can help with sleep, and there are several types of sleeping medications that can be useful. Sleeping pills, however, may have side effects, cause dependency, or have reduced effectiveness over time.

Diet

There has been controversy over the possible role of diet or diet supplements in the treatment of depression. You may have seen books or pamphlets with claims that diet changes can cure depression. We are much more cautious about recommending diet or diet supplements as a path to recovery, but there are scientific findings worth noting. Some of the possible diet modifications that may have some merit include use of the "Mediterranean diet," fish oil supplements, and vitamin D (see Chapter 11 for details).

CAUTION
- Lifestyle changes such as exercise and diet supplements can be valuable parts of an overall plan for recovery from depression.
- But we don't recommend that people rely completely on lifestyle changes for treatment of depression.
- A comprehensive plan that includes one or more of the core, evidence-based treatments such as CBT or antidepressant medication should be considered for people who suffer from significant major depression.

Substance Misuse or Abuse

Many people with depression fall into the trap of using alcohol or street drugs to "self-medicate." Although the substances can seem to temporarily take some of the pain away, the ultimate outcome is to worsen symptoms and to make it harder to recover. If you are having issues with alcohol or drugs, you will need to confront this problem. Otherwise, your other efforts to overcome depression may be in vain.

Light Therapy

Seasonal depression, or "seasonal affective disorder" (SAD), is a type of depression that occurs when the days grow shorter and there is less sunlight. There is plenty of scientific evidence that light therapy can work for seasonal depression. The treatment that we explain later in the book uses a "light box" for about 30 minutes a day to stimulate brain chemicals involved in depression.

FAST FACT   Light therapy can be effective for seasonal depression, a type of depression that occurs when days grow shorter and there is less sunlight.

Do you think that any of these ideas for lifestyle change could be part of your path out of depression? Could changes in any of these areas help you in other ways? Almost all

---

EXERCISE 3.8   ## My Interest in Using the Lifestyle Path

Instructions: Place a mark on the ruler to indicate your interest in using the lifestyle path to overcome depression.

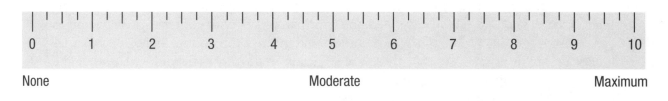

None   Moderate   Maximum

of the people we see in clinical practice have one or more good opportunities for working on their lifestyle as they move toward recovery.

The Spiritual Path

Most people describe themselves as having a spiritual side even if they don't have religious beliefs. And when depression strikes, their spiritual dimension can either become part of the problem or offer potential solutions for fighting the condition. In an earlier book, *Getting Your Life Back: The Complete Guide to Recovery from Depression,* Dr. Monica Basco and I (JHW) offered a definition of spirituality that is based on the work of Dr. Fredrick Luskin from Stanford University and Dr. Roger Walsh, author of *Essential Spirituality.* Do you identify with any of these common elements of spirituality?

1. Having meaning and purpose in life.
2. Having faith in a higher power and/or a greater good or purpose.
3. Being connected to life and people; giving to others.
4. Feeling that mind, body, and spirit are unified and whole.

When Depression Darkens the Spirit

Just as depression can drain your energy, deplete your interest, or lower your self-esteem, it can erode your spiritual underpinnings. Kate withdrew from many things in her environment, including her church activities and the people who used to be such a vital part of her life. As her depression worsened, she became more dispirited and found that her sense of meaning and purpose was diminishing. She was able to put one foot in front of the other and get to work—she had to keep her job to keep her finances afloat. But her usual drive was gone. She was starting to ask herself "What's the use?" When she got out of bed to start the day, it seemed that there was nothing to inspire her, nothing to make her feel truly alive and connected.

The questions in Exercise 3.9 can help you see whether any spiritual issues could be considered as you work to overcome depression.

Spirituality in the Fight against Depression

There are a number of different ways to use spiritual resources to combat depression. Here are two of the paths that people have taken.

Search for Increased Meaning and Purpose in Life

Viktor Frankl, a highly influential Austrian psychiatrist, developed a form of psychotherapy called logotherapy that focuses on efforts to enhance one's sense of meaning. He had endured the horrors of a concentration camp during World War II and found that having a deep sense of meaning, even in the face of some of the worst circumstances imaginable,

EXERCISE 3.9	Depression and Spirituality Checklist

Instructions: Use this checklist to identify spiritual concerns that you may want to address in your path toward overcoming depression.

Concern	Not a concern for me	A minor concern for me	A moderate concern for me	A major concern for me
Feeling that my life lacks a full sense of purpose				
Feeling distant from a higher power				
Being uninvolved in what's really important in life				
Wanting a greater spiritual underpinning to give my life more direction				
Having feelings of emptiness				

From *Breaking Free from Depression*. Copyright 2012 by The Guilford Press.

helped him avoid despair. In Chapter 12 we share Frankl's inspiring ideas with you as you follow your path to recovery.

Draw Strength from Religious Beliefs and Practices

If you have a religious faith, you may want to think of ways to tap this strength as you work to overcome depression. Disconnecting from religious practices that have been an important part of one's life can contribute to the downward spiral of depression, but a reengagement in these activities may offer comfort, support, and increased hope.

Is There Scientific Evidence for the Spiritual Path?

Spiritually oriented approaches to depression have been researched much less heavily than biological treatments, evidence-based psychotherapies such as CBT and IPT, and lifestyle changes such as exercise and light therapy. Thus we don't recommend that the spiritual path be the only method that people use to try to overcome significant major depression. Spiritually oriented activities can be used to augment other treatments such as CBT or antidepressants that have been researched extensively and found to be effective.

| EXERCISE 3.10 | **My Interest in Using the Spiritual Path** |

Instructions: Place a mark on the ruler to indicate your interest in using the spiritual path to overcome depression.

```
| | | | | | | | | | | | | | | | | | | | | | | | | | | | | | | | | | | | | | | | |
0       1       2       3       4       5       6       7       8       9      10
```

None   Moderate   Maximum

The research that has been done on the effects of spiritually oriented practices has generally been positive. For example, several studies have shown that people who have a strong sense of meaning and purpose in life have a substantially reduced risk for depression.

Although involvement in religious practices hasn't been studied as a specific treatment for depression, surveys have found that people who attend religious services may have a decreased rate of depression and suicide. The benefits of involvement in religious practices may also extend to improving physical health and increasing the life span.

The broad definition that we gave for spirituality leaves room for people of different backgrounds to consider how depression might be affecting their spiritual life and how they might use spiritually oriented avenues in the recovery process. Are you getting any ideas for using the spiritual path?

The Mindfulness Path

The last path for coping with depression that we describe in this book is mindfulness meditation. This method was pioneered by Drs. Mark Williams, John Teasdale, Zindel Segal, and Jon Kabat-Zinn, who blended mindfulness practices derived from ancient Buddhist traditions with the more modern principles of CBT to develop a treatment program they call "mindfulness-based cognitive therapy." Their approach enhances people's ability to stay "in the moment" and to fully experience and appreciate the good things in their lives. Achieving a state of mindfulness can help people stay away from the dark road to depression.

FAST
FACTS
- Mindfulness teaches people to focus their attention in a way that helps calm their emotions, relieve stress, and reduce negative thinking.

- Mindfulness changes negative thinking in a different way than traditional CBT.

Instead of directly challenging negative thoughts, meditative techniques are used to enhance positive emotions such as feelings of kindness and self-compassion while quieting worrisome or self-condemning thoughts.

Research on mindfulness meditation has shown that it can substantially reduce the risk of relapse into depression. In one study, people who participated in the mindfulness-based cognitive therapy program had about 50% fewer episodes of depression after treatment than those who didn't have the mindfulness-oriented treatment. Therefore mindfulness-based cognitive therapy is typically recommended for people who have had more than one episode of depression. Investigators also have found that people who received mindfulness-based cognitive therapy reported improved quality of life, better interpersonal relationships, and an ability to accept that negative thinking is a part of depression and not an accurate representation of themselves.

Despite these potential benefits, *a note of caution is needed*. Researchers on mindfulness-based cognitive therapy typically recommend that it *not* be used as a treatment for acute or severe depression. Instead, it is usually implemented when people have either recovered or made significant progress with other treatments and are trying to resolve residual symptoms. The meditative practices that are a core element of this approach may require levels of concentration and attention that are hard to achieve if you are deeply depressed. Because of these limitations, we offer the following recommendations:

- Do not use mindfulness as a stand-alone treatment for acute or severe depression.
- Use mindfulness only if this approach appeals to you and you find that the practices outlined in Chapter 13 are enjoyable and helpful.
- Use mindfulness methods primarily as a way to enhance quality of life and to reduce the risk for relapse.

To give you a brief preview of the mindfulness methods described in Chapter 13, we'll outline three features of the mindfulness path.

1. *Learn how to shift from the "doing mode" to the "being mode."* Most of us spend the majority of our days in the "doing mode." Our minds are churning with thoughts about accomplishing tasks, how we are measuring up, how we are going to manage lists of things yet to be accomplished, and how we might handle the other stresses of the day. Although the doing mode is critically important for getting things done, we can get so consumed by having our minds in this mode that our senses can be dulled to the pleasures and joys of life.

Mindfulness exercises build up your ability to enter the "being mode" in which you become fully aware of sensations such as the tastes of the food that you eat, calming feelings in your body, and positive emotions about important people in your life. Achieving a good balance between the being mode and the doing mode can enhance quality of life because you become more open to experiences of happiness and acceptance while paying less attention to unproductive self-talk and negatively toned ruminations.

A Mindfulness Questionnaire

Instructions: Answer these questions to explore how a mindfulness-based approach might help you cope with depression. If you answer yes to the first question and to three or more of the other questions, you may want to add the mindfulness path to your plan for wellness.

Question	Yes	No	Comment
Are you at the point where your depression is in fairly good control and you think you could concentrate on learning to use mindfulness practices?			
Have you had more than one episode of depression and you want to find ways to cut the chances of depression returning?			
Do you get preoccupied with negative or worrisome thinking and have trouble putting these thoughts aside?			
Do you think you need to open yourself up to an increased sense of self-acceptance and self-compassion?			
Do you often find yourself engaging in "mindless" activities in which you are not fully aware of the richness of your life experiences?			
Do you need to work on ways to be less stressed?			
Have you ever tried meditation and found it helpful?			
Would you like to learn more about mindfulness as a way of improving quality of life and controlling depression?			

2. *Learn about the downsides of "mindlessness."* In Chapter 13, you'll have the opportunity to take an inventory to see whether you have fallen prey to some of the common features of mindlessness, such as:

- Daydreaming or letting your mind drift when you could be appreciating good things that are "right under your nose."
- Listening to someone with one ear while doing something else at the same time.
- Worrying about the past or future without having much awareness of the present moment.
- Driving your car or doing other routine activities while on "automatic pilot"—then realizing that you had little memory of what happened while you were engaged in that activity.

Spotting these types of "mindless" activities can help you develop a more centered and mindful way of engaging in activities of everyday life.

3. *Learn how to use basic meditation methods.* Simple meditation practices such as paying attention to your breath or other sensations in your body are part of the mindfulness-based cognitive therapy program. You don't have to have extensive training in meditation to gain help from these practices, so we suggest some easy-to-use methods for building meditation skills in Chapter 13. If you find these practices helpful and wish to expand your knowledge and application of mindfulness, you might consider starting more formal training in meditation.

Exercise 3.11 on the previous page might help you identify some reasons to explore the mindfulness path as part of your plan for overcoming depression.

After answering these questions, you should have a better sense of how much you want to use the mindfulness path in your journey out of depression. So take a moment now to rate your interest using Exercise 3.12.

EXERCISE 3.12	**My Interest in Using the Mindfulness Path**

Instructions: Place a mark on the ruler to indicate your interest in using the mindfulness path to overcome depression.

```
|ı|ı|ı|ı|ı|ı|ı|ı|ı|ı|ı|ı|ı|ı|ı|ı|ı|ı|ı|ı|ı|ı|ı|ı|ı|ı|ı|ı|ı|ı|ı|ı|ı|
0     1     2     3     4     5     6     7     8     9     10
```

None   Moderate   Maximum

Charting a Course to Recovery

Our next step is to pull all of your ratings together to get a "dashboard" display of the paths that you might want to take to overcome depression. To do Exercise 3.13, just leaf back through this chapter to retrieve the interest scores that you gave to each of the paths. If you have any specific ideas about things you would like to try or questions that you want to answer as you read this book, you can write these down in the comments column.

Before you complete the exercise, we want to return for a moment to the concept of using evidence-based treatments. In discussing the possible paths to recovery, we have suggested many different ideas for charting an effective course. The scientific evidence is greater for some of these approaches than for others, so in our clinical work we typically recommend one of the biological treatments and/or psychotherapies that have been demonstrated to be effective in a large number of studies. The other strategies, such as lifestyle changes or using the spiritual and/or mindfulness paths, can then be used to augment the basic treatment initiatives. So, if your symptom rating on the Patient Health Questionnaire–9 (PHQ-9) introduced in Chapter 1 indicates significant depression, we suggest that you get professional help in using one of the very well-established, scientifically proven treatments.

To help organize your work in the book, you may want to work first on chapters that discuss paths that you think might be the most helpful. The chart below shows which chapters discuss each path.

Chapter Organization
Breaking Free from Depression: Pathways to Wellness

Path to recovery	Chapter numbers	Title
The thoughts–action path	4	Fighting Negative Thinking
	5	Restoring Energy and Enjoying Life
	6	Building Self-Esteem and Using Strengths
	7	Enhancing Well-Being
The biology path	8	Getting the Most from Antidepressants
The relationship path	9	The People in Your Life: How Relationships Can Influence Recovery from Depression
	10	Managing Relationship Problems to Improve Depression
The lifestyle path	11	Lifestyle Changes
The spiritual path	12	Using Spiritual Resources
The mindfulness path	13	Mindfulness

My Interest in Using the Paths to Wellness

Instructions: Record the interest ratings you made for each of the paths to wellness here. Then make some notes about how you might like to use the paths.

Path to recovery	Interest score	Comments
Thoughts–action path		
Biology path		
Relationship path		
Lifestyle path		
Spiritual path		
Mindfulness path		

From *Breaking Free from Depression*. Copyright 2012 by The Guilford Press.

Summary

The path to recovery can focus on using a single approach such as an antidepressant or a proven form of psychotherapy. But people who want to develop a more diverse and multitextured path can select from a range of potentially useful strategies. In this chapter we suggest that you choose at least one of the evidence-based approaches that has been shown to be effective for depression and that you strengthen your plan by drawing from the rich resources of other paths to wellness. As you work through the remaining chapters in this book, you'll be able to learn about many powerful methods for putting depression behind you.

THE THOUGHTS–ACTION PATH

4

Fighting Negative Thinking

> ## Chapter Highlights
>
> ▶ Negative thinking in depression
>
> ▶ Spotting automatic thoughts
>
> ▶ Challenging automatic thoughts
>
> ▶ Modifying automatic thoughts

When you're depressed, do you think less about the good times in your life? Do you find it hard to shut off your worries? Do you put yourself down? Is it hard to be upbeat about the future? If your answer to any of these questions is yes, you are not alone. Most people with depression have a shift in their thinking style that is part of the problem—but it also can be part of the solution.

In Chapter 3 you were introduced to the thoughts–action path and completed a brief checklist of some negative thoughts that people commonly have when depressed. In this chapter, you'll learn how to spot depressive thinking, challenge distorted or unproductive thoughts, and make changes in your thinking style that will help you overcome depression.

Negative Thinking in Depression

To become skilled at changing depressive thinking, it can help to learn about how thoughts—or *cognitions*, to use the term from CBT—become negatively biased in depression.

DEFINITION *Cognition* is a word used to describe our thinking. Examples of cognitions are thoughts, ideas, and conclusions that we have reached.

Self-Talk

The great majority of our thoughts are not expressed out loud. Think for a minute about the percentage of your thoughts that are part of your self-talk or your inner dialogue. When people become depressed, their self-talk usually changes. It can become more doubting, self-critical, or pessimistic, as illustrated in the following example.

Ted

When Ted, a middle-aged man who works as a sales agent for a construction equipment company, isn't depressed, his self-talk during meetings at work is usually centered on finding solutions for business problems. Even if his mind drifts to other topics, such as looking forward to playing in an amateur soccer league match after work or remembering an interesting movie he saw over the weekend, the tone of his inner dialogue is generally positive, or at least neutral. And he can quickly focus his thoughts back on the agenda at hand—being an effective participant in the business meeting.

Ted's self-talk when he is depressed has a very different quality. Here is what Ted was thinking at a recent meeting.

"My new sales campaign is like everything else in my life—it's going nowhere. If I don't get something accomplished soon, the whole thing will fall apart. Everybody else is doing fine, but I just mess everything up."

Did you notice that Ted is using strongly negative, absolute terms to describe his situation? Perhaps his problems at work and the rest of his life are really that bad. But if depression is influencing his thinking, Ted might be able to start feeling better by spotting the negative thoughts, challenging them, and modifying his thinking style to be more realistic and balanced. Even if he isn't doing as well with his job as usual, the self-condemning thoughts aren't doing him any good. He would be better off if he could accurately assess any problems, give himself credit for his strengths, and then focus his energies on finding ways to manage the situation more effectively.

Another example, one with a humorous twist, also shows how negative self-talk can drive people further down. In the cartoon on the facing page, Charles Schulz, the creator of Peanuts, gives a good illustration of how negative self-talk can breed depressed mood and depressed behavior. Charlie Brown is offered a seemingly wonderful opportunity—to go down the "grocery aisle of life" and choose anything he wants to put in his cart. But, his response—"I think I have six items or less"—has the classic ring of depressive thinking. As Charlie puts himself down and minimizes his potential, his body language shows a sagging mood and a sense of defeat and helplessness.

Your Self-Talk

Did either of these examples stimulate you to think of some of your own self-talk? Are you like Ted in shifting to more negative or self-critical self-talk when you get depressed? Could you be like Charlie Brown, who has a pessimistic view of himself and his life prospects?

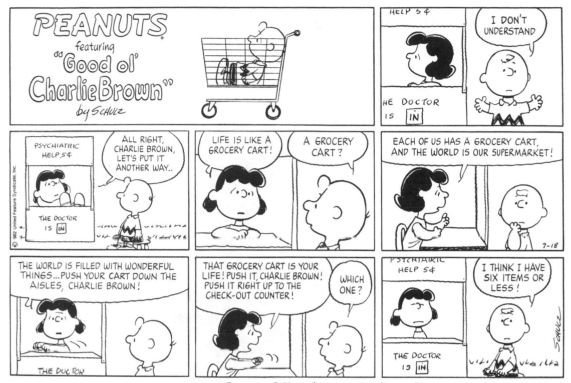

Peanuts. © United Feature Syndicate, Inc. Reprinted by permission.

When Ted started CBT, his therapist suggested a simple exercise (shown on the next page) to help him understand the impact of self-talk on depression. After you see Ted's responses, you can do the same exercise yourself.

This exercise showed Ted that there was a distinct change in his thinking style when he became depressed, and the exercise set the stage for his learning to use other self-help methods to spot and change his negative thoughts. After you view Ted's example, you can draw some pie graphs to start analyzing your self-talk.

Automatic Thoughts

One of the most important characteristics of self-talk is that many of our thoughts have an automatic quality. They just pop into our heads and stir up emotions without our stopping to fully evaluate them to see whether they are true. During periods of depression or anxiety, thoughts often become more automatic and less rational. In some cases they just roll through people's heads like a runaway train, causing lots of emotional distress and diverting energy into unproductive and self-defeating behavior. An example of automatic thoughts is when Ted was invited to go bowling with a friend. As soon as his friend mentioned the idea during a phone call, Ted thought "He's just trying to be nice ... I'm such a drag, nobody would really want to go anywhere with me ... I'd be miserable all night long ... I better make an excuse so I can stay home."

Ted's Analysis of His Self-Talk

Step 1: Draw a pie graph that shows how much of your self-talk has a negative, worried, or self-critical tone when your depression is *most severe*. Also, note how much of your self-talk is in the neutral or positive/pleasurable categories.

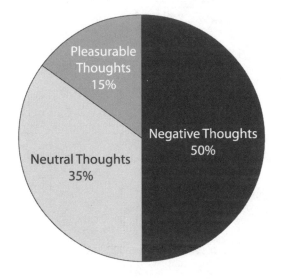

Step 2: Draw a pie graph that shows how much of your self-talk has a negative, worried, or self-critical tone when you are *not* depressed (or before you became depressed). Also, note how much of your self-talk is in the neutral and positive or pleasurable categories.

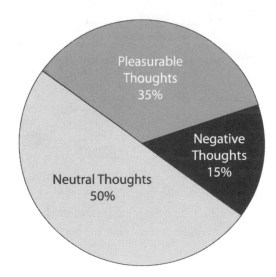

My Self-Talk When I Am Depressed
and When I Am Not Depressed

Instructions: Draw pie graphs to show your thinking style when your depression is most severe and when it has totally gone away (or before you became depressed). If you have been depressed for many years and have trouble thinking of a time when you were not depressed, try to imagine what your thinking would be like if the depression went away.

Step 1: Draw a pie graph that shows how much of your self-talk has a negative, worried, or self-critical tone when your depression is *most severe*. Also, note how much of your self-talk is in the neutral and positive or pleasurable categories.

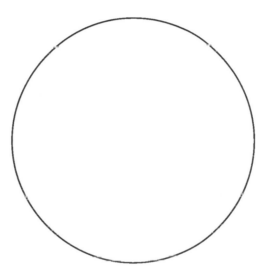

Step 2: Draw a pie graph that shows how much of your self-talk has a negative, worried, or self-critical tone when you are *not* depressed (or before you became depressed). Also, note how much of your self-talk is in the neutral and positive or pleasurable categories.

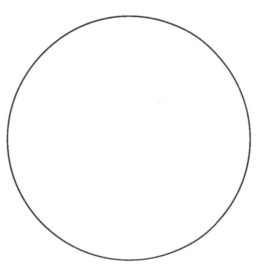

SCIENCE
CORNER

- Studies have found dramatic increases in negative automatic thoughts when people become depressed.
- Research on CBT has shown that this treatment has a marked effect in reducing negative automatic thoughts.
- In one study performed by Jesse Wright, an author of this book, and his associates, treatment with CBT reduced negative automatic thoughts to about a third of their pretreatment level.

Another example of automatic thoughts is shown in a Peanuts comic strip of Charlie Brown working at the chalkboard in his classroom.

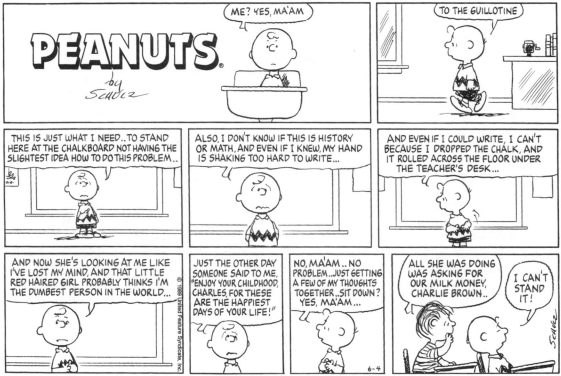

Peanuts: © United Feature Syndicate, Inc. Reprinted by permission.

Key Features of Automatic Thoughts

Some of the key features of automatic thoughts are:

1. Everybody has automatic thoughts.
2. Automatic thoughts are more common and more likely to be negatively biased when people are depressed.
3. Although automatic thoughts are typically under the surface of our thinking, and

we may not be fully tuned in to them, they have a strong impact on our emotions and our behavior.

4. People can learn to spot negative automatic thoughts and change them.
5. Changing negative automatic thoughts is an especially valuable skill for overcoming depression.

What If Your Automatic Thoughts Are True?

You may be thinking "I have real problems ... It's not just that I'm having negative automatic thoughts." Of course, most people with depression face real problems. They can have marital or family conflicts, financial difficulties, health issues, job stresses, or other problems that may have played a role in triggering symptoms or are making it hard to get over the depression. Someone might think "I'm bound to lose my job" when the likelihood of being laid off or getting fired is actually quite high. Or another person who is waiting for his wife to come home and is thinking "I'm sure she is having an affair" might later find that she is being unfaithful.

The CBT strategy for working with automatic thoughts is first to recognize that they are occurring and then to check them out to see if they are true. When automatic thoughts are negatively biased and are part of the depression, as is so often the case, efforts are made to develop more rational thoughts. For example, if Ted thinks "He's just trying to be nice ... I'm such a drag, nobody would really want to go anywhere with me" when his friend genuinely wants Ted's company, there is a great opportunity for helping Ted by changing his automatic thoughts. When automatic thoughts are true or have a reasonable chance of being accurate, however, the therapy focuses on building ways to cope with the problem.

? **Are you having automatic thoughts that may be true?**

If so, you can write down some of these thoughts here:

_____

_____

_____

_____

What can you do to cope?

- Don't try to ignore automatic thoughts that are true or "sweep them under the rug." They need to be recognized so that an effective coping plan can be developed.

- See the section on "coping cards" later in this chapter and other action-oriented strategies for problem solving described throughout the book. These methods can help you take practical steps to manage your real-life problems.

- Even if some of your automatic thoughts are true, you probably have some other negatively biased or distorted automatic thoughts that can be prime targets for CBT. Changing these types of thoughts can often help relieve depression and anxiety.

How Do Automatic Thoughts Affect Emotions and Behavior?

In describing the thoughts–action path in Chapter 3, we explained the close link between thoughts, emotions, and actions. Because this is such an important concept, we'll briefly review it here.

Just for a moment, flip back to the cartoon of Charlie Brown in the "grocery store of life." When Charlie had the negative automatic thought "I think I have six items or less," what happened to his mood? His facial expression certainly didn't show much happiness or pleasure. Instead he looked downcast and depressed, and it seemed unlikely that he would respond in a positive way to Lucy's invitation. The link between triggering events, automatic thoughts, emotions, and behavior is shown in the next example.

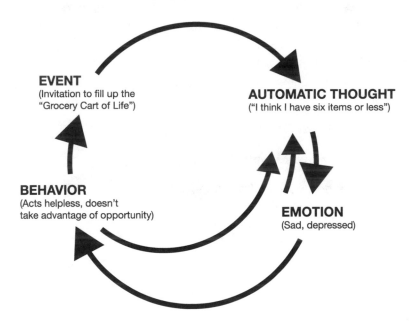

EVENT
(Invitation to fill up the "Grocery Cart of Life")

AUTOMATIC THOUGHT
("I think I have six items or less")

EMOTION
(Sad, depressed)

BEHAVIOR
(Acts helpless, doesn't take advantage of opportunity)

FAST FACTS

- Automatic thoughts and other cognitions are a driving force behind our emotions.
- An advantage of spotting automatic thoughts is that it can give you a way to learn to control or reduce painful emotions.

? **Do you understand the difference between a thought and an emotion?**

Write down an example of one of your thoughts or cognitions:

_____

_____

Then write down the emotions associated with this thought:

_____

_____

If you have trouble figuring out the differences between thoughts and emotions, these points may help:

- Thoughts are ideas, evaluations we make of ourselves or situations, or conclusions we reach.

- If you said to yourself "I feel worthless," you would actually be stating a thought about yourself—not a feeling or an emotion. But if you did have a thought like "I feel worthless," it would likely stir up some emotions such as sadness or anger toward yourself.

- Emotions are feelings—such as happiness, sadness, anxiety, fear, anger, pleasure, ecstasy, irritability, tension, and calmness.

To practice recognizing the link between automatic thoughts and emotions, try to find the correct answers in the quiz in Exercise 4.2.

Spotting Automatic Thoughts

The three steps that you will use to change negative thinking are:

Spot ▶ **Challenge** ▶ **Modify**

If you can tune in to your negative thinking and spot automatic thoughts, you will be well on your way to change. Simply recognizing that your thinking has taken a twist in an unhelpful direction is often enough to start the process of getting back to a healthier way of seeing yourself and your future.

You already completed some self-help exercises in the first part of this chapter that have probably helped you recognize some of your automatic thoughts. But now we want to introduce you to one of the most powerful methods from CBT—thought recording. This technique helps you identify the automatic thoughts that are the most troubling and most relevant to your depression.

Automatic Thoughts and Emotions

Instructions: Choose the emotion(s) that you think would be most likely to be stimulated by each of the automatic thoughts. There is only one correct answer for each automatic thought.

Automatic Thoughts:

1. (Ted) He's just trying to be nice ... I'm such a drag, nobody would really want to go anywhere with me. _____

2. (A person having a panic attack) I can't get my breath. I'll have a heart attack or a stroke. _____

3. (A person who is having an argument with his partner) She never listens to a thing I say ... I might as well be talking to the wall ... Nobody gives a ##!! about me. _____

4. (A person who has manic symptoms and has grandiose ideas about a new business idea) I can't miss on this one ... It's sure to be a huge success. _____

5. (A person who is studying for an exam) This is too much for me ... I'll mess up for sure ... I can't seem to do anything right. _____

Emotions:

a. Fear, sadness

b. Anger, sadness

c. Happiness, euphoria

d. Sadness

e. Anxiety

Answers:

1. d

2. e

3. b

4. c

5. a

FAST
FACTS
- Thought recording is an excellent method from CBT for spotting, challenging, and modifying automatic thoughts.
- If you practice thought recording regularly, you will probably gain powerful skills for changing negative thoughts and overcoming depression.

Thought Recording

In the first stage of using a thought-recording log you:

1. Identify specific events or triggers for negative automatic thoughts.
2. Write down the automatic thoughts on the log.
3. Record and rate the emotions that are stimulated by the automatic thoughts.

Ted used a thought-recording log to tune in to the negative cognitions that were a large part of his depression. One of his logs from when he was most depressed showed a flurry of negative automatic thoughts that were causing very painful emotions.

You might be wondering how writing down automatic thoughts could possibly help. Wouldn't paying attention to the negativity that is in much of Ted's thought-recording log make him feel more depressed, tense, and nervous? Although there is some risk that looking at negative automatic thoughts could deepen a depression (especially if the thinking remains fixed and the person concludes that the situation is hopeless), research on CBT has shown that logging methods work very well for most people. Writing down the thoughts and the emotions brings them out in the open, where they can be questioned and changed. As we show in the next section of the chapter, CBT thought-recording methods can be expanded to work on developing rational, healthy thoughts that help with coping instead of driving people further into depression.

Before you try your hand at thought recording, it may be helpful for you to review Ted's log to answer these questions:

1. Can you spot two or three examples of particularly strong wording that suggests that Ted's automatic thoughts could be distorted and not entirely accurate? One of the characteristics of negative automatic thoughts is that they often use very strong or absolute terms.

Ted's automatic thoughts that are worded in an absolute manner:
1.
2.
3.

Ted's Thought-Recording Log

Event *Write down an event or situation, or a memory of an event, that triggered automatic thoughts.*	Automatic thoughts *Record the automatic thoughts that occurred while you were experiencing or thinking about this event.*	Emotions *Identify emotions such as sadness or anger that were stimulated by the automatic thoughts. Rate the intensity of the emotions on a 0–100 point scale where 100 = the most extreme emotion.*
My wife gets upset as I'm trying to pay the bills. She is worried about our finances because I haven't been making as many sales as usual.	*I'm failing again. If this keeps up, she's bound to leave me. My life is falling apart. I don't know what to do.*	*Sad 90* *Anxious 90* *Tense 80*
I call one of my old customers. He isn't interested in buying any construction equipment now.	*This is a catastrophe. This business is going straight downhill.*	*Anxious 95* *Sad 70*
Watching my son's soccer game.	*I really love soccer. It's great to see him playing. He's a terrific kid. But my life is full of trouble. I could lose everything.*	*Happy (at least for a while) 70* *Calm (for the first part of the game) 40* *Then tense (75), anxious (80), and sad (80)*

2. The last entry in the log is an example of a mixture of positive or adaptive thoughts and negative automatic thoughts. Try to help Ted with this one. What might you say that could help him retain the positive feelings for a longer time and avoid slipping into the negative thinking of depression?

Tips for Ted:

1.

2.

3.

Thought-Recording Log

Instructions: Identify at least one situation in which you had troubling automatic thoughts and emotions. You can also use the log to record positive thoughts and emotions.

Event *Write down an event or situation, or a memory of an event, that triggered automatic thoughts.*	Automatic Thoughts *Record the automatic thoughts that occurred while you were experiencing or thinking about this event.*	Emotions *Identify emotions such as sadness or anger that were stimulated by the automatic thoughts. Rate the intensity of the emotions on a 0–100 point scale where 100 = the most extreme emotion.*

Using Your Emotions to Spot Automatic Thoughts

Because automatic thoughts almost always trigger emotions, a good way to learn to spot automatic thoughts is to first recognize strong surges in feelings such as sadness, anxiety, irritability, or anger. Then you can step back to identify the thoughts that went through your mind just before you started having the more intense feelings. An example of the value of using strong emotions as markers of automatic thoughts are the anxiety attacks that Angelina has been trying to overcome.

Angelina

Angelina suffers from both depression and anxiety. When she has a sudden bout with anxiety, it seems like it "comes out of the blue" and there is no way to control it. During a treatment session with one of us, she said that she couldn't remember any thoughts that she was having before her waves of anxiety.

To help Angelina find out what thoughts might be preceding the spells of anxiety, she was asked to first remember all she could about the emotions she felt during one of these attacks. Next she was asked to imagine herself back in the anxiety spell and to think about what she was doing right before the spell began. Her answers helped pave the way for helpful work on overcoming the anxiety. The dialogue between Angelina and Dr. Wright went like this:

Angelina: I don't have any thoughts. I just feel so anxious I can't stand it. Then I will do anything I can to get away by myself, where I can try to settle down.

Dr. Wright: Even though it seems like the emotions come "out of the blue," I wonder if we are missing something here. Could we try an exercise to see if we can find out more about what is going on?

Angelina: Sure.

Dr. Wright: Okay. Try to put yourself back in the situation and describe your emotions in as much detail as possible. Can you imagine yourself having your last anxiety attack?

Angelina: I was feeling fairly good, but then I got real tense, and I was full of fear.

Dr. Wright: What else?

Angelina: I got short of breath, I felt dizzy, and I was sure I would pass out.

Dr. Wright: What could you have been thinking about that could have made you so anxious? Can you imagine yourself back in the time before the anxiety began to build? What were you thinking?

Angelina: I was thinking "I'm totally overwhelmed ... It's too much for me ... I'm losing control ... I've got to get out of here."

? Are you having difficulty identifying automatic thoughts? If so, you can try these strategies:

- Use your emotions as avenues to understanding. After you recognize a surge of emotion, try to imagine yourself right before the emotion increased. What were you doing? What were you thinking?

- Sometimes automatic thoughts can take the form of mental images instead of words. If you can get in touch with a mental image that seemed to set off an emotional reaction, try to put this image into words. An example is when Ted couldn't think of any specific thoughts at first but could see an image of himself getting very tense at a dinner party with some friends. After describing the image, he was able to recognize some upsetting thoughts such as "Everything is going great in their lives, mine is a disaster . . . I'll never be happy."

Using a Checklist to Spot Automatic Thoughts

In Chapter 3 we introduced you to negative thinking in depression by having you complete a brief checklist. Now that you've learned much more about depressive thinking, we want you to use another checklist to see whether you have any commonly occurring automatic thoughts that you would like to target for change. The checklist on the next page is a shortened form of the scale called the Automatic Thoughts Questionnaire that is used by doctors and therapists in clinical practice of CBT and also has been used extensively in research studies in depression. You can use the checklist to spot automatic thoughts and also to measure your progress in overcoming depression. Blank checklist forms are available on the publisher's website (*www.guilford.com/breakingfreeforms*), or you can make several photocopies of the form that follows, so you can check your scores as you work through the book.

Challenging Automatic Thoughts

After you spot some automatic thoughts, the next step is to check them out to see whether they are being influenced by the negative mind-set of depression. In a way, you need to act like a scientist and be very objective. You need to ask yourself questions that can sort out accurate, true thoughts from ones that are colored by depressive thinking.

You can challenge or test your automatic thoughts in several very useful ways:

1. Turn off the automatic pilot.
2. Recognize your strengths.
3. Examine the evidence.
4. Look for thinking errors.

Automatic Thoughts Checklist

Instructions: This list contains a variety of automatic thoughts that just pop into people's heads. Use the list to indicate how frequently each of the thoughts occurred to you over the past week.

	Never	Sometimes	Moderately often	A great deal of the time	All the time
1. I wish I were a better person.	0	1	2	3	4
2. No one understands me.	0	1	2	3	4
3. I can't get things together.	0	1	2	3	4
4. I feel like I'm up against the world.	0	1	2	3	4
5. I've let people down.	0	1	2	3	4
6. Nothing feels good anymore.	0	1	2	3	4
7. I'm so disappointed in myself.	0	1	2	3	4
8. I can't get started.	0	1	2	3	4
9. I hate myself.	0	1	2	3	4
10. I'm so helpless.	0	1	2	3	4
11. My life is a mess.	0	1	2	3	4
12. I'm worthless.	0	1	2	3	4
13. My future is bleak.	0	1	2	3	4
14. It's just not worth it.	0	1	2	3	4
15. I can't finish anything.	0	1	2	3	4

Add columns: _____ + _____ + _____ + _____

Total:

Adapted with permission from Hollon, S. D. & Kendall, P. C. (1980). Cognitive self-statements in depression: Development of an automatic thought questionnaire. *Cognitive Therapy and Research, 4*, 383–395.

Turning Off the Automatic Pilot

If your thinking has been on automatic pilot, and you have been having lots of automatic thoughts that you haven't fully questioned or checked out, it's time to take the controls. Unlike flying a plane, you don't need special training to do this. Just pause for a brief while to *think about your thinking*. Take a time-out to ask yourself some questions about your automatic thoughts.

QUICK
TIPS

- When you go off automatic pilot, you are making a conscious decision to check out your automatic thoughts.
- The great teacher of ancient times, Socrates, asked his students questions that stimulated them to think about situations in fresh and creative ways. This helped them avoid getting into ruts of thinking in the same way over and over. You can do the same thing for yourself.
- You can ask yourself questions such as these:
  ○ "What other ways could I view this situation?"
  ○ "What would a good friend say about my thinking? What positive or encouraging things might he tell me?"
  ○ "If I wasn't depressed, how might my thinking change? How would my automatic thoughts be different?"

Recognizing Your Strengths

Depression is often a thief of self-esteem. It seems to rob people of abilities to see their strengths, to give themselves credit for good things they have done, or to remember contributions they have made. It also makes people minimize their potential for using their strengths in the future. By identifying your strengths, you can challenge negative automatic thoughts and develop a more balanced thinking style.

When Ted was depressed, his flaws and shortcomings seemed to stand out in bold relief, while his positive features faded into the background. It was almost as if all of his previous successes in his business, his hard-won education, everything he had poured into building a life for his family, and the strong support and love that his family had for him were from another planet. On one level he was aware of all of these things, but he became so consumed with the depressive thinking that he mostly ignored his strengths.

Not all people with depression become as negatively preoccupied as Ted. Perhaps your self-esteem is still fairly robust, and you are aware of many of your strengths. But even if you still can give yourself credit for many of your positives, it could help to take some time to catalog your strengths and think of how you might use them to build your power over depression.

Ted did the exercise on page 77 to counter his negative automatic thoughts and also to identify some of his attributes that could be used to fight depression.

Does seeing Ted's strengths inventory stimulate you to think of some of your own

| EXERCISE 4.5 | **Going Off Automatic Pilot** |

Choose an automatic thought from the Thought-Recording Log or the Automatic Thoughts Checklist. Write this thought down here:

_____

_____

_____

Now go *off* automatic pilot. Look at this thought from different angles. Ask yourself questions that make you think about your thinking. Write down some alternatives here:

_____

_____

_____

_____

_____

_____

_____

_____

strengths? You can use the same inventory now to record some of your positive features that will help you challenge negative automatic thoughts and work toward recovery from depression.

Examining the Evidence

People with depression usually don't stop very often to question their negative thoughts. They accept the negative thoughts as proven facts despite evidence to the contrary. To develop the kind of healthy thinking style that can help you overcome depression, you need to move three key words into a very prominent part of your vocabulary. The three words are:

WHAT'S THE EVIDENCE?

Ted's Inventory of Strengths

Some of my strengths as a friend are:

I'm loyal to my friends. They can always trust me. I'll go out of my way to help them.

Some of my strengths as a family member are:

I really love my wife and my kids. I'd do anything for them. They seem to love me and stick by me, even when I'm not at my best. I get along well with my parents and my brother. We have always had a close family.

Some of my skills as a worker are:

I know all of the basics of my job. I've been a sales leader many years in the past. I am honest with my customers and keep their best interests in mind. I've weathered many downturns in the business cycle before.

Some of my skills in coping with stress are:

I've exercised in the past—this helped with stress. When I am feeling better, I can have a pretty good sense of humor. Helping with my son's soccer league has been good for me.

Some of my best attributes are:

I care about other people. I like to help other people. I worked my way through school and got a good education. I've worked steadily for over 20 years. People can count on me.

Some of my interests or hobbies are:

I played sports in school and used to enjoy tennis. At one time, I read a fair number of books. I like to read about and take care of cars.

Some of my other strengths are:

My spiritual beliefs. I am a fairly good cook, and when I am feeling well, I do a lot of the cooking for my family. Even though I get down, I don't give up.

My Strengths Inventory

Instructions: Try to lift the veil of depression and identify some of the strengths that you have had during your life or strengths you might be able to develop further in the future. You may need to think back to before you became depressed, or imagine that the depression is gone, to generate full answers to these questions.

Some of my strengths as a friend are:
Some of my strengths as a family member are:
Some of my skills as a worker are:
Some of my skills in coping with stress are:
Some of my best attributes are:
Some of my interests or hobbies are:
Some of my other strengths are:

Letting these three words be your guide, you can start to challenge negative automatic thoughts by using CBT methods for examining the evidence. Self-help exercises to examine the evidence are one of the most useful CBT tools. To use this method, you act like a wise and thoughtful judge who wants to collect all of the key evidence before coming to a conclusion. Angelina learned how to use this technique in her CBT sessions and then applied it in everyday life. An example of one of her evidence-examining exercises is shown below.

Ted also did an evidence-examining exercise. Check his responses and see whether you can think of anything else to add in the "evidence against" column. (Hint: review Ted's strengths inventory for ideas.)

If you reviewed Ted's strengths inventory, you might have noticed several entries that could have been added to the "evidence against" his automatic thought about his life falling apart and not knowing what to do. Another thing that you could do to help Ted with this exercise is to look carefully at the things he wrote in the "evidence for" column. When people first start using this self-help exercise, they often write down "evidence for"

Examining the Evidence: Angelina's Example

Automatic thought: *I'm totally overwhelmed ... It's too much for me.*

Evidence for automatic thought	Evidence against automatic thought
I have frequent anxiety attacks.	*I'm full of fear, but I survive these attacks.*
I get so tense that I can't think straight.	*I'm starting to learn to cope with depression and anxiety.*
My life isn't going so great right now.	*It's not as bad as I tell myself. I start using real strong words like "totally overwhelmed," and it makes the situation worse.*
	I've handled tough things in the past. I can keep fighting and get this under control.
	If I get my mind on something else, the anxiety starts to fade.

Alternative thoughts: *The anxiety is very upsetting, but I can tolerate it while I learn to manage it better.*

that seems convincing to them but is actually false evidence. Could you poke any holes in the second entry in Ted's "evidence for" his automatic thought? He fell into the trap of writing down some other negative automatic thoughts in this column.

It's your turn now to do a personal example of this exercise. (You may find that you want to do this exercise with automatic thoughts that you want to challenge in the future, in which case you can print out the blank form from the publisher's website, *www.guilford.com/breakingfreeforms*, or make photocopies.)

Looking for Thinking Errors

One of the most important things you can do to challenge and change automatic thoughts is to look for thinking errors. These errors in the logic of thought are very common in depression. They often act to validate negative automatic thoughts and to perpetuate symptoms.

Examining the Evidence: Ted's Example

Automatic thought: *My life is falling apart. I don't know what to do.*

Evidence for automatic thought	Evidence against automatic thought
My wife is really upset about the financial stress that we are facing.	*My wife and the rest of the family are still behind me. It's normal for all of us to be stressed by the financial situation.*
My business is going straight downhill. Everything seems like it is out of control.	*My boss is still supporting me. He knows I'm having a struggle now, but he reassured me that he thinks that business will get better before too long. He tells me I'm a great member of the team.*
My sales were off 15% in the last quarter.	*Most of the others also are seeing a downturn. The economy is tough right now.*

Alternative thoughts: *I'm under a lot of stress, but I'm still working steadily and I have good support. I need to hang in there until things improve.*

Examining the Evidence

Instructions: Write down an automatic thought that you want to challenge. Then try to identify any *evidence for* the validity of the thought and any *evidence against* the validity of the thought. If you conclude that there is enough evidence against the automatic thought, then write out some alternative thoughts.

Automatic thought:

_____

Evidence for automatic thought	Evidence against automatic thought

Alternative Thoughts:

_____

SCIENCE CORNER
- Everybody has thinking errors. Who among us is always completely logical and rational?
- However, studies have shown that when people are depressed they have about three times as many thinking errors as when they are not depressed.

To get started with recognizing some of your own thinking errors, take a few minutes to read and study the definitions in this list.

DEFINITIONS OF THINKING ERRORS*

- **All-or-nothing thinking:** Have you ever had thoughts like these? "Nothing ever goes my way ... There's no way I could handle it ... I always mess up ... She's got it all ... Everything is going wrong." These thoughts are examples of one of the most damaging of the thinking errors—*all-or-nothing thinking*.

    When you let *all-or-nothing thinking* go unchecked you see the world in absolute terms. Everything is completely black or completely white—all good or all bad. You believe that others are doing great and you are doing just the opposite.

    All-or-nothing thinking also can interfere with your working on tasks. Imagine what would happen if you thought you had to achieve 100% success or you shouldn't even try at all. It's usually better to set reasonable goals and to realize that we are rarely complete successes or total failures. Most things in life are not totally black or white but fall somewhere in between.

- **Jumping to conclusions:** Depressed people often *jump to conclusions*. They immediately think of the worst possible interpretations of situations. Once these negative images come into their minds, they become certain bad things will happen. Another form of *jumping to conclusions* is the tendency to immediately think that others see you in a negative light. Have you ever done this? If you *jump to conclusions,* you may feel overwhelmed or hopeless and give up trying.

- **Ignoring the evidence:** When you *ignore the evidence,* you make a judgment (usually about your shortcomings or about something you think you can't do) without looking at all the information. This thinking error has been called "the mental filter" because you filter, or screen out, valuable information about topics such as (1) positive experiences from the past, (2) your strengths, and (3) support that others can give. Instead of looking at a full range of information about the situation and your resources, you dwell on a negative feature or on a single flaw.

- **Magnifying or minimizing:** One of the most common thinking errors is *magnifying or minimizing* the significance of things in your life. When you are depressed, you often *magnify* your faults and *minimize* your strengths. You can also *magnify* the risks or difficulties in situations and *minimize* the options or resources that you have to manage the problem. Can you think of examples of times when you have done this?

*Adapted with permission from *Good Days Ahead: The Interactive Program for Depression and Anxiety* by Jesse H. Wright, Andrew S. Wright, and Aaron T. Beck. Copyright 2003, 2010 by Mindstreet; Copyright 2011 by Empower Interactive.

An extreme form of *magnifying* is sometimes called "catastrophizing." When you catastrophize, you automatically think that the worst possible thing will happen. If you are having an anxiety attack, your mind races with thoughts like "I'm going to have a heart attack or stroke" or "I'm going to totally lose control." Depressed persons may think they are bound to fail or that they are about to lose everything.

One of the ways to fight depression is to spot your tendency to *magnify* and *minimize*.

- **Overgeneralizing:** Sometimes we can let a single problem mean so much to us that it colors our view of everything in our lives. We can give a small difficulty or flaw so much significance that it seems to define the entire picture. This type of cognitive error is called *overgeneralizing*.

- **Personalizing:** Another way to make things worse is to get caught up in taking personal blame for everything that seems to go wrong. When you *personalize*, you accept full responsibility for a troubling situation or problem even when there isn't good evidence to back your conclusion. This type of thinking error undermines your self-esteem and makes you more depressed.

    Of course, you need to accept responsibility when you make mistakes. Owning up to problems can help you start to turn things around. However, if you can recognize when you are *personalizing*, you can avoid putting yourself down unnecessarily, and you can start to develop a more effective style of thinking.

We'll practice looking for thinking errors briefly in Exercise 4.8. You'll be able to get more experience in spotting thinking errors later in the chapter.

QUICK TIPS
- When you try to spot thinking errors in Exercise 4.8, don't worry if you don't make the exact same selections as we did.
- There is considerable overlap in the definitions of thinking errors, and often it is a judgment call to select the errors involved in an automatic thought.
- It can help a lot just to recognize that *any* thinking errors are occurring.
- When you look for thinking errors in your own automatic thoughts, just try to write down any errors that you think might be giving you trouble. Taking this step can give you a big boost in your progress in changing negative automatic thoughts.

Next you can try to look for thinking errors in some of your own automatic thoughts in Exercise 4.9.

Modifying Automatic Thoughts

We've been working on the *challenging* phase of changing automatic thoughts for a while, so it might help to stop briefly for a reminder about the three steps used to change automatic thoughts. The three steps are:

Looking for Thinking Errors

Instructions: Review the definitions of thinking errors and then try to spot some of these errors in Ted's automatic thoughts. Place a check mark beside the thinking errors that you believe may be involved in each automatic thought.

Automatic thoughts	All-or-nothing thinking	Jumping to conclusions	Ignoring the evidence	Magnifying or minimizing	Overgeneralizing	Personalizing
If this keeps up, she (wife) is bound to leave me.						
My life is falling apart. I don't know what to do.						
This business is going straight downhill.						

Suggested answers:

If this keeps up, she (wife) is bound to leave me.

This automatic thought is loaded with thinking errors such as jumping to conclusions (that she is bound to leave him), ignoring the evidence (that his wife is still very supportive), magnifying the problem, overgeneralizing (letting the financial problem color his view of his entire marriage and life), and personalizing (taking excessive blame for the problems at work, when there is an economic downturn and most of the others are also struggling).

My life is falling apart. I don't know what to do.

This thought also is laced with cognitive errors such as all-or-nothing thinking (stating the problem in black-and-white or absolute terms), ignoring the evidence (that he has many positives at work and at home and he has coped with economic downturns before), magnifying the problem and minimizing his strengths, and overgeneralizing.

This business is going straight downhill.

This automatic thought is a classic case of all-or-nothing thinking. Ted is also jumping to conclusions (about what will happen with his business), ignoring the evidence (for example, of his boss's support and encouragement), and magnifying the extent of the problem at work.

Spot ▶ Challenge ▶ Modify

You've already done a good deal of the work you'll need to do to change automatic thoughts by spotting them and challenging them. In fact, we suspect that you have already made good progress toward being able to change your automatic thoughts. In this last stage of changing automatic thoughts we'll teach you some extra methods that can help you "seal the deal" on breaking out of a depressed thinking style. First we'll revisit the thought-recording method to add some useful elements to this powerful technique.

EXERCISE 4.9	Looking for Thinking Errors

Instructions: Write down one or more of your automatic thoughts that you would like to change. Then try to spot some of thinking errors in your automatic thoughts. Place a check mark beside the thinking errors that you believe may be involved in each automatic thought.

Automatic thoughts	All-or-nothing thinking	Jumping to conclusions	Ignoring the evidence	Magnifying or minimizing	Overgeneralizing	Personalizing

Thought Change Records

Earlier in this chapter you used a thought-recording log to spot some of your automatic thoughts. By expanding this log to five columns, you'll have a valuable, scientifically tested method from CBT to modify negative thoughts.

The key actions that you will take in using thought change records are:

1. Record events, automatic thoughts, and emotions just as you did in the earlier thought recording log.
2. Rate the degree of belief in the automatic thoughts at the time they occurred. This rating will tell you how strong the automatic thoughts were before you tried to change them.
3. Challenge negative automatic thoughts by going off automatic pilot, examining the evidence, and looking for thinking errors.
4. Then write out some rational alternatives to the negative automatic thoughts.
5. Rate your degree of belief in the rational alternatives.
6. Finally, rerate the intensity of your emotions after you have modified the automatic thought. Also, record any changes in your behavior. Are you coping better? What are you doing differently as a result of changing your automatic thoughts?

To get familiar with this method, let's look at an example. After Ted spotted some automatic thoughts, turned off his automatic pilot, examined the evidence, and found some thinking errors, he completed the thought change record on the facing page.

We strongly recommend that you complete Thought Change Records (TCRs) on a regular basis. If you want to build skills in recognizing and changing automatic thoughts, the TCR is a basic tool to help you do the job. In Exercise 4.10, you can complete your first TCR. This form is available in an electronic version on the publisher's website (*www. guilford.com/breakingfreeforms*), or you can make several photocopies so that you can practice using this especially valuable worksheet.

Generating Rational Alternatives

When you're working to change automatic thoughts with challenging techniques or TCRs, rational alternatives may become obvious to you. But sometimes it may be harder to generate rational alternatives, especially when you're facing significant life challenges or issues. Maybe you're thinking that there are few or no rational alternatives to some of your automatic thoughts.

> **?** **Do you have trouble generating rational alternatives for your TCR?**
>
> **Could you have difficulty finding alternatives to other automatic thoughts?**

Ted's Thought Change Record

Event	Automatic Thought(s)	Emotion(s)	Rational Response	Outcome
My wife gets upset as I'm trying to pay the bills. She is worried about our finances because I haven't been making as many sales as usual.	I'm failing again. 95 If this keeps up, she's bound to leave me. 50 My life is falling apart. 100 I don't know what to do. 95	Sad 90 Anxious 90 Tense 80	I'm magnifying the problem and jumping to conclusions. There is plenty of all-or-nothing thinking here. It is okay for both of us to get upset about the financial crunch. But I'm not a failure. I just am going through a tough time. 100. There's no evidence that she will leave me. We've had a strong marriage for more than 20 years. 95 I'm under stress, but there are many parts of my life that are actually going well—relationship with kids and parents, physical health, volunteer work at church, etc. 95 I know how to do my job. I need to hang in there until things improve. 95.	Sad 50 Anxious 30 Tense 15 I feel much more comfortable talking with my wife about our finances and working together to manage the problem. We are working on a plan to get through this pinch.
I call one of my old customers. He isn't interested in our new product.	This is a catastrophe. 100 This business is going straight downhill. 90	Anxious 95 Sad 70	I'm jumping to conclusions again and using all-or-nothing thinking. It's a negative that the customer wasn't interested, but we have other leads. I've had plenty of customers say no in the past. Hearing no is part of this business. 100 Our business is down this year, but we have gone through downturns before. The long-term prospects are pretty good. 90 I need to see the problem for what it is instead of magnifying it. 100	Anxious 40 Sad 40 I am more optimistic about being able to get through this downturn. I'm trying to work steadily to make more contacts.

Thought Change Record

Event	Automatic Thought(s)	Emotion(s)	Rational Response	Outcome
Write down an event or situation, or a memory of an event, that triggered automatic thoughts.	*1. Record the automatic thoughts that occurred while you were experiencing or thinking about this event.* *2. Rate how much you believed the thought at the time it was happening. Use a 0–100 scale where 100 = complete belief.*	*1. Identify emotions such as sadness or anger that were stimulated by the automatic thoughts.* *2. Rate the intensity of the emotion on a 0–100 point scale where 100 = the most extreme emotion.*	*1. Challenge the automatic thoughts by going off automatic pilot, examining the evidence, looking for cognitive errors, or other methods.* *2. Write out some rational alternatives to the automatic thoughts.* *3. Rate your belief in the rational alternatives using a 0–100 scale.*	*1. Specify and rate subsequent emotions using a 0–100 scale.* *2. Describe changes in behavior.*

Write down any such automatic thoughts here:

_____

_____

_____

_____

If rational alternatives don't come easily to mind, you might find these strategies helpful:

1. Open your mind to the possibilities.

2. Brainstorm.

3. Learn from others.

Open Your Mind to the Possibilities

Use the technique of thinking from the perspective of another person. For example, you could imagine that you are a very effective coach, doctor, clergyperson, or therapist who is giving you positive and constructive feedback. Or you could try to think like a detective who makes a habit of trying to avoid jumping to conclusions or ignoring evidence. Another perspective that might help is to think like a best friend or a trusted family member who is giving you sound advice about rational ways to see things.

Brainstorm

Effective brainstorming involves freeing up your mind to consider a variety of options. Because you are trying to get the creative juices flowing, you want to avoid crossing off possibilities immediately because they seem to be impractical. At least in the beginning of the brainstorming exercise, you should try to take the "but" out of "yes, but." Sometimes an alternative that seems to be impossible at first may actually be worth considering—at least to stir up other ideas that might work out for you. Also, overdrawn alternatives will sometimes stimulate other thoughts that have merit.

When Angelina brainstormed for alternatives to an automatic thought "My life is out of control," she wrote down options such as these:

1. There aren't any problems with my life, it is just my depression.

2. Everything is actually under control. Don't worry about it.

3. Most of my life is in fairly good control (for example, my job is going okay and my

relationships are mostly in good shape). It is the depression and anxiety attacks that need attention.

4. If I could be less of a procrastinator, my life would be in much better control.

5. I probably think too much about having to have everything in perfect control. Maybe I could learn to be more accepting of things that I can't control or are hard to control.

6. I must be in control.

Which of the options from Angelina's brainstorming list do you think might work the best for her or give her good opportunities for making positive changes? Before reading our suggestions below, circle the alternatives that you would suggest she use. You can also make a few notes on what you think the positive or adaptive features of your choices might be. Write these down in the exercise below.

We think that numbers 1 and 2 seem to be inaccurate and misleading. She would be kidding herself if she accepted these alternatives. Number 3 appears to be a balanced alternative that cuts through her thinking errors such as magnification and ignoring the evidence, and it points her in a positive direction to work on managing her depression and anxiety. Number 4 also has a good deal of appeal. She is being honest with herself that she has a problem with procrastination, and she is recognizing that she needs to do something about it. Number 5 is an especially helpful alternative because it could lead her

| EXERCISE 4.11 | Helping Angelina with Brainstorming |

Instructions: Look at the alternatives that Angelina generated from her brainstorming exercise. Enter the numbers of the alternatives you think would work the best for her in the table. Then write out a few comments on how you believe the alternative might help her change.

The most helpful alternatives for Angelina to consider are:	This alternative might help Angelina to:

to make meaningful changes in her need to always be in control. However, number 6 is going in the wrong direction. It is a very demanding and unrealistic alternative.

Learn from Others

People who are depressed can turn inward and brood about their problems and close themselves off from hearing opinions of others. This tendency would seem to be self-protective. After all, if you feel you are in a weakened state, and your self-confidence is ebbing, it might make sense to not ask others for feedback. Perhaps other people would confirm your fears or dash your hopes.

Yet asking trusted people to give you feedback can sometimes be very helpful in checking out the validity of automatic thoughts and generating rational alternatives. Ted was able to show his brother his TCR and to ask him whether the changes he was making in his thinking made sense. He also asked his brother if he had any other ideas for rational thinking that could help him overcome depression.

EXERCISE 4.12   **Brainstorming to Find Alternatives to Automatic Thoughts**

Instructions: Write down one of your automatic thoughts in the box below. Then try to brainstorm at least three alternative thoughts. Free up your imagination to come up with some creative and interesting possibilities.

An automatic thought I want to change is:

_____

Brainstorming helped me find these alternatives:

1.

2.

3.

4.

5.

6.

There can be risks in asking others to help you find alternative ways of seeing things, so we suggest that you ask yourself these questions before using this strategy: "What are the possible risks and benefits of asking this person for feedback?" "How much can you trust this person to tell you the truth and still be supportive?"

Putting Changes into Action

To help make your modifications in automatic thoughts stick, you will need to put them into action. Unless you practice using your more adaptive thoughts in real-life situations, you may find yourself slipping back into an automatic style of negative thinking. Another very important reason to put the changes into action is that your healthier, rational thoughts can be a big help in coping with the problems in your life.

So how do you move from doing the exercises in this book to applying your knowledge in everyday life? These strategies could help you put the lessons to work:

1. Keep a self-help notebook.
2. Set up experiments to try out your changed thinking.
3. Use coping cards.

Keep a Self-Help Notebook

A good way to remember, rehearse, and solidify your changes in thinking is to create a notebook to store and review the key self-help exercises from this book (and from therapy if you are seeing a professional counselor). You can make copies of the exercises that seemed helpful, and you can go online (*www.guilford.com/breakingfreeforms*) to download electronic versions of some of the forms so that you can complete additional self-help exercises. When you review exercises or do new ones, you can circle the most important changes that you want to put into action, and you can write yourself notes on how you could apply the changes to manage your problems and fight depression.

Set Up Experiments to Try Out Your Changed Thinking

When people are receiving professionally administered CBT, their doctors or therapists often suggest homework assignments to help them practice things they have learned from treatment and to gain skills and experience in applying CBT principles in everyday life. Even if you are not involved in professional treatment, you can develop similar assignments or projects for yourself. Exercise 4.13 will help you learn how to do this.

Use Coping Cards

Another very helpful strategy for putting changes into action is to write out a coping card. This device is very simple but very powerful. All you need is an index card of any size (3

Setting Up an Experiment
to Try Out Changed Thinking

Instructions: Review a Thought Change Record or other exercise from this chapter. Try to find an example of changes in your thinking that could pay off if you could apply these changes in specific situations in your life. Then follow the steps below.

Write down an example of negative automatic thoughts and changes you have made in these thoughts.

Automatic thoughts:

_____

_____

Changes I have made in these automatic thoughts:

_____

_____

Describe a specific situation in which you will put these changes into action:

_____

_____

How do you think this experiment will work out? What are your predictions for positive benefits? Could anything get in the way of your carrying out the experiment? Could there be any downsides?

_____

_____

_____

(cont.)

If you identified barriers to having success with the experiment or any downsides, do some brainstorming about things you could do to improve the chances of success. Write these ideas down here:

_____

_____

_____

_____

Complete the experiment and record the results here. What did you learn? How could you continue to put changed thinking into action in other life situations?

_____

_____

_____

_____

by 5 inches is a commonly used size, but a business card size can be used if you want to keep the card small to slip into your wallet or purse) and a pen or pencil. On one side of the card you write down a problem or a situation that is giving you trouble. On the other side you write down the principal changes in your thinking that you want to apply to cope with the problem. You can also write down any behaviors or actions that could help you cope. You'll learn much more about developing effective behavioral strategies for depression in Chapter 5, but if you have any ideas for behavior changes that could be useful, you can add them to the coping card now.

Before you work on writing out one of your own coping cards, we'll show you an example. Ted wrote out the card on the facing page to help him manage his discouragement and fear at work.

Do you think the coping card method could work for you? In our clinical practices we find that coping cards are some of our patients' favorite self-help exercises. Many of them develop a series of cards and keep them close at hand to coach themselves on ways to handle their problems.

Ted's Coping Card

Problem: *I am trying to work to build my contacts and make new sales, but I start getting negative thoughts like "This business is going straight downhill." Then I feel like I won't be able to make it—that I should give up.*

Coping Strategies:

- *Remind myself that everybody is being affected by the economic downturn. It's not just me.*

- *Remember I have support from my boss, who thinks we will be okay if we keep plugging along.*

- *Remind myself that business is off only about 15%. It's not a disaster. I've gotten through similar times in the past.*

- *Just put in the time at my desk. Go to work every day, make at least three calls a day. Don't get down on myself if the sale doesn't go through.*

- *Take care of myself when I am not at work. Get back to exercising at least three times a week. Do fun things with family. Try to lighten up a bit and still enjoy some things in life.*

EXERCISE 4.14 | **Building a Coping Card**

Instructions: Use this form to write out a coping card. Try to record positive changes in your thinking that will help you cope, and note any effective actions that you can take to manage the problem or situation.

Problem:

_____

_____

Coping Strategies:

_____

_____

_____

_____

_____

Summary

Most people have a distinct shift in their thinking style when they become depressed. Their negative automatic thoughts become much more frequent, and these thoughts are often loaded with thinking errors. These doubting, self-critical, worried, or despairing thoughts are frequently a large part of the downward spiral of depression. But fortunately, methods from CBT can reverse this trend for negative thinking and offer a hopeful path to wellness. In this chapter you learned how to *spot, challenge, and modify* negative automatic thoughts. In the next chapter, you'll practice employing these core CBT methods to build your self-esteem and use your strengths to overcome depression.

5

Restoring Energy and Enjoying Life

Chapter Highlights

⬧ Has my behavior changed?

⬧ Waiting for recovery versus taking action now

⬧ Action prescriptions

⬧ Activity scheduling

⬧ Motivational enhancement

⬧ The step-by-step approach

Low energy and reduced interest are part of the downward spiral of depression. If you feel fatigued, the natural inclination is to do less. And if you are feeling depressed and aren't enjoying your usual activities, you will probably be less likely to get involved in doing the things that used to give you pleasure. Unfortunately, becoming less active often makes the problem worse. Most people need to engage in stimulating, enjoyable, or meaningful activities to feel good about themselves and about life.

Some people have such severe depression that their activity levels seem to come almost to a standstill. They may have trouble getting out of bed, going to work, or carrying out any of their normal routine. Even if symptoms are not this severe, most people with depression notice definite changes in their energy and ability to enjoy pleasurable activities. In this chapter, we draw from the scientifically tested methods of CBT to show you effective methods for getting your energy back and reengaging in enjoyable activities that can help you pull out of depression.

Has My Behavior Changed?

Have you noticed changes in your activity levels that seem to be part of depression? To identify behaviors that you may want to modify, complete the checklist below.

Waiting for Recovery Versus Taking Action Now

If you identified several problems in Exercise 5.1, you might be thinking "I would need to be less depressed before I could make any changes in these problems—it's the depression that is holding me back." In a way, this assumption is correct. Behavioral changes such as the ones in the checklist are classic symptoms of depression. If medications or other treatments relieved the depression, you would probably be able to return to a more active,

EXERCISE 5.1	Depressive Behaviors Checklist

Instructions: Put a check mark in one of the boxes (none, a little, moderate, a great deal) to indicate how much each of the problems has been affecting you in the past 2 weeks.

Problem	None	A little	Moderate	A great deal
Low energy				
Reduced pleasure in activities				
Avoidance of usual activities				
Helplessness				
Procrastination				
Spending too much time alone				
Having difficulty completing effortful tasks				
Being overwhelmed by challenges				

engaged, and productive lifestyle. On the other hand, many studies have shown that people who participate in CBT and use the behavioral methods described in this chapter can make changes in their activity levels that will help relieve depression. So you can wait until other treatments lift depression. But if you want to take advantage of the effective methods of CBT, you can take action now to increase energy and enjoy life. Yes, struggling with low energy and low interest can make this tough, but if you give it a chance, you'll see that the extra effort often pays off.

SCIENCE CORNER More than 300 studies have demonstrated the effectiveness of CBT. Some of these studies, such as one done by Drs. Dimidjian, Hollon, and associates, have shown that *"behavioral activation"* (using specific CBT methods to increase involvement in stimulating and pleasurable activities) *by itself, without any other treatment components*, can relieve symptoms of depression.

Do you remember Kate from Chapters 1 and 2? To refresh your memory, here's an excerpt from Chapter 1.

As so often happens with depression, Kate gradually pulled away from many of the activities and relationships that used to give her enjoyment and a sense of purpose. It was as if the depression were driving her into a shell.

Kate was still able to go to work, but when she came home she spent much of her time alone, staring at the TV or doing "mindless" tasks. After Kate had made repeated excuses for avoiding social activities, many of her friends either called her only infrequently or had stopped calling her altogether. As the gloom of depression intensified, Kate began to think of herself as a "failure" and a "loser."

Prior to becoming depressed, Kate had led a fairly healthy lifestyle. She took yoga classes, rode a bicycle two or three times a week, or went to the gym to do aerobic exercise. She sang in a choir and attended church services regularly. Now, however, the only activity she enjoyed outside of work was having dinner with her family on Sunday evenings.

Kate seemed to be stuck in a deep depression, but the key behavioral strategies from CBT were very helpful in her recovery. We'll show you how Kate used these methods—*action prescriptions, activity scheduling, motivational enhancement*, and the *step-by-step approach*—so that you can apply these techniques in your own life.

Action Prescriptions

When Kate started treatment, we recognized from the first session that the behavioral changes that were such a large part of her depression were gripping her in a "vicious cycle." The inactivity, social isolation, and lack of stimulation were making her feel worse about herself. And the worse she felt about herself, the more she seemed to back away from social opportunities and other activities that used to be a routine part of her life. So we decided to ask Kate to work with us in designing an action prescription.

> *Dr. Wright:* You've been telling me about how much your life has changed since you've been depressed—how you haven't been able to exercise and how you spend so much time alone not really enjoying anything. But you also seem to want to start turning things around. Could you think of one step that you could take in the next week—a step that would make you feel better if you could take it? This step wouldn't have to be a big challenge, just something to get you going in a more positive direction.
>
> *Kate:* Well, I've been thinking about starting to exercise again. Maybe I could try that.
>
> *Dr. Wright:* What would be a reasonable goal just for the next week?
>
> *Kate:* I haven't been on the bike or to the gym for a couple of months. I guess I liked yoga classes the most, and they would get me back in touch with some people I know.
>
> *Dr. Wright:* Okay. I have a prescription pad here. We usually write down prescriptions for medications, but sometimes taking a behavioral action is just as important. For some people, it can be even more important. Would you be willing to write out your own action prescription?
>
> *Kate:* Sure [*takes the pad, thinks for a few moments, writes down "Attend yoga class twice next week," and signs the prescription*].

This bit of dialogue shows how you and your therapist can work together as a team in CBT. With Kate, we went on to briefly discuss any problems she might encounter in carrying out the action prescription and to troubleshoot some solutions so she could begin to overcome the inertia of depression. We wrote down these ideas on the back of the action prescription.

To write an action prescription with the greatest possible chance of success, follow these guidelines:

1. *Make the plan specific.* Just like a medication prescription that tells you exactly what type of medication and dosage will be used, an action prescription should give a clear plan for taking a behavioral step toward recovery.

2. *Keep it simple and doable.* If Kate had written down "Get back to my old exercise routine," she probably would have been tackling too much, too fast.

3. *Choose an action that you want to do (at least in part).* If you wrote down "clean the basement," and this seemed like a particularly unpleasant task that you didn't really want to do, you might struggle to complete it. Because action prescriptions

Kate's Action Prescription

An action that I want to take in the next week:

Attend yoga class twice next week

Potential problems and solutions in carrying out the plan:

Possible barriers or roadblocks	Possible solutions
I call to schedule class but find that it is full or won't be held next week.	*Go on waiting list for next available class or check for other classes that might be held next week. If this fails, try to ride bike for at least 30 minutes twice next week.*
I have second thoughts about attending the class.	*Remind myself that it would really help me to get involved again and that resuming enjoyable activities would be good for me. Think about how good I used to feel after practicing yoga.*
I feel so tired, I don't think I can get through the class.	*Realize that I am out of shape from not going to class or exercising for several months. Go easy at the beginning. Don't choose an advanced class. Explain the situation to the instructor and take a break in a relaxation pose or leave early if needed. If I can't get through an entire class, don't criticize myself—accept any attempt at getting moving again as a positive.*
I'm not able to attend any yoga class or do any exercise.	*Try not to get down on myself. Regroup and try again. Talk it over with my sister and ask her to go to yoga with me or to exercise with me.*

are often designed as first steps to get people going again, they work best when there is a genuine interest in making the change and the plan offers a good chance for a positive outcome.

4. *Build in troubleshooting elements.* Because it isn't always easy to implement action prescriptions, and depression can interfere with taking the actions that you know will help you, it can help to plan in advance for possible barriers or roadblocks. You can use Kate's troubleshooting plan to get ideas for your own plan. Please remember to give yourself a break if you have difficulty completing an action prescription. Learn from the experience and give it another try.

Are you ready to write your own action prescription? You can write out as many of these as you wish by copying this form or downloading it from *www.guilford.com/ breakingfreeforms.*

My Action Prescription

Name: _____ Date: _____

✎ **An action that I want to take in the next week:**

_____

_____

Potential problems and solutions in carrying out the plan:

Potential barriers or roadblocks	Potential solutions

Signed: _____

QUICK
TIP Watch out for the "Yes ... but" trap in trying to implement action prescriptions. The "yes" part of you may be saying that the action prescription makes a lot of sense. Depression, however, often seems to amplify the *but*s in our thinking ("but I just don't have the energy ... but it wouldn't make any difference anyway ... but I don't have the time to do this"). Remembering the lessons from Chapter 4, spot automatic thoughts and thinking errors that could interfere with your giving a good action prescription a chance to work.

Activity Scheduling

Have you thought about how your daily schedule might influence your energy, your mood, and your self-esteem? Could your choices of activities be playing a role in keeping you depressed? Are there any opportunities for adjusting your schedule so that your energy increases and you experience more pleasure in life?

Although depression typically interferes with having an active and fulfilling daily schedule, CBT research has shown that there is much to be gained by making efforts to change daily routines. Start by assessing your current daily schedule to see how you rate your current activities on two important dimensions: (1) your sense of mastery (how well you think you accomplished a task) and (2) your sense or pleasure or enjoyment.

QUICK
TIP One of the key principles of CBT, recording thoughts or behaviors by completing logs or worksheets, journaling, or any other method of recording, is at work in activity scheduling. Depression tends to improve when people keep a record of thoughts or behaviors. You completed Thought Change Records in Chapter 4. Now we recommend that you keep a schedule of your daily activities.

To get an idea of how activity scheduling can help you, let's take a look at a schedule that Kate completed for two days of her life (see pages 104 and 105). One of the days was a workday, and another was on a weekend. Kate's job is in the human resources department of an appliance manufacturer, so much of her workday is scheduled fairly tightly. But there is still room for adjustments that might be useful to her in overcoming depression.

As you review Kate's schedule, see if you can find any patterns of activities that you think might be playing a role in keeping her depressed. Also, see if you can identify any opportunities for positive change. Are there activities that seem to drag her down that she might deemphasize? Are there any activities that seem to give her at least a bit of enjoyment that she might try to build up?

In our work with patients who are experiencing depression, we almost always find that at least some ability to experience mastery and pleasure is retained—even when

Kate's Activity Schedule

Instructions: Write down your primary activities for each of the hours in the schedule below. Then rate each activity for mastery (M = 0–10, where 0 = no mastery and 10 = full mastery of the activity; mastery = how well you performed the activity) and pleasure (P = 0–10 where 0 = no pleasure and 10 = maximum pleasure).

Hour	Day of Week _Tuesday_	Day of Week _Saturday_
7–8 A.M.	Shower, breakfast, drive to work M = 6, P = 2	Read newspaper, breakfast M = 7, P = 3
8–9 A.M.	Office time, trying to get organized for the day, paperwork on benefit claims M = 6, P = 2	TV M = 3, P = 1
9–10 A.M.	Daily meeting with benefits team M = 8, P = 4	Walked down street to farmers' market M = 8, P = 8
10–11 A.M.	More paper work in office M = 7, P = 2	Called sister and told her I bought some nice vegetables at the market, planned to meet for coffee this afternoon M = 9, P = 7
11 A.M.–Noon	Appointments with employees M = 7, P = 5	Worked in yard, cut grass M = 7, P = 4
Noon–1 P.M.	Lunch by self in office; read some benefit manuals M = 3, P = 2	TV and lunch M = 5, P = 2
1–2 P.M.	Teleconference with other benefit offices in company (just listened to presentation) M = 6, P = 2	Nap M = 4, P = 3
2–3 P.M.	Appointments with employees M = 7, P = 5	Tried to read, mind wandered off M = 2, P = 2

Hour	Day of Week _Tuesday_	Day of Week _Saturday_
3–4 P.M.	Appointments with employees $M=7, P=5$	Met sister for coffee $M=8, P=8$
4–5 P.M.	Office time, wrap-up work for day, planning for rest of week $M=6, P=3$	Grocery shopping $M=7, P=4$
5–6 P.M.	Drive home, stop for gas, pick up some fast food for dinner $M=5, P=1$	Prepared some food for dinner including things from market while I listened to music $M=7, P=6$
6 7 P.M.	Dinner, watch TV $M=4, P=1$	Dinner, read a magazine $M=7, P=4$
7–8 P.M.	Did some laundry and picked up house $M=4, P=2$	TV $M=5, P=2$
8–9 P.M.	Internet, e-mails, and some contacts with friends $M=8, P=6$	TV $M=5, P=1$
9–10 P.M.	TV $M=5, P=2$	TV $M=5, P=1$
10–11 P.M.	TV, get ready for bed $M=5, P=2$	TV, get ready for bed $M=5, P=2$

Kate's Activity Scheduling:
Generating Ideas for Change

When Kate talked with us about her depression, she described herself as "not enjoying anything anymore." The negative thinking style of depression described in Chapter 4 was probably influencing Kate's view of her daily activities and how she was responding to them. In reviewing Kate's schedule, can you identify some enjoyable activities that might help her challenge the notion that she is "not enjoying anything anymore?" This could help Kate focus on positive activities that she could expand. Make a list here of five or more activities that she associated with at least a moderate degree (P ≥ 5) of pleasure or enjoyment.

_____

_____

_____

When Kate isn't at work, she devotes a lot of time to watching TV alone. How do her mastery and pleasure ratings change when she gets involved in more stimulating activities such as going to the farmers' market, spending time with her sister, or communicating with friends? What is her average pleasure rating for watching TV alone compared to the five most stimulating and enjoyable activities that she recorded?

_____

_____

_____

Kate seems to be performing fairly well at work. She typically rates her mastery in the 6–8 range, and her pleasure ratings are definitely higher than when she watches TV while she is alone at home. She doesn't have much room to change her work schedule, but there might be some opportunities for enhancing her sense of mastery and pleasure. Do you have at least one suggestion for her?

_____

_____

_____

Before Kate became depressed, she had an active lifestyle. She met frequently with friends and family, exercised regularly, sang in a choir, and participated in a number of other meaningful activities that were an important part of her weekly routine. There isn't a switch that can be flipped to help her immediately resume all of these activities or to engage in a variety of new pursuits that will reverse depression. But there may be some ways for her to start changing her daily and weekly schedules to improve her sense of mastery and pleasure. What preliminary ideas do you have for helping Kate begin to change?

_____

_____

_____

CAUTION
- Please note that a brainstorming list may contain many more ideas than you will have the energy or time to implement right away.
- Kate was able to generate a large number of ideas, but she chose to do only some of them in the first week.
- When you brainstorm your list of activities to build into your schedule, put a check mark beside the ones that make the most sense to try now. Be realistic and don't do too much too fast.
- You can save the brainstorming list and draw from it as you gradually try to do more things that make you feel better.

it seems that all of the enjoyment in life has disappeared. Activity schedules can help people like Kate see that choices of how to spend their time can significantly influence their mood. We suspect that you were able to recognize that the amount of pleasure that Kate felt was a lot higher when she spent time with her sister or communicated with friends on the phone or Internet. And at work she rated face-to-face meetings with people higher than paperwork and other tasks, so she clearly takes more pleasure in personal interaction than in other kinds of work. Kate also seemed to get a significant lift from getting involved in interesting activities such as visiting a farmers' market, going shopping, and cooking with fresh ingredients. Plus, there were signs that doing some chores such as cutting the grass gave her at least a modest amount of pleasure and that reading could sometimes make her feel better than spending long hours in front of the TV.

With these observations in hand, Kate did some brainstorming and came up with a list of activities that might stimulate a greater sense of mastery and pleasure. This list is shown on page 108.

Kate built up her daily schedule over several weeks by trying some of the activities on her brainstorming list. And she used other ideas that surfaced as she began to pay special attention to the choices she made about how to spend her time. Examples of an evening weekday schedule and a Saturday schedule from about a month after Kate started activity scheduling (see pages 108 and 109) show how much she was able to benefit from this method.

Can you follow Kate's lead and put activity scheduling to work? The next four exercises could provide excellent opportunities for you to increase your energy and experience more enjoyment in your life. You can complete activity schedules for as many days of the week as you like. Some people find that working on just a day or part of a day at a time works best. Others can benefit from sketching out a whole week's activities. We provide a worksheet for two days of the week. Make copies of the worksheet or download it at *www.guilford.com/breakingfreeforms* if you want to write out schedules for more days.

After you complete a baseline activity schedule that shows what your days are like before making changes, do some brainstorming. Identify some possible areas for positive changes. When you brainstorm, let your mind run free. Open it up to a full range of possibilities. Maybe you are already doing some things that could be increased or enhanced. Perhaps there are hobbies, sports, musical interests, or activities you did with friends in the past that could be brought back into your life. Could you recycle some old ideas—ones that might still have some potential? Have you automatically rejected ideas

Kate's Brainstorming Exercise
Positive Activities I Could Build Into My Schedule

Instructions: Review your activity schedule and then try to generate a list of at least 10 ideas for positive changes. Do some brainstorming to come up with options that may involve a little change and some that may be more extensive. Then choose at least five of the ideas to put into action. Circle the activities that you want to implement now.

1. Call friends at least three times a week.

2. Try to plan at least one event with friends (go out for coffee, see a movie, etc.) a week.

3. Try to arrange a larger number of meetings with coworkers during the workday—increase contact with people and decrease time alone in office.

4. Go to farmers' market every Saturday.

5. Do something during my lunch hour at work that is more stimulating than sitting alone (eat with coworkers; take a walk out to a local place to eat, preferably with someone from work; read something interesting that will make for good conversation with others).

6. Attend yoga at least three times a week.

7. Start to attend church again.

8. Go to special events at church such as concerts and dinners.

9. Treat myself by downloading some new music and taking the time to enjoy listening to it.

10. Ask a friend or my sister to go shopping and stop for a light dinner while we are out.

11. Read some humorous books.

12. Go to a softball game to watch friends play.

13. Limit my time watching TV alone to no more than 2–3 hours a day.

---

for things you have never tried? Are there some really interesting and stimulating things to do that you haven't considered previously—ones that might lift your mood and bring some fun back into your life?

Would it help you to push yourself a bit to become more active, even if it seemed like you were just "going through the motions" in the beginning? Sometimes it can help to "fake it until you make it"—meaning that you participate in activities that don't initially make a big difference because you are feeling depressed, but after a while begin to feel more natural and more fulfilling. As you complete this brainstorming exercise, try to generate a list of many options. Then you can decide which ones have the most appeal or may seem most reasonable to try. Also, you can consider some activities that you might

Kate's Activity Schedule after She Made Changes

A WORKDAY EVENING

Hour	Day of Week _Tuesday_
5–6 P.M.	Drove home, stopped at bookstore, and picked up some interesting travel literature; browsed in the bookstore _M = 8, P = 6_
6–7 P.M.	Dinner, started reading the travel book _M = 7, P = 5_
7–8 P.M.	Called a friend who suggested we go bowling with a church group on Saturday night; did some laundry and sorted mail _M = 8, P = 6_
8–9 P.M.	Internet, e-mails to friends, updated Facebook with some photos, looked at some travel sites (window shopping for places I'd like to visit) _M = 8, P = 7_
9–10 P.M.	Called sister, did some planning for a family picnic; watched some TV _M = 8, P = 4_
10–11 P.M.	TV, get ready for bed, read for about 30 minutes before going to sleep _M = 7, P = 5_

A SATURDAY

Hour	Day of Week _Saturday_
7–8 A.M.	Read newspaper, put away clean dishes, worked in garden briefly, pulling a few weeds _M = 8, P = 4_
8–9 A.M.	Took a walk in neighborhood and talked with some neighbors _M = 7, P = 5_

(cont.)

Kate's Activity Schedule after She Made Changes (*cont.*)

9–10 A.M.	*Farmers' market with sister and a friend; had breakfast there* M=9, P=9
10–11 A.M.	*Still at market for a while, then came home and put away fruits and vegetables* M=9, P=7
11–Noon	*Cut grass* M=7, P=4
Noon–1 P.M.	*Lunch* M=6, P=4
1–2 P.M.	*Did some work at home, caught up with some special project work* M=8, P=3
2–3 P.M.	*Downloaded some new music, updated my music files and relaxed while listening; sang along with some of the choral music* M=10, P=7
3–4 P.M.	*Watched softball game for a brief time before yoga class* M=8, P=6
4–5 P.M.	*Yoga class* M=7, P=9
5–6 P.M.	*Grocery shopping for week* M=7, P=4
6–7 P.M.	*Listened to music, got ready to go out* M=8, P=6
7–8 P.M.	*Pizza with church group before bowling* M=9, P=8
8–9 P.M.	*Bowling* M=3, P=7
9–10 P.M.	*Bowling* M=3, P=7
10–11 P.M.	*TV, get ready for bed* M=8, P=4

Instructions: Write down your primary activities for each of the hours in the schedule below. Then rate each activity for mastery (M = 0–10, where 0 = no mastery and 10 = full mastery of the activity; mastery = how well you performed the activity) and pleasure (P = 0–10 where 0 = no pleasure and 10 = maximum pleasure).

Hour	Day of Week _____	Day of Week _____
7–8 A.M.		
8–9 A.M.		
9–10 A.M.		
10–11 A.M.		
11 A.M.–Noon		
Noon–1 P.M.		
1–2 P.M.		

(cont.)

Hour	Day of Week _____	Day of Week _____
2–3 P.M.		
3–4 P.M.		
4–5 P.M.		
5–6 P.M.		
6–7 P.M.		
7–8 P.M.		
8–9 P.M.		
9–10 P.M.		
10–11 P.M.		

EXERCISE 5.5	**Positive Changes I Could Make in My Activity Schedule**

Instructions: Review your activity schedule and then try to generate a list of at least 10 ideas for positive changes. Do some brainstorming to come up with options that may involve a little change and some that may be more extensive. Then choose at least five of the ideas to put into action. Put a check mark beside the activities that you want to implement now.

1. _____

2. _____

3. _____

4. _____

5. _____

6. _____

7. _____

8. _____

9. _____

10. _____

have to stretch to complete but could have a positive payoff in helping you move from depression to wellness.

If you have difficulty thinking of ideas or you want to expand the list of possibilities, you might find a "Pleasant Events Checklist" helpful. These types of inventories list a very large number of activities that people have reported to have been pleasurable to them. Pleasant events checklists that contain many hundreds of activities are available on the Internet at sites such as *www.healthnetsolutions.com*. We provide an abbreviated list in Exercise 5.6 to help stimulate your thinking about the wide variety of activities that can be pleasurable. Your interest may vary over time; to use the checklist again in the future, photocopy it or download it from *www.guilford.com/breakingfreeforms*.

We hope these exercises have stimulated some good ideas for modifying your daily schedule to participate in more activities that are "depression lifters" instead of depression reinforcers. To wrap up our work on activity scheduling, we recommend that you

Pleasant Events Checklist

Instructions: Try to keep an open mind as you scan through this list of activities that have given people pleasure. Maybe there are activities you have never tried that could spark your interest. Or there could be activities you have done in the past and could be brought back into your life. Also, there could be things that that you are doing infrequently but could become a larger part of your daily or weekly schedule. Rate your interest in engaging in each of the activities by putting a check mark in one of the columns. Then circle at least three activities that you will consider emphasizing more in your life.

Activity	No interest	Little interest	Moderate interest	High level of interest
Listening to music				
Using my sense of humor				
Doing crosswords or puzzles				
Driving				
Spending time with pets				
Walking				
Volunteering				
Playing a sport				
Watching movies				
Going to a concert or play				
Planning a trip				
Shopping				
Being at the beach or mountains				
Reading magazines or books				
Fixing up my house or apartment				
Taking a shower or bath				
Singing or playing a musical instrument				

(cont.)

Activity	No interest	Little interest	Moderate interest	High level of interest
Woodworking				
Spending time with friends				
Going to religious services				
Writing				
Going out to lunch or dinner				
Water sports				
Cooking				
Being intimate				
Gardening				
Saying prayers				
Yoga				
Doing crafts				
Being with family				
Personal grooming				
Exercise				
Bowling				
Knitting or other needlework				
Dancing				
Going to the zoo or to a park				
Bicycling				
Wearing new clothes				

(*cont.*)

Activity	No interest	Little interest	Moderate interest	High level of interest
Listening to the radio				
Appreciating nature				
Playing cards or board games				
Watching birds				
Using the Internet				
Giving gifts				
Fishing or hunting				
Going to the beautician or barber shop				
Talking with neighbors				
Photography				
Going to yard sales or auctions				
Reading cartoons				
Eating a good meal				
Hiking or camping				
Going to a health club				
Talking on the telephone				
Going to a museum or show				
Getting a massage or backrub				
Skiing				
Meditation				
Playing pool, darts, or Ping-Pong				
Giving things to others				

Activity Schedule after Making Changes

Instructions: Write down your primary activities for each of the hours in the schedule below. Then rate each activity for mastery (M = 0–10, where 0 = no mastery and 10 = full mastery of the activity; mastery = how well you performed the activity) and pleasure (P = 0–10 where 0 = no pleasure and 10 = maximum pleasure).

Hour	Day of Week _____	Day of Week _____
7–8 A.M.		
8–9 A.M.		
9–10 A.M.		
10–11 A.M.		
11 A.M.–Noon		
Noon–1 P.M.		
1–2 P.M.		

(cont.)

Hour	Day of Week _____	Day of Week _____
2–3 P.M.		
3–4 P.M.		
4–5 P.M.		
5–6 P.M.		
6–7 P.M.		
7–8 P.M.		
8–9 P.M.		
9–10 P.M.		
10–11 P.M.		

implement some of your ideas for change and then record the effects of these actions on your experiences in feeling mastery and pleasure. You can come back to complete more activity schedules at any time, by photocopying the worksheet or downloading it from *www.guilford.com/breakingfreeforms*. This basic method is used throughout CBT to help people move toward recovery.

Motivational Enhancement

Motivational speakers and writers are in great demand for good reason. Lots of people have difficulty getting motivated and staying motivated to complete tasks and reach their goals. Unless you are a supermotivated person who is always productive, never wastes time, and unfailingly attains goals (we've never met anyone who truly functioned on this level), you have probably struggled with motivation from time to time and have experienced bouts of procrastination. Although we have been able to complete projects such as writing this book, we too have had times of lowered motivation and have caught ourselves procrastinating when action is needed.

We don't have the ultimate answer to becoming fully motivated or banning procrastination from our lives. (If we did, we would have used it on ourselves.) But we have learned some motivational enhancement methods from CBT and a therapeutic approach called "motivational interviewing" that can help people get unstuck and get things done.

When you are depressed and are trying to use techniques such as action prescriptions or activity scheduling, a bit of a boost from motivational enhancement might be just what you need to start breaking out of a depressive behavioral pattern. To learn how these methods might work for you, let's first see how Kate increased her motivation to change.

Kate sketched out a reasonable action prescription to get back into the habit of going to yoga classes, and she wrote out a great plan for her activity schedule, but the depression seemed to be conspiring to pull her back into a rut of inactivity and isolation from others. So we suggested that she could benefit from highlighting and reinforcing her positive motivators for change.

Kate: I kept up most of the new activity schedule for about a week, but I hate to admit that it just seemed easier to plunk myself down in front of the TV and spend hours there without making calls to friends or doing much else.

Dr. Wright: You're not alone in having this type of reaction. Almost everybody has had problems carrying out plans to change—even when the plans seem to make perfect sense. I wonder if it would help if we could figure out what might motivate you to get back in there and keep trying. Could we try to list some positive reasons to carry out your plans? Then we can try to build up these motivators.

Kate: Well, I guess the number-one thing is that doing these things could make me feel less depressed.

Dr. Wright: And how much do you believe that carrying out a new activity schedule could help you feel better?

Kate: Close to 100%. I know that I need to get into a regular exercise routine and get out with people.

Dr. Wright: Okay. If we start a list of motivators for change, we can write down that you believe strongly that making positive changes in your activity schedule will help relieve depression. Can we generate a longer list and then see what we can do to keep these motivators at the top of your mind?

Kate: Sure.

During this CBT session, they used a worksheet to develop a list of motivators and demotivators (things that might interfere with staying the course in making changes) and then worked out a way to highlight the motivators and deal with the demotivators. Kate's list is shown on the facing page.

In completing this exercise, Kate was able to draw from a tip list that we have developed for building motivation and combating procrastination. We gave this tip list to Kate and asked her to use it as a self-help exercise to strengthen her motivational enhancement plan. As you read the list, you may get some ideas for how you could use motivational enhancement strategies in your own life.

Motivational Enhancement Strategies

Set specific, well-defined goals for change: Vague or overly general goals (such as "get my life in gear" or "be happy again") won't give you much guidance or be very effective motivators. Specific, attainable goals, if partnered with some of the other methods on this tip list, will probably do a better job of helping you make meaningful changes.

Be realistic: Choose targets that are reasonable and within your capacity for change. Take your current level of depression into consideration. If energy and concentration are significant problems, it may be best to plan activities that are doable now instead of stretching too far, too fast to make extensive changes. You can expand your goals for change after you start to feel better and gain strength.

Devote time to work on your goal: Make a commitment to carve out the time needed to work on making planned changes. One of the common mistakes in getting motivated and staying motivated is neglecting to find time in a busy schedule for the activity. For example, if you decided to start an exercise program but didn't plan ahead to have specific times for the workouts, you might be more likely to procrastinate and not follow through with your plans. We use the principle of scheduling ahead a great deal in our own planning. We set aside time for exercise, writing, socializing, and other activities that are very important to us and are "musts" in our weekly schedules.

Get into a routine: Most people seem to do better and to more regularly complete activities and tasks if they follow a routine. If you commit to a yoga class on Mondays and Thursdays from 6:00 to 7:00 P.M. and Saturdays from 2:00 to 3:00 P.M., you probably will attend many more classes than if you just hoped to work a few classes into your schedule when you had the time, energy, and motivation. You could wait for a long time before all of these factors seemed to be in the ideal place to help you get to a class.

Post the goal: To keep your goal in top-of-the-mind awareness, write it down and place it where you will be sure to read it several times a day.

Kate's Motivational Enhancement Worksheet

Instructions: Select a goal that is specific and attainable. Then list some of the key motivators that could help you make the planned changes. Next, write down any demotivators that could interfere with your plan. Finally, list some actions you could take to boost the motivators and cope with the demotivators.

Goal or action to take: *Sticking with positive changes in an activity schedule—carry out at least 5 positive changes a week.*

MOTIVATORS:

* *There is a very strong chance that following an activity schedule will help relieve depression.*
* *Exercise and yoga will help me get back in shape and will build my energy.*
* *I will get back into life and enjoy being with friends and family.*
* *Participating in activities at church is very important to me. I will feel much better about myself if I attend regularly.*
* *My friends will stick with me. If I keep avoiding them, they could drift away.*
* *If I get out of my rut, I could eventually meet someone and start a new relationship. I don't want to be alone the rest of my life.*

DEMOTIVATORS:

* *I get tired and just want to stay by myself and not do anything.*
* *I start to think that nothing will make a difference.*
* *Friends or family don't call me. I start to think that people don't want to be around me.*

ACTIONS I CAN TAKE TO BUILD UP MOTIVATORS AND MAKE THEM WORK FOR ME:

* *Post the list of motivators on my refrigerator and on my bathroom mirror. Read the list at least three times a day.*
* *Try to get excited about making these changes. Think of all of the good things that could come my way.*
* *Talk with my sister about the activity schedule. Call her every evening to review the day and to get her support and feedback.*
* *Realize that there can be ebbs and flows in levels of motivation and being able to carry out plans. If it doesn't work well for a day or more, don't panic and give up. Remind myself of the reasons to change and try again!*

ACTIONS I CAN TAKE TO COPE WITH DEMOTIVATORS AND MAKE THEM LESS OF A PROBLEM:

* *Commit to a regular time to go to yoga. Make this a priority. Be sure that the time commitment is realistic and that I can do it when scheduled.*
* *Even if I am tired, push myself to attend yoga. Think of how good I will feel after I go to the class.*
* *If I have negative thoughts such as "nothing will work" or "I don't have any energy to do these things," recognize that they are automatic thoughts that are part of the depression. Challenge the negative thoughts and replace them with more reasonable thoughts.*
* *If I don't get a call from friends or family, avoid catastrophizing and thinking that they don't care or I am bound to be alone. Realize that I haven't been responding much to their calls and I need to get back into the swing of things. I have good friends and am close to my family. If I contact them, they will probably be interested in doing things with me.*

Set a start date: Some people find that setting a start date helps to build anticipation and excitement for change. Prior to the start date you can try to motivate yourself for making change by doing things like reading about the goal, doing Internet searches, and refining your plans for reaching the goal.

Get support: Although some people like to "do it alone," the support of family, friends, or others can often be a big help. Kate reached out to her sister. We supported each other in writing this book, and we received excellent support from our editor, our families, and our friends. Are there people who could support your efforts to change? Maybe an exercise "buddy" would give you more motivation to stick with a plan. Perhaps a book group would help you get back into reading again. Could online support groups play a role in enhancing your motivation?

Use CBT methods to counter negative thoughts: Negative automatic thoughts such as "I'll never be able to stick it out," "Nothing will help," or "I've failed so many times—what's the use?" can quickly undermine your motivation and derail efforts to change. The methods you learned for identifying and modifying automatic thoughts earlier in this book are some of the most powerful ways to enhance motivation and stick with plans until you reach your goals. Try using methods such as thought records, examining the evidence, and looking for cognitive errors to stop the erosion of motivation and to get the dose of confidence that you will need to sustain your efforts.

Take an inventory of your procrastinating behaviors: Procrastination is such a common problem that it enters into almost everybody's lives. Who hasn't put off a task while managing to find time to do other things? One way to build your motivation is to look procrastination "in the eye." Be honest with yourself and make a list of the main things that you do to procrastinate. Could it be spending big hunks of time surfing the Internet without any clear focus or intention? Could it be getting distracted by loads of TV programs that you don't really enjoy very much or give you any sense of fulfillment? Could it be spending excessive time on household chores that don't really need to be done as carefully or frequently? After you list your procrastinating behaviors, make a contract with yourself to reduce the amount of time you spend in these activities. For example, if you are currently surfing the Internet as a procrastinating behavior about 3–4 hours a day and you are doing this off and on throughout the entire day, you could commit to limiting the total time to no more than an hour a day and bracketing this in a time slot from 8:00 to 9:00 in the evening.

Reward yourself: The rewards for making changes will probably show up in the list of motivators that you will complete in the next exercise. You might gain energy, rebuild friendships, lose weight, or have other positive outcomes of working toward your goals. However, you might think of building other rewards into your plan. Would it help motivate you to decide to go to a free concert, buy a new outfit, do some window-shopping, or take a weekend break if you stayed the course in working toward a goal?

Keep track of your progress: Logging or monitoring is a very useful tool to increase and sustain motivation. Kate completed activity schedules for several weeks until she was feeling much better and the changes became a routine part of her life. Other people we have known have used computerized systems for recording calories consumed and the effects on weight, have joined health clubs that have electronic recording methods for exercise and give encouraging feedback on progress, or have used simple methods such as keeping a diary or journal. Seeing evidence of progress or spotting problems with sticking with a plan can help you stay focused on making the changes you desire.

To practice ways of increasing motivation, we suggest that you choose a goal and then complete Exercise 5.8. (You might want to do this exercise more than once as you work toward recovery from depression; photocopy the worksheet or download it from *www.guilford.com/breakingfreeforms.*)

Motivational Enhancement Worksheet

Instructions: Select a goal that is specific and attainable. Then list some of the key motivators that could help you make the planned changes. Next, write down any demotivators that could interfere with your plan. Finally, list some actions you could take to boost the motivators and cope with the demotivators.

Goal or action to take: _____

_____

MOTIVATORS:

1.

2.

3.

4.

5.

DEMOTIVATORS:

1.

2.

3.

4.

5.

ACTIONS I CAN TAKE TO BUILD UP THE MOTIVATORS AND MAKE THEM WORK FOR ME:

1.

2.

3.

4.

5.

ACTIONS I CAN TAKE TO COPE WITH DEMOTIVATORS AND MAKE THEM LESS OF A PROBLEM:

1.

2.

3.

4.

5.

The Step-by-Step Approach

Another CBT method that Kate used for behavioral change was the step-by-step approach. This commonsense method is such a frequent part of everyday life for most people that you may wonder why we emphasize it as a tool to counter depression. Yet many people who are mired in depression seem to forget or lose touch with the principle of breaking down large or challenging tasks into manageable pieces that can be taken one at a time.

If you wanted to run a 5-mile race and were totally out of shape and not running at all, it wouldn't be such a good idea to try to pound out a mile or two the first time you put on your running shoes. In fact, you would probably not be able to accomplish this feat, and you could get discouraged and back away from your goal or even injure yourself. A better approach would be to prepare for starting this type of exercise by acquiring proper equipment, checking your health status with your doctor, and reading about how to train to do some jogging or running. Then you might start with running brief distances such as a few blocks, alternating with some walking. As you built up your strength and endurance, you could gradually increase the length of time that you ran until you were able to cover the full 5 miles without straining or hurting yourself.

The step-by-step approach can be a big help when you feel overwhelmed by tasks, have tried to make headway but seem to be stuck in the starting gate, or are facing an especially demanding or challenging project. You have almost certainly used this strategy to good effect previously in your life, but you may not be tapping its full strength now.

Basics of the Step-by-Step Approach

- Select a problem or task that seems difficult or has been hard to accomplish.
- Break the problem down into manageable chunks or steps. Make the steps quite small if needed.
- Sometimes steps may need to be subdivided into even smaller pieces. For example, if a step in "getting finances in order" is to "organize and pay outstanding monthly bills," it might be necessary to sketch out substeps such as (1) sort mail into junk mail that can be thrown away versus bills that need attention, (2) balance the checkbook, (3) prioritize bills and decide which ones need to be paid now.
- Take it a step at a time. You can build confidence and a sense of accomplishment as you gradually take on each step.

Kate identified a problem with her condo as a candidate for the step-by-step approach. As she had become more depressed, a tendency to let things pile up had grown to the point that she described her home environment as "a total mess." She wasn't a hoarder, but she did have stacks of unopened mail, boxes that had arrived from mail-order companies that had never been opened or she had intended to return, a big backup of laundry, and a garage that was so full of stuff that she couldn't park her car inside. When Kate came home from work, just opening the door to her stuffed house seemed to depress her. And she was avoiding asking friends to visit her because she was "embarrassed to let them see how I live."

We suggested she use a "Step-by-Step Worksheet" to organize and implement a plan of attack on her condo. In the example on pages 126 and 127, Kate had done the first three steps and had noted progress. The rest of the plan appeared to be reasonable and had a good chance of success.

> **?** **Have you had trouble sticking with step-by-step plans? Does a step-by-step plan sound too difficult or complex to work for you? If you have concerns about using a step-by-step plan, consider these perspectives:**
>
> - You don't need to develop a full plan with many steps such as Kate's to benefit from this approach. Perhaps organizing your efforts into just a few steps would yield results.
>
> - Keep it simple if you are just starting to use the step-by-step approach as a depression fighting tool. Choose a single problem that is not too complex—a problem that can be addressed with some straightforward steps.
>
> - View the step-by-step approach as a learning opportunity. You could build skills by organizing a step-wise approach to a task.
>
> - If you have difficulty following the plan, stand back and reassess the strategy. Can you make some changes (slow it down, get some help, change directions, etc.) that would help you succeed?
>
> - Review the motivational enhancement strategies on pages 120 and 122 for suggestions on how to keep going with behavioral change plans when you confront difficulties or need a boost.

What tasks or challenges are you facing that might be managed effectively with a step-by-step plan? You can use one copy of the worksheet to develop an overall plan; or if the task is complex and multifaceted, you can use several copies of the worksheet to divide the big problem into separate categories that can be targeted with the step-by-step approach; photocopy it or download it from *www.guilford.com/breakingfreeforms*.

Summary

Low energy, lack of interest, difficulties experiencing pleasure, and problems completing tasks are some of the major behavioral changes that occur in depression. You can directly address these problems with evidence-based methods from CBT, or you can wait for other treatments to possibly reverse the symptoms. We recommend a multipronged approach in which you try to make changes in your behavior while also working on other fronts such as changing negative thoughts and considering biological treatments. In the next chapter, you'll learn additional CBT methods that can help you build your self-confidence and draw more power from your strengths. As you move ahead in the book, please also keep in mind the lessons we covered here on how to restore energy and enjoy life. We think these lessons can be an important key to success in overcoming depression.

Step-by-Step Worksheet: Kate's Example

Instructions: (1) Identify a task or challenge that is giving you difficulty. (2) Make a list of manageable steps—ones that you could accomplish in a gradual, step-by-step manner. (3) Rate the steps for degree of difficulty on a scale of 0–10 (0 = no difficulty, 10 = maximum difficulty). (4) If steps seem too difficult, break them down into smaller steps. (4) Write down any special plans that you have for accomplishing the step. (5) Log your progress in following the steps and modify the plan if necessary to meet your goal.

Task I want to accomplish: Get my condo back in order so that I feel good when I come home and I can invite friends over for dinner.

Step #	Step description	Degree of difficulty	Plans and comments	Progress
1	Sort mail and throw out any mail that doesn't need a response or doesn't interest me.	2	Spend 15 minutes every day this week until job is done.	No problem doing this one.
2	Pay any bills that are due.	4	Do this on Sunday afternoon after I get all mail sorted out. It is difficult, but I really need to get it done. It is hanging over me.	I had to push myself to get it done, but the bills got paid.
3	Open boxes from mail-order companies, take an inventory of what has come in the mail in the last few months.	4	Be prepared to be stuck with some things that I would like to return but can't because it is too late. Take the hit of being unable to return some things, but get all of the boxes organized. Don't order anything else until I take care of this backlog.	I got a bit down when I found four shipments that I couldn't return. One was okay because it was a coffee pot I needed. Another had some clothes that fit well. But there were two shipments of clothes that didn't fit or didn't look right. I'll have to take the losses and move ahead.
4	Prepare boxes for shipping and take them to UPS.	3	Get tape and mailing labels from store.	Pending

Step-by-Step Worksheet (*cont.*)

Step #	Step description	Degree of difficulty	Plans and comments	Progress
5	Tackle the unwashed laundry. Do the current needs first, then wash the bedspreads and guest towels and sheets that haven't been used for months.	5	Start with sorting all of the laundry. Do it one load at a time, about one per day. Dry and fold each load each day as it is completed and put it away.	Pending
6	Keep up with laundry each week by setting goal of having all laundry completed by Sunday evening before I start the work week.	6	I don't really enjoy this. Download some music on Monday evening if I have taken care of the week's laundry.	Pending
7	Make a list of all of the things that are congesting my garage. Rate them in categories (definitely want to save, can be given to friends or family if they want it, can be given away to charity, or junk).	5	This can be delayed until I get the inside of the house in better order. Slur I In about 3 weeks. Do on a Saturday or Sunday when I have plenty of time. Can be done 30 minutes or an hour at a time over several weeks if needed.	Pending
8	Ask my brother-in-law to help me haul away the junk. He has a pickup.	6	He will probably do this. He is usually willing to help.	Pending
9	Organize the stuff I will give to charity; make a list so I might get a tax deduction for some of it. Call charities to see if any of them have Saturday pickups. If they don't pick up on Saturday, ask brother-in-law to help again.	7	This will take a lot of work because there are many things that I have just piled up in the garage. I will need to take my time with it.	Pending
10	Find space to store any things I want to save from the garage. If I have too much stuff, make another donation to charity.	8	I really need to pare down the stuff that I keep in my condo. It will be good for me to get rid of things I really don't need or use.	Pending

Step-by-Step Worksheet

Instructions: (1) Identify a task or challenge that is giving you difficulty. (2) Make a list of manageable steps—ones that you could accomplish in a gradual, step-by-step manner. (3) Rate the steps for degree of difficulty on a scale of 0–10 (0 = no difficulty, 10 = maximum difficulty). (4) If steps seem too difficult, break them down into smaller steps. (4) Write down any special plans that you have for accomplishing the step. (5) Log your progress in following the steps and modify the plan if necessary to meet your goal.

Task I want to accomplish: _____

_____

Step #	Step description	Degree of difficulty	Plans and comments	Progress
1				
2				
3				
4				
5				

(cont.)

Step #	Step description	Degree of difficulty	Plans and comments	Progress
6				
7				
8				
9				
10				
11				
12				

6

Building Self-Esteem and Using Strengths

Chapter Highlights

▶ Core beliefs: the roots of self-esteem

▶ Identifying core beliefs

▶ Changing negative core beliefs

▶ Tapping your strengths to overcome depression

When people become depressed, they usually experience a drop in self-confidence and have difficulty seeing and using their strengths. If your self-esteem could use a lift or you haven't fully recognized and used your strengths in overcoming depression, this chapter could help you learn powerful methods for change.

Core Beliefs: The Roots of Self-Esteem

In Chapter 4 you practiced ways of recognizing and modifying automatic thoughts. There is another, deeper layer of our thinking that is often an important part of depression. We all have core beliefs about what kind of person we are. These core beliefs (or *schemas*, to use the technical term from CBT) define our self-concept, guide how we respond to stress, and shape our coping behaviors. Some positive or adaptive examples of core beliefs are "I'm a good friend," "I can handle stress," "I'm intelligent," and "I can figure things out." Negative or maladaptive core beliefs could include "No matter how hard I try, I'm bound to fail," "I'm never good enough," "I'm a loser," and "I'm stupid."

The terms *positive* and *adaptive* are used interchangeably by therapists to describe core beliefs that support healthy self-esteem and effective functioning. These types of beliefs help people *adapt* to life circumstances and to have an accurate and balanced view of themselves—not to be irrationally happy or to have unrealistically high estimates of their strengths. The terms *negative* and *maladaptive* are used interchangeably to describe core beliefs that can be damaging to self-esteem and interfere with effective behavior.

Some core beliefs have mixed positive (adaptive) and negative (maladaptive) features. If you had a belief that "I must be in control," you might work very hard to organize your life and to achieve success. But the belief might lead to problems such as driving yourself and others to extremes, having difficulty trusting coworkers and family to complete tasks, and getting depressed or anxious when life situations make it difficult for you to maintain control.

Core beliefs start developing in childhood and continue to evolve throughout life. They are shaped by many influences, including genetics, relationships with parents and other important figures, and experiences with school, peers, dating, partners and children, work, and spiritual activities. For example, an adaptive core belief such as "I can handle stress" could be rooted in parental messages of confidence, in addition to multiple experiences of coping with challenges throughout childhood, adolescence, and adulthood. Perhaps there were especially memorable events such as family crises or job problems that seared this adaptive belief into the person's mind. Conversely, a maladaptive belief such as "I'm never good enough" could have resulted from early experiences in which this person couldn't seem to please his parents, teachers, and others. "Rejections" such as broken romantic attachments later in life could have reinforced this negative belief.

What Is the Difference between Automatic Thoughts and Core Beliefs?

Automatic thoughts and core beliefs are both part of our self-talk, and identifying and changing both types of cognitions is one of the primary goals of CBT.

The difference between these two levels of thinking is:

Automatic thoughts are the thoughts that just pop into our heads about specific situations in our lives. Ted had the automatic thought "He's just trying to be nice" when his friend called and suggested they go bowling. The phone call stimulated the automatic thought.

Core beliefs are enduring basic views of oneself. They serve as *rules* for understanding reactions and responses of other people and for guiding behavior. When Ted participated in CBT, he discovered that one of his negative core beliefs was "I'm no good at social situations." Thus when he was feeling depressed and was invited to do things with others, he had negative automatic thoughts about the invitation and often declined to participate.

What Is the Relationship between Core Beliefs and Depression?

One of the basic theories of CBT is that negative or maladaptive core beliefs can lie dormant or be relatively inactive when people are well. But when they are depressed, negative beliefs become much more active and believable. Also during a depression, positive or adaptive core beliefs may be hard to remember and fade into the background of your thinking. So efforts to recall, strengthen, and use the adaptive beliefs and to change or dampen the negative beliefs can help you gain power over depression.

Identifying Core Beliefs

Because core beliefs can often be below the surface of our thinking, people can have difficulty spotting them and putting them into words. It may be especially challenging to articulate positive core beliefs. Because modesty is a highly regarded virtue, people often downplay their strengths and coach themselves not to think much about their positive attributes. Also, depression typically acts like a dark cloud that hides positive or adaptive core beliefs from us.

We don't want to encourage you to use self-flattery or to develop unrealistically positive self-assessments, but we do want you to be honest with yourself and give yourself credit for the things you do well. We also want you to recognize the key maladaptive beliefs that may be holding you back from recovery from depression.

Identifying Positive Core Beliefs: Some Questions to Ask Yourself

A good way to uncover core beliefs is to ask yourself some questions that may stimulate your thinking and help you search for the rules that govern your self-concept. Ted used the next exercise to spot some of his most important core beliefs.

Are you getting some ideas about your own positive core beliefs? If so, you can write them down now.

? **Are you having trouble recognizing positive core beliefs? If so, try these strategies for identifying positive core beliefs:**

1. Use the checklist in the next part of the chapter to get ideas about adaptive beliefs.

2. Ask a trusted family member or friend to discuss some of your adaptive attributes and to coach you on recognizing and holding on to these attitudes or rules.

3. Think back to when you weren't depressed or were much less depressed. Try to imagine how you were thinking about yourself then without the negative influence of depression.

4. Search for positive rules in many areas of your life, for example, in your relationships with others, in your skills, in your interests and hobbies, in your work, in your intimate life, in your spiritual life, in your physical life.

Questions about Positive Core Beliefs: Ted's Example

Instructions: Respond to these questions by writing down some positive core beliefs that you may have.

What positive rules help define who you are?

What positive rules about yourself have you learned from your parents, grandparents, or other people in your life?

What positive rules about yourself could you be forgetting or ignoring now?

Some of my positive core beliefs are:

I love my family and would do anything for them.

I have been a good athlete, and I still have some athletic skills.

I usually can "remain calm in the eye of a storm" and stay clear-headed and focused even when trouble strikes.

Others can trust me.

I have a good education and know a lot about how to do my job.

I am usually a good person. I never intentionally hurt others.

I am loved by my family.

I often have a good sense of humor.

I like to do things for others when I can.

I can be a good listener with family and friends.

I am usually interested in life, in trying out new things.

I'm good at working with my hands, doing mechanical things like wiring and plumbing. If you give me a manual, I can usually learn how to do a mechanical task.

EXERCISE 6.1   **Questions about Positive Core Beliefs**

Instructions: Respond to these questions by writing down some positive core beliefs that you may have. You can use an additional piece of paper if you identify more positive beliefs than will fit in the box.

What positive rules help define who you are?

What positive rules about yourself have you learned from your parents, grandparents, or other people in your life?

What positive rules about yourself could you be forgetting or ignoring now?

Some of my positive core beliefs are:

Using a Checklist to Spot Positive Core Beliefs

To get more ideas on positive core beliefs that you have now or would like to develop, complete the next checklist. The list will not cover all the core beliefs that are part of your self-concept, but it may include some that you will want to consider emphasizing as you move toward wellness. You can fill out this checklist periodically if you like; photocopy it or download it from *www.guilford.com/breakingfreeforms*.

Positive Core Beliefs Checklist

Instructions: Use this checklist to recognize positive core beliefs. Check "No" if you don't have the belief, "Maybe" if it is possible that you have this belief or could develop this belief, and "Yes" if you are sure that you have this belief.

Positive Core Beliefs	No	Maybe	Yes
No matter what happens, I can manage somehow.			
When I work hard at something, I can master it.			
I'm a survivor.			
Others trust me.			
I'm a solid person.			
People respect me.			
They can knock me down, but they can't knock me out.			
I care about other people.			
I usually do better when I prepare in advance.			
I deserve to be respected.			
I like to be challenged.			
There's not much that can scare me.			
I'm intelligent.			
I can figure things out.			
I'm friendly.			
I can handle stress.			
The tougher the problem, the tougher I become.			
I can learn from my mistakes and be a better person.			
I'm a good spouse (and/or parent, child, friend, lover).			
Everything will work out all right.			

We hope you've been able to identify some positive core beliefs, and the exercises have given you ideas about how you can use these attributes in overcoming depression. In the last part of this chapter we'll suggest some methods for applying these adaptive beliefs and tapping your strengths to reduce symptoms. But now let's turn our attention to the other side of your thinking—the negative or maladaptive beliefs that could be leading to depression and/or blocking your progress toward recovery.

FAST FACT   Negative or maladaptive core beliefs are usually associated with behavior patterns that are consistent with the belief. For example, if you believed that "I'm no good at social situations," you might get tense whenever you had to socialize and try to avoid as many stressful social situations as possible. As a result, you wouldn't have the chance to practice or build social skills. To change this pattern, you would need to work on modifying the core belief and also on building up your social skills.

Identifying Negative Core Beliefs

To get started on spotting your maladaptive beliefs, ask yourself the same types of questions we used for positive beliefs. An example (see the facing page) might help you tune in to your negative beliefs.

Did you notice that Ted's negative beliefs have absolute, self-condemning, or fear-inducing qualities? Later in the chapter, you'll learn how to take the sting out of such beliefs and to modify them in ways that will help you break free from depression. But for now try Exercise 6.3 on page 138 to see what you can learn about your thinking. We don't want you to dwell on negative thinking, but we do want you to recognize some of the key beliefs that you might want to target for change.

? **Is it getting you down to list some of your maladaptive core beliefs?**

Sometimes people feel somewhat worse at first when they search within themselves and find negative rules or beliefs. If the exercises for spotting maladaptive beliefs seem upsetting, try to remember these points:

1. Most people have a mixture of positive and maladaptive core beliefs. If you recognized some negative beliefs, you are not alone.

2. Maladaptive core beliefs often can be changed. People can learn to think and act differently, and in doing so they can build their confidence and their effectiveness in everyday life.

3. Exercises from CBT that are included in this book can help you modify your negative beliefs.

4. One of the core principles of CBT is that revising maladaptive beliefs can help prevent people from slipping back into depression once they feel well.

Questions about Maladaptive Core Beliefs: Ted's Example

Instructions: Respond to these questions by writing down some negative or maladaptive core beliefs that you may have.

> **What maladaptive rules about yourself could be lowering your self-esteem or promoting ineffective behavior?**
>
> **What maladaptive rules about yourself have you learned from experiences growing up and in your adult life?**
>
> **What maladaptive rules may be under the surface of your thinking but still exert a negative influence on you?**

Some of my maladaptive core beliefs are:

1. *I'm no good at social situations.*

2. *All of the people in our family have had job problems. I'm bound to fail.*

3. *I've always just faked it. I don't know what I'm doing.*

4. *I've always had to try harder than others. Nothing comes easily to me.*

5. *I'm unattractive.*

6. *No matter how hard I try, I'm sure to end up a financial ruin.*

Using a Checklist to Spot Maladaptive Core Beliefs

The checklist on page 139 contains some of the negative core beliefs commonly seen in people with depression. You may recognize some of your own rules of thinking in this list. As with positive core beliefs, your negative or maladaptive core beliefs may change over time. To use the worksheet more than once, photocopy it or download it from *www.guilford.com/breakingfreeforms*.

QUICK TIPS
- To recall and use your positive core beliefs and to target specific negative core beliefs for change, it can help to create a *core belief log.*

- You can review your core belief log on a regular basis to remind yourself of your adaptive attributes and to stay focused on changing the key maladaptive beliefs that may be knocking down your self-esteem or holding you back from recovery.

| EXERCISE 6.3 | Questions about Maladaptive Core Beliefs |

Instructions: Respond to these questions by writing down some negative or maladaptive core beliefs that you may have.

> **What maladaptive rules about yourself could be lowering your self-esteem or promoting ineffective behavior?**
>
> **What maladaptive rules about yourself have you learned from experiences in growing up and in your adult life?**
>
> **What maladaptive rules may have been under the surface of your thinking but are still exerting a negative influence on you?**

Some of my maladaptive core beliefs are:

Keeping a Core Belief Log

You can use the core belief log in Exercise 6.5 to help organize your efforts to make positive changes in your thinking. Start your log now. You can come back to it later to revise the entries as you make progress in strengthening your positive beliefs and changing your maladaptive beliefs.

Maladaptive Core Beliefs Checklist

Instructions: Use this checklist to see if you might have any core beliefs that could be part of depression or part of your way out of depression. Check "No" if you don't have the belief, "Maybe" if it is possible that you have this belief, and "Yes" if you are sure you have this belief.

Maladaptive Core Beliefs	No	Maybe	Yes
I must be perfect to be accepted.			
If I choose to do something, I must succeed.			
I'm stupid.			
Without a woman (man), I'm nothing.			
I'm a fake.			
Never show weakness.			
I'm unlovable.			
If I make one mistake, I'll lose everything.			
I'll never be comfortable around others.			
I can never finish anything.			
No matter what I do, I won't succeed.			
The world is too frightening for me.			
Others can't be trusted.			
I must always be in control.			
I'm unattractive.			
Never show your emotions.			
Other people will take advantage of me.			
I'm lazy.			
If people really knew me, they wouldn't like me.			
To be accepted, I must always please others.			

Instructions:

1. Review your responses to Exercises 6.1 (Questions about Positive Core Beliefs) and 6.3 (Questions about Maladaptive Core Beliefs). Write down on this log any of the positive beliefs that you want to single out to remember and any of the maladaptive beliefs that you would like to change.

2. Now review Exercises 6.2 (Positive Core Beliefs Checklist) and 6.4 (Maladaptive Core Beliefs Checklist). You can circle the beliefs that you think are most important or are giving you the most trouble and then record them on this Core Belief Log.

Positive core beliefs	Maladaptive core beliefs

Changing Maladaptive Core Beliefs

Because you learned how to modify negative automatic thoughts in Chapter 4, you should have an excellent head start on developing skills for changing maladaptive core beliefs. You can work on revising negative core beliefs by (1) going off automatic pilot, (2) examining the evidence, (3) looking for thinking errors, and (4) putting changes into action.

Going Off Automatic Pilot

By identifying some negative beliefs and writing them down in the first part of this chapter, you have already started to go off automatic pilot. Putting core beliefs into words, logging them, and looking at them in the "cool light of day" can often start the process of change. For example, when Angelina wrote down the belief "I must be in control" on a log, she began to question herself about the impact of holding this belief. How was it increasing her anxiety and tension? How did it affect relationships with her family and her coworkers? Although the belief did tend to make her work hard, what price was she paying for being so rigid about requiring control in every corner of her life?

Examining the Evidence

You can use the same two-column method that you learned for examining the evidence for automatic thoughts to check out the validity of maladaptive core beliefs. To gain experience in using this valuable technique, help Ted work on changing two of his negative core beliefs. First, you'll need some more background information on Ted.

Two of Ted's negative core beliefs about how life might work out for him in the future ("All of the people in our family have had job problems ... I'm bound to fail" and "No matter how hard I try, I'm sure to end up a financial ruin") didn't seem to have much impact when he wasn't depressed. The beliefs stayed relatively weak when things were going well at work and at home. However, when there was an economic downturn and Ted's business declined, he became depressed, and the maladaptive core beliefs gathered much more force.

Ted's father and his uncle had indeed had some work problems that had been upsetting to the whole family and had caught Ted's full attention as he was growing up. His father was a contractor who remodeled and built homes, and his uncle had a related business as a plumber. The two of them often worked together on building projects. During an earlier economic recession, Ted's father had to declare bankruptcy when the houses that he had built didn't sell, and he was stuck with carrying the interest payments for more than a year. His uncle was also felled financially by this recession and had to temporarily close his plumbing business and lay off all of his employees.

Ted was 11 and 12 years old during this stressful time for his family. He remembered being ashamed that he didn't have money for sporting equipment, clothes, and

Going Off Automatic Pilot

Instructions: Choose a maladaptive core belief from your log. Write it down in the box below. Then ask yourself questions to help you understand the impact of the negative core belief on your mood and your behavior. You can repeat this exercise multiple times for different core beliefs.

A negative core belief I want to change:

How is this belief affecting my life? How does it influence my moods and behavior? Does it affect my behavior in any positive or productive ways, or does the belief have a completely negative impact?

What ideas do I have now for changes in this belief that could help me think and act in a healthier way?

---

other things that his classmates seemed to have no trouble getting. And he remembered that his father and mother were very tense and distressed during this time in their lives.

Although Ted's father and his uncle were eventually successful in reestablishing their construction businesses, the difficult times during the bankruptcy left a mark on Ted. As he considered various careers, Ted decided against any options that would involve his owning or being responsible for a business. He thought that he had chosen a very secure career as a sales agent for a heavy construction equipment company. But it turned out that this business was not immune to economic downturns.

Ted's core belief stated that "all of the people in my family have had job problems ... I'm bound to fail." Yet his father and his uncle didn't "fail" over the long run. In fact, they showed considerable resilience and an ability to manage their lives in the face of adversity. Also after the bankruptcy, Ted's mother went back to school to complete a teaching degree and went on to have a satisfying career as an educator. Ted's brother had been laid off from a management job in a grocery store chain about 6 years ago, but he had since found another job in the same field that had more responsibility and paid better. His sister was a successful administrator for a health plan, and both of his grandfathers held steady jobs (one as a machinist and the other as store manager) throughout their lives. So the absolute nature of Ted's core belief didn't fit with the facts of his life.

The core belief "No matter how hard I try, I'm sure to be a financial ruin" also seemed to have been shaped by Ted's early experiences with seeing his family struggle with bankruptcy and trying to make ends meet when their income plummeted. However, his family made it through this crisis and actually seemed to grow stronger as time went by. His father and uncle regrouped as the recession eased, and both formed somewhat smaller companies that continue to be functioning well to this day. Ted's mother found a meaningful career that contributed greatly to his parents' eventual financial security. Although his family hasn't been rich, they have had a good quality of life and have a reasonably solid financial footing.

EXERCISE 6.7	**Examining the Evidence for Core Beliefs:** **Ted's Example**

Instructions:

1. Use this worksheet to write down any evidence that may support Ted's maladaptive core beliefs.

2. Then write down any evidence against these negative core beliefs.

3. Finally, try to write down any realistic modifications in these beliefs that you think might help Ted be less depressed and cope better with his stresses.

(cont.)

Core belief 1: "All of the people in my family have had job problems ... I'm bound to fail."

Evidence for belief	Evidence against belief

Rational alternatives to this belief:

- _____

- _____

- _____

(cont.)

Core belief 2: "No matter how hard I try, I'm sure to have financial ruin."

Evidence for belief	Evidence against belief

Rational alternatives to this belief:

* _____

* _____

* _____

QUICK TIPS
1. To find rational alternatives to maladaptive core beliefs, you can use the same methods that you learned to generate rational alternatives to automatic thoughts. These methods include opening your mind to the possibilities, brainstorming, and learning from others.
2. When you *open your mind to the possibilities*, you try to step outside the narrow thinking style of depression to look at yourself from different perspectives. You can imagine yourself in the place of a trusted friend or a great coach who is giving you realistic but affirming advice on how you can see yourself in a better light and change negative thinking.
3. When you *brainstorm*, you try to give your mind free rein to consider many different options, even if they seem to be a stretch at first glance. Just write down a wide variety of possible changes. Then you can select some that seem to offer the most promise.
4. When you *learn from others*, you actually talk with people you can trust to weigh the merits of possible changes in your rules of thinking. Others may be able to see potentials for change that are not apparent to you or can give you valuable feedback on some ideas you're considering.

To give you an illustration of the effective use of examining the evidence, we'll show you a completed worksheet for one of Ted's negative core beliefs.

Helping Ted examine the evidence has probably "primed the pump" for using this exercise to challenge and change some of your own maladaptive core beliefs. You can use the worksheet on page 148 to modify a number of your core beliefs. Just make photocopies of the form or go to the publisher's website (*www.guilford.com/breakingfreeforms*) to print out extras.

Looking for Thinking Errors

In Chapter 4 you learned about the different types of thinking errors that can make automatic thoughts seem so believable:

- All-or-nothing thinking
- Jumping to conclusions
- Ignoring the evidence
- Maximizing or minimizing
- Overgeneralizing
- Personalizing

If you've been trying to spot thinking errors in your automatic thoughts, you can use the same tool for developing rational and healthy core beliefs. In fact, you may already have spotted some of the thinking errors in the examples of negative core beliefs used in

Examining the Evidence for Core Beliefs: Ted's Example

Core belief: "All of the men in my family have had job problems ... I'm bound to fail."

Evidence for belief	Evidence against belief
My father went bankrupt and lost his business.	My father eventually recovered and built a successful business.
My uncle also had to shut down a business.	My father didn't really fail—he had business problems that were largely due to a recession. He is a good person who has had problems in life, but has been able to overcome them. My uncle had the same type of problems and has also put his life back together.
My brother lost a good job.	The fact that my father went bankrupt and lost a business doesn't predict what will happen in my life. In fact, I know my job well and have good support from my boss.
	My mother went back to school when times were tough and has had a good career as a teacher. My sister is an administrator and single mother who is doing just fine. Both of my grandfathers had good careers. My brother lost a job but is now back on his feet and doing better than ever. There is really no evidence from my family that any of us are "bound to fail."

Rational alternatives to this belief:

- My father and uncle had difficult times in business but weathered the storms. I can ride storms out and find ways to manage problems.

- I have lots of positive models of how to handle adversity.

- I am skilled at my work. Even if I lost my current job, I could cope with the blow and regroup to have success.

- Having a problem in life doesn't mean that you are a "failure." I have had many successes and will have more in the future.

Examining the Evidence for Core Beliefs

Core belief: _____

Evidence for belief	Evidence against belief

Rational alternatives to this belief:

- _____

- _____

- _____

this chapter. The next exercise asks you to identify thinking errors in one of Ted's and one of Angelina's negative core beliefs.

As noted in Chapter 4, there's considerable overlap between the different types of errors in thinking. Because it's unlikely that all observers will agree on which thinking errors are involved or spot all of the thinking errors, we want to emphasize that you don't have to make all the correct choices to benefit from exercises such as these. Recognizing any thinking errors can help you develop healthier core beliefs.

We believe that Ted's core belief has an *absolutistic* quality because he says that "all" of the people in his family have had job problems and that he is *jumping to conclusions* because he predicts that he is "bound to fail." He is also *ignoring the evidence* that he has good job skills and support from his boss and family that should help him through his period of difficulty. Did you think that Ted was *magnifying* the problem and *minimizing* his strengths to cope with it? We believe this classic form of thinking error was perpetuating his negative core belief. Finally, Ted was *personalizing* when he said to himself that "I'm bound to fail." He seemed to be taking too much personal responsibility for the challenging economic conditions and blaming himself excessively for all of his troubles.

Looking for Thinking Errors in Core Beliefs: Ted's and Angelina's Examples

Instructions: Place a check mark beside any of the thinking errors that you believe might be involved in the negative core belief.

Ted's core belief	All-or-nothing thinking	Jumping to conclusions	Ignoring the evidence	Magnifying or minimizing	Overgeneralizing	Personalizing
All of the people in my family have had job problems ... I'm bound to fail.						

Angelina's core belief	All-or-nothing thinking	Jumping to conclusions	Ignoring the evidence	Magnifying or minimizing	Overgeneralizing	Personalizing
I must be in control.						

Angelina's core belief about control is very *absolutistic*. Any time words such as "must," "always," or "never" are used to qualify core beliefs, absolutistic thinking is very likely to be influencing core beliefs. We believe that she is probably *magnifying* her need for control and *minimizing* her abilities to cope with situations in which she doesn't have full control. *Overgeneralizing* is another thinking error that could be giving Angelina problems. Could she be overgeneralizing her wish for control to a broad sweep of all of her activities and involvements? Angelina may also be *ignoring the evidence* that she doesn't want or need to have complete control in some areas of her life.

EXERCISE 6.9	**Looking for Thinking Errors in Core Beliefs**

Instructions: Write down one or more of your core beliefs that you would like to change. Then try to spot some of the thinking errors in your core beliefs. Place a check mark beside the thinking errors that you believe may be involved in each core belief.

Core beliefs	All-or-nothing thinking	Jumping to conclusions	Ignoring the evidence	Magnifying or minimizing	Overgeneralizing	Personalizing

Putting Changes into Action

Have you ever heard the term "armchair philosopher"? This term is used to describe someone who has lots of ideas but doesn't put them into action. If you want to make changes in negative core beliefs that stick with you and will make a real difference in your life, you can't be just an armchair philosopher. You will need to try out the changes in real-life situations, learn from the experiences, make adjustments if needed, and get lots of practice in acting in ways that are consistent with your changed rules of thinking. The three most important words in making effective changes in maladaptive core beliefs are:

PRACTICE, PRACTICE, PRACTICE

To illustrate methods of practicing changes in real-life situations, we'll describe how Angelina worked on her belief "I must be in control."

Angelina came to realize that her core belief about control was causing a great deal of difficulty in her life and that change was needed. After doing some brainstorming, she chose these changes as her best options. Both of these statements seemed rational and acceptable to her.

1. I want to learn to be more accepting of things that I can't control or are hard to control.

2. I don't need to control everything in my life. I can make priorities and then work to be more effective and more efficient in the areas that I really want to control better (for example, exercise regularly, keep the house reasonably clean and in order, get my work done on time most of the time)

Next, Angelina needed to find ways to break out of the behavioral patterns that were driven by the old core belief (for example, seeking control "across the board," getting very tense and driven when she felt out of control, and procrastinating and then believing that her life was out of control). She used the worksheet on page 153 to plan some ways to practice putting her changed core belief into action.

?   **Does it seem challenging to think of ways to put changed core beliefs into action?**

Could it be difficult for you to take the steps to put changes into action?

If so, these tips and suggestions may help:

1. Try to select specific, practical, and reasonable steps that you can take.

2. If you are not ready to take an action, delay it until you build your confidence and skills.

3. The self-help methods you learned in Chapter 4 can help with putting changed core beliefs into action. For example, you could do a Thought Change Record to spot and modify any

negative automatic thoughts that may be interfering with progress. Or you could write out a coping card to assist you with putting your plans to work.

4. Take advantage of your strengths and your positive core beliefs in your action plans. You can review the strengths list that you developed in Chapter 4 and the list of positive core beliefs from this chapter to get ideas.

5. Several chapters in this book will teach you additional methods that you can apply to changing core beliefs. Examples include learning CBT methods to reduce procrastination (Chapter 5), acquiring skills for generating feelings of well-being (Chapter 7), and using mindfulness techniques (Chapter 13) to reduce tension and anxiety.

6. It can be highly beneficial to have a doctor or therapist guide you in changing core beliefs. If you are receiving professional treatment, you can share the exercises you are doing in this book with your doctor or therapist. If you are not working with a professional and are having difficulty making changes, it might be time to consider the option of starting therapy.

Try the exercise on page 154 to get some experience in taking action to make changed beliefs a solid and enduring part of your life. After you have read further in the book, you can come back to this exercise to add more detail or include other self-help methods in your plan. If you need additional copies of the worksheet, photocopy the form or go to the publisher's website (*www.guilford.com/breakingfreeforms*).

Tapping Your Strengths to Overcome Depression

One of the problems that we often see in our jobs as medical educators (JHW teaches psychiatry residents and practicing clinicians, and LWM teaches primary care physicians) is that doctors can fall into the trap of focusing only on their patient's illnesses or pathologies, instead of recognizing and fully utilizing patients' personal strengths in the recovery process. Patients also typically focus on their difficulties, not their positive experiences or potentials, when they come to appointments with their doctors.

There are many good reasons to pay attention to the positive side of your life when you are trying to work your way out of depression:

1. Adaptive core beliefs, such as the ones you identified in Exercises 6.1, 6.2, and 6.5, can counter negative core beliefs, enhance healthy self-esteem, and provide effective thinking rules for your path to wellness.

2. Other strengths, such as the ones you listed in Exercise 4.5, can be highlighted and drawn upon as you work toward overcoming depression. Later in the chapter, you'll see how Ted worked out a plan to use specific strengths such as his sense of humor, his volunteer work, and his ability to "remain calm in the eye of the storm" in his path to recovery.

Putting Changed Core Beliefs into Action: Angelina's Example

Instructions:

1. Write down a maladaptive core belief.

2. Record a changed version of this belief.

3. Then list at least two ways that you could practice behaving in a way that is consistent with the new belief and will help you make the changes stick. Be specific and plan some activities that you think you can actually carry out.

Maladaptive core belief:

I must be in control.

Changed belief:

I don't need to control everything in my life. I can make priorities and then work to be more effective and more efficient in the areas that I really want to control better.

Things I will do to put the changed belief into action:

1. *Identify at least three areas of my life where I can learn to greatly reduce my need for control and to accept that full control is not possible. Examples are (1) how my daughter does her homework, (2) how quickly my sister responds when we are planning family activities, (3) the productivity of coworkers who are doing projects with me.*

2. *Choose no more than three areas of my life that I believe could use more "healthy control." In this case, "healthy control" will mean that I am working in an organized and productive way. But I will not get down on myself if I am not achieving "perfect control." It will be fine if I have selected some targets and am working toward my goals.*

3. *The first target for "healthy control" will be to exercise for at least 30 minutes, three times a week.*

4. *I will keep a journal of my efforts to do 1, 2, and 3 above, will identify any problems that I have in taking these actions, and will brainstorm for solutions to make the plans work. I'll also discuss the plans and the results with my doctor.*

Putting Changed Core Beliefs into Action

Instructions:

1. Write down a maladaptive core belief.

2. Record a changed version of this belief.

3. Then list at least two ways that you could practice behaving in a way that is consistent with the new belief and will help you make the changes stick. Be specific and plan some activities that you think you can actually carry out.

Maladaptive core belief:

⬇

Changed belief:

⬇

Things I will do to put the changed belief into action:

1.

2.

3.

4.

5.

---

3. Striving for balanced thinking, in which you make an honest appraisal of the problems that confront you while you also take note of your adaptive life skills and your positive core beliefs, can help dispel the pessimism and hopelessness of depression.

4. Building up your use of adaptive core beliefs and other strengths can help you reverse the overwhelmed and helpless feelings that are so common in depression.

5. Engaging in activities or behaviors based on adaptive core beliefs and other personal strengths can lift your mood and help you experience positive emotions such as compassion, calmness, satisfaction, happiness, and a sense of well-being.

? **Are you wondering "How can I pay attention to my strengths and use them effectively when depression is sapping my energy and eroding my self-confidence?" "If I wasn't depressed, I wouldn't have so much of a problem using my strengths!"**

If you are having thoughts such as these, you are correct in concluding that depression often gets in the way of recognizing and using strengths.

Maybe if you waited until an antidepressant or some other treatment relieves symptoms, you could more easily get back on track to put your strengths to work in managing your problems. Yet if you want to use a multifaceted path to recovery, you can make some decisions now to channel your positive attributes in the direction of wellness.

Consider these suggestions:

1. At least review your list of strengths from Exercise 4.5 and your list of positive core beliefs in Exercise 6.5 as a reminder of your adaptive attributes and potentials.

2. As symptoms improve with the use of other treatments such as medications, CBT methods, exercise, or other approaches, take advantage of your strengths to escalate the rate of recovery. For example, increase your involvement in positive activities that play to your strengths.

3. Think of ways to employ your strengths as you learn about other paths to wellness in later chapters in this book. Perhaps a key relationship could help in your recovery plan. Or you might have spiritual beliefs that could give you hope and bolster your self-acceptance.

4. Learn from Ted's example described in the next section of this chapter and try to use the same type of strategies for harnessing the power of your own strengths and capacities.

Ted used the exercise on pages 156 and 157 to focus on some of his adaptive attributes that he thought might be especially useful in his efforts to get well.

As you read other chapters in this book, we hope that you'll be stimulated to think of many ways to use your positive core beliefs and other strengths. But we suspect you're at a point now where you can use the next worksheet to organize some plans to capitalize on your strengths to reduce symptoms and take positive steps toward wellness. To modify this plan, make photocopies of the worksheet or download the form from *www.guilford. com/breakingfreeforms*.

Summary

We all develop core beliefs through our lifetimes that help define our self-concept and provide rules to guide our actions. We all have a blend of adaptive and maladaptive core beliefs. But in depression the negative, maladaptive beliefs often gain momentum, and it may be difficult to remember positive core beliefs or put them to use. This chapter has focused on learning ways to change maladaptive core beliefs, or minimize their impact, and learning methods to identify and build up your positive core beliefs and other personal strengths. The strategies are drawn from CBT and are part of the thoughts–action path toward recovery from depression. The next chapter will help you go farther along the thoughts–action path as you learn ways to enrich your life with a sense of well-being.

Using My Strengths and Positive Core Beliefs to Fight Depression: Ted's Example

Instructions:

1. Review your list of personal strengths from Chapter 4 and your list of positive core beliefs from this chapter. Circle any entries that you think could be particularly helpful in working toward recovery from depression.

2. Next select three to five of these positives and sketch out some specific plans for using them.

3. Log examples of times you put these positives into action.

Strength or positive core belief	Ways I could use this positive to help me fight depression	Examples of times that I actually used this positive
I really love my family, and they love me. We have a close family.	Do more activities with my wife, kids, and parents, even if I don't have too much motivation to get out of my shell. Go to kids' ball games, have "date nights" with my wife, play cards with my parents, etc. Reach out to my parents and my brother and sister for support.	I have made an effort to do at least one activity with my children every day, go out with my wife once a week, and get together with parents once a week. I had coffee with my brother and talked about the stresses I am facing.

(cont.)

Using My Strengths and Positive Core Beliefs to Fight Depression (*cont.*)

Strength or positive core belief	Ways I could use this positive to help me fight depression	Examples of times that I actually used this positive
My volunteer work at the church has been a positive contribution that has always made me feel better in the past.	I could gradually resume some of this work. I need to be careful not to promise too much because they can expect a lot from me. And I might not be able to fully deliver until I am feeling better.	I helped cook for a church supper. I think that I will try to help out with a Spring Clean-up in the grounds outside the church. It is good for me to get back to being involved in these activities.
I usually can "remain calm in the eye of a storm" and stay clear-headed and focused even when trouble strikes.	Since I became depressed, I seem to have forgotten this belief. I tend to get rattled and think about the worst things that could happen. To resurrect and reinforce this belief, I'll write out a coping card for times at work when I am worrying about the low volume of sales. The card will remind me of this positive belief plus state some concrete steps I can take to stay on track to make the sales that are possible.	I did write out the coping card and I have it stored in my wallet. I look at it when I start to get tense about business problems. It helps me calm down and work effectively. I use it to remind myself that I actually do have lots of experience in staying the course through rough times.
I often have a good sense of humor.	This is another trait that seems to elude me when I am really down. But there is no question that humor can lighten my mood and help me cope. Some things that I could do are to rent a funny movie, read a humorous book, and especially try to laugh with my family and friends whenever I have the opportunity. Depression isn't humorous, but maybe some well-placed humor could relieve some of my depression.	I've watched two comedies and made a special effort not to watch really dark, violent, or disturbing films. I've tried to lighten up with my family and to search again for the humor in situations. They have commented that it is good to see me back to my "old self" and not being so tense and preoccupied with all of my worries.

**Using My Strengths and Positive Core Beliefs
to Fight Depression**

Instructions:

1. Review your list of personal strengths from Chapter 4 and your list of positive core beliefs from this chapter. Circle any of the entries that you think could be particularly helpful in working toward recovery from depression.

2. Next select three to five of these positives and sketch out some specific plans for using them.

3. Log examples of times you put these positives into action.

Strength or positive core belief	Ways I could use this positive to help me fight depression	Examples of times that I actually used this positive

7

Enhancing Well-Being

Chapter Highlights

⯈ What can well-being therapy add to CBT?

⯈ A well-being checkup

⯈ Monitoring well-being

⯈ Building and sustaining well-being

⯈ Acceptance as a path to well-being

⯈ The thoughts–action path in your plan for wellness

You've probably had times in your life that have been marked by a sense of well-being. But these times may have been shorter than you wished. Problems and concerns may have intruded to sap the good feelings, or days of depression may have left you largely devoid of feelings of well-being. Fortunately, methods have been developed to help people generate and hold on to a sense of well-being. You'll learn about these alternative methods for overcoming depression in this chapter.

Well-being therapy was developed in Italy by Dr. Giovanni Fava as a method of helping people who still had lingering symptoms of depression after antidepressant therapy, for those who may have rid themselves of a lot of the symptoms of depression but still lacked a sense of well-being, and for those who wanted to reduce the risk of relapse. Dr. Fava based his theories and techniques on a growing recognition in the field of psychology that the presence of well-being is as important to ongoing resilience and mental health as the absence of illness. Well-being therapy uses the general principles of CBT but adds a dimension that specifically enhances well-being. If you seem to be stuck in a rut of continued depression, dwell on the negative, and have difficulty appreciating the things around you, the methods of well-being therapy may offer excellent opportunities for change.

What Can Well-Being Therapy Add to CBT?

As discussed earlier in this book, CBT has been found to be highly effective in treating symptoms of depression. If standard CBT methods have completely relieved

> **DEFINITION: WHAT IS WELL-BEING?**
>
> - One level of well-being is the experience of positive emotions such as happiness, joy, tenderness, gratitude, satisfaction, compassion, and respect.
> - Well-being is much more than the pursuit of pleasure. People who have healthy states of well-being typically can accept themselves for both their strengths and weaknesses, show care and concern for others, and have a sense of direction or purpose in life.

depression for you, there may be no need to go further. Dr. Giovanni Fava and other researchers have, however, found that well-being therapy can be a valuable addition to CBT because it reduces vulnerability to future adversity that can continue to interfere with optimal functioning and leave you at risk of relapse. Besides using CBT techniques you've already learned, such as modifying negative automatic thoughts (Chapter 4) and activity scheduling (Chapter 5), well-being therapy uses exercises that stimulate people to recognize the feeling of well-being in their life and look for opportunities to promote it. Whereas CBT focuses primarily on relieving psychological distress (excessive self-criticism, low energy, inability to experience pleasure, etc.), well-being therapy focuses primarily on building positive emotional experiences.

Before moving ahead, we want to explain that a full course of well-being therapy with a professional therapist would likely use exercises similar to the ones in this chapter. It would also include in-depth experiences with enhancing a variety of dimensions of well-being such as self-reliance, personal growth, positive relations with others, and meaning and purpose in life. Our focus in this chapter is on introducing you to some of the most accessible and practical ways to increase and sustain feelings of well-being. You'll find individual aspects of well-being covered elsewhere in the book: building self-esteem and using your strengths in Chapter 6, improving relationships in Chapters 9 and 10, searching for meaning in Chapter 12, and experiencing the richness of life's moments in Chapter 13.

SCIENCE CORNER

- A study by Dr. Fava and his associates found that well-being therapy was effective for people who had not fully responded to previous treatment with antidepressants. Treatment led to a significant improvement in depression scores in addition to increased ratings of well-being and personal growth.

- A study of people who had experienced many previous relapses of depression found that a combination of CBT and well-being therapy was much more successful in preventing further relapses than standard clinical treatment (with no CBT). The relapse rate was more than 2 times higher for those who received standard treatment than for those who received the package of CBT and well-being therapy.

- Another study found that well-being therapy was effective for people who had initially responded to antidepressants but then had a return of symptoms.

A Well-Being Checkup

What is your current state of well-being? Do you participate in activities every day that seem to stimulate a sense of well-being? Can you look forward to events, people you will see, things you will do for others, or other involvements associated with positive emotions? Do you often think that your life has a good sense of direction and purpose? Let's do a brief well-being checkup, and then we'll show you some exercises from well-being therapy that might help you turn your life in a more positive direction.

We hope that Exercise 7.1 will show you that you already do have a sense of well-being about some of the things in your life and that it will stimulate some thoughts about how you might begin to search for ways to enhance those feelings. Later in the chapter we'll try to help you organize your efforts to promote well-being. But first we'll take a look at how Roberto's level of well-being seemed to be holding him back from full recovery from depression.

Roberto

When Roberto became depressed, he was in the middle of a downturn in his insurance business that had triggered a number of negative automatic thoughts such as "This new campaign is like everything else in my life—it's going nowhere. If I don't get something accomplished soon, the whole thing will fall apart. Everybody else is doing great, but I just mess everything up."

After starting CBT, Roberto experienced steady improvement. His score on the PHQ-9 (see Chapter 1) had dropped from 20 (top score is 27) to 8, but he hadn't yet achieved a full recovery (a score of 4 or less on the PHQ-9 is a typical target for recovery), and he frequently felt he wasn't in "top form." So his therapist introduced concepts from well-being therapy and suggested that Roberto do the Well-Being Checkup.

You'll probably notice that there are gaps between Roberto's rating of his well-being *now* and his *goals* for well-being in all of the areas in the exercise (see page 163). Also, the exercise demonstrates that he felt he clearly had greater levels of well-being earlier in his life. When Roberto began to think about the ratings and discussed them with his therapist, he started to see some opportunities for change. For example, he realized that he wasn't relating to his family and friends in a way that would build his sense of well-being to the optimal level. His depression had made him pull into himself and become

A Well-Being Checkup

Instructions: Rate your overall sense of well-being and your well-being in some key areas of life using 0–100 point scales (0 = no sense of well-being and 100 = maximum sense of well-being). Place an *N* on each scale to mark your sense of well-being *Now*. Place a *B* to mark the *Best* place on the scale you have been during your life. And then place a *G* on each scale to mark a realistic *Goal* for the sense of well-being that you would like to reach.

My overall sense of well-being:

| 0 | 10 | 20 | 30 | 40 | 50 | 60 | 70 | 80 | 90 | 100 |

My sense of well-being about my interests in life:

| 0 | 10 | 20 | 30 | 40 | 50 | 60 | 70 | 80 | 90 | 100 |

My sense of well-being about my relationships with others:

| 0 | 10 | 20 | 30 | 40 | 50 | 60 | 70 | 80 | 90 | 100 |

My sense of well-being about my purpose in life and/or spiritual activities:

| 0 | 10 | 20 | 30 | 40 | 50 | 60 | 70 | 80 | 90 | 100 |

My sense of well-being about my physical activities and health:

| 0 | 10 | 20 | 30 | 40 | 50 | 60 | 70 | 80 | 90 | 100 |

My sense of well-being about accepting myself and my life:

| 0 | 10 | 20 | 30 | 40 | 50 | 60 | 70 | 80 | 90 | 100 |

My sense of well-being about my personal growth:

| 0 | 10 | 20 | 30 | 40 | 50 | 60 | 70 | 80 | 90 | 100 |

Well-Being Checkup: Roberto's Example

My overall sense of well-being:

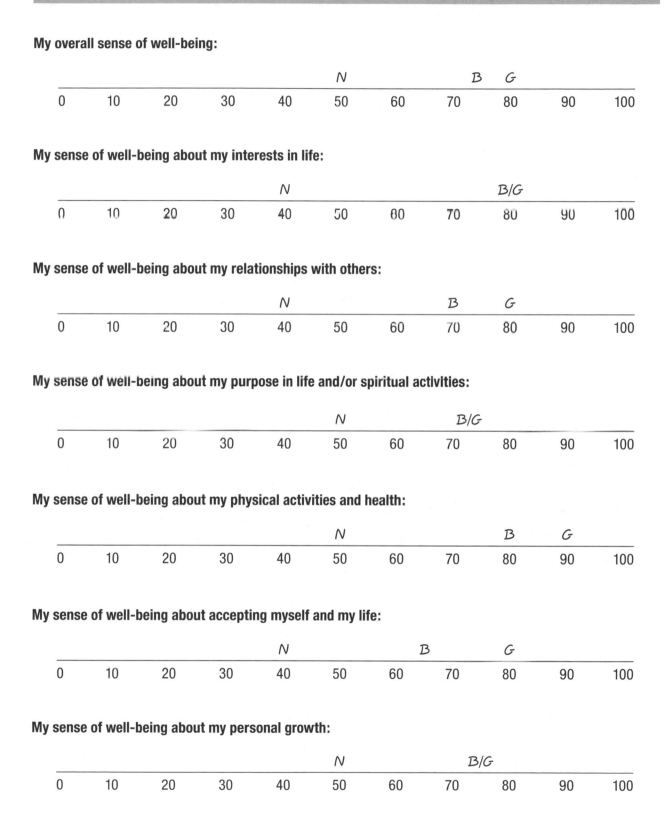

					N		B	G		
0	10	20	30	40	50	60	70	80	90	100

My sense of well-being about my interests in life:

			N			B/G		
0	10	20	30	40	50	60	70	80	90	100

My sense of well-being about my relationships with others:

				N		B	G			
0	10	20	30	40	50	60	70	80	90	100

My sense of well-being about my purpose in life and/or spiritual activities:

					N		B/G			
0	10	20	30	40	50	60	70	80	90	100

My sense of well-being about my physical activities and health:

					N		B	G		
0	10	20	30	40	50	60	70	80	90	100

My sense of well-being about accepting myself and my life:

				N		B	G			
0	10	20	30	40	50	60	70	80	90	100

My sense of well-being about my personal growth:

					N		B/G			
0	10	20	30	40	50	60	70	80	90	100

more self-absorbed (a common and understandable byproduct of depression) than he had been in the past. He hadn't been helping others out as much as usual. Maybe he was feeling better enough now to pay more attention to other people and to give more of a helping hand when needed. Also, he began to think that he wasn't tuning in as much as he might to the kind things that others were doing for him and to the richness of his important relationships.

If your own ratings in Exercise 7.1 showed a gap between your current level of well-being in your relationships and how you would like it to be, you can tap the ideas in Chapters 9 and 10 as part of your plan to enhance well-being. In a similar way, Chapters 4 and 6 can help you better accept yourself and your life circumstances while trying to find ways to stimulate well-being. Chapter 5 can help you look for activities that may uncover and strengthen positive emotions. Chapters 12 and 13 can help you open doors to layers of thinking and experience that many others have used to build a sense of purpose and well-being. And lessons from many of these chapters can be used in paths that lead to personal growth.

Monitoring Well-Being: How an Ancient Method Has Relevance in Today's World

The current methods of well-being therapy have their roots in the practices and writings of the Roman philosopher Seneca, who lived from 3 B.C. to A.D. 65. He realized that many potential experiences of well-being can go by unnoticed or underappreciated, especially when people are preoccupied with the concerns of everyday life. So he recommended that people keep a diary of instances of well-being. The diary served to draw people's attention to a full range of experiences, even those that were very small and seemingly unimportant, that could be associated with a sense of well-being. By attending to these cues for well-being and learning to hold on to them and savor them, people could develop a richer, more satisfying, and more meaningful life.

Roberto's therapist suggested that he start a well-being log and that he try to find three or more life experiences in the next week that gave him at least a small amount of well-being. He was instructed to look especially for things he might have missed if he wasn't paying attention—things that he might have ignored if he was thinking only of the tasks ahead or regrets from earlier days. As you can see, Roberto's log shows a number of very astute observations. Many of the entries relate directly to the gaps in well-being that were identified in Exercise 7.1.

To further explore how well-being logs can help with depression, try to answer the questions in Exercise 7.2.

We thought Roberto did a great job in his first attempt to complete a well-being log. The exercise seemed to help him draw attention to many everyday activities that could stimulate positive emotions. Even a routine shopping trip that ordinarily would have been unappealing to him turned out much better when his senses were directed at looking for

Roberto's Well-Being Log

Situation	Experiences and feelings of well-being	Intensity (0–100)
My daughter helped me do the dishes.	It was good to work shoulder-to-shoulder with her, even for a few minutes. She's a good kid. She didn't need to do that.	40
I shopped for a new pair of pants and a shirt. The clerk was very nice to me. He made a good suggestion.	Sometimes people go out of their way to be friendly. It must be hard to do that when you have to stand all day and meet all kinds ot customers.	30
I heard a song on the radio that was popular when I first started dating my wife.	I let the good feelings wash over me. I really love my wife. We have had so many good times together.	70
I was watching my daughter's softball game.	I am really fortunate to be able to sit here watching a healthy daughter who is having a great time	45
I was with a client and talking about his insurance needs. I wasn't trying to push things he doesn't need—just helping him make the decisions that are best for him.	My job isn't terrific, but I can actually help people. It is good to work with people in a straightforward, honest way.	40
I prepared a new recipe for a family dinner. It went over very well.	I'm often happier when I am in the kitchen and trying new things. It's especially nice when the family sits down to a meal and everybody seems to enjoy it. I really liked the tastes in the meal.	60

sources of well-being. However, the ratings were typically in the moderate range except for a few special moments with his family. And it's likely that there were plenty of other possibilities that he hadn't yet recognized for capturing a sense of well-being. Later in this chapter, we'll show you some ways that Roberto could benefit more from the well-being logging method. But first we suggest that you complete one of your own well-being logs (Exercise 7.3). To use it again in the future, photocopy the form or download it from *www.guilford.com/breakingfreeforms*.

EXERCISE 7.2	Reviewing Roberto's Well-Being Log

Instructions: Look over Roberto's log and use these questions to stimulate your thinking about how it could make a difference in your own life.

How do you think the well-being log may have helped Roberto move closer to the goals he set in his well-being checkup?

_____

_____

_____

List at least three instances in which Roberto may have paid special notice to things that previously could have been ignored or undervalued.

_____

_____

_____

What tips could you give Roberto for how he might learn from his experiences in completing this log as he searches for other opportunities to build well-being?

_____

_____

_____

List at least three ideas you have now for things you could do in your own life to promote a sense of well-being.

_____

_____

_____

Well-Being Log

Instructions: Check over the goals you set in Exercise 7.1. Then use this log to write down at least five instances in which you felt positive emotions associated with a state of well-being. Try to spot at least two little things that you may have ignored if you weren't paying attention to a full range of well-being experiences.

Situation	Experiences and feelings of well-being	Intensity (0–100)

> **?** **Are you having difficulty identifying events that stimulate a sense of well-being?**
>
> If so, you can try these things:
>
> • Review the exercises you completed in Chapter 5. Activity schedules can be used to plan events that generate feelings of well-being. The pleasant events checklist might give you some additional ideas for ways you could put a greater sense of well-being into your life.
>
> • Take a "time-out" from the concerns and burdens of the day. Allow yourself at least 15 minutes to engage in an activity that might be associated with positive emotions and feelings of well-being.
>
> • Give your senses of sight, hearing, smell, and/or taste full rein. Zone in on a life experience while attempting to fully appreciate it. For example, study the patterns of clouds, the feel of the air, and the sounds of nature as a thunderstorm approaches.
>
> • Look in unlikely places. Maybe it seems like your work is mostly drudgery, or you are thinking of ways to avoid an upcoming social event. Could there be a way to find some sense of well-being in activities such as these? Don't rule out areas of your life that seem to have little chance of providing feelings of well-being. The "tunnel vision" of depression may be interfering with your seeing opportunities for having well-being suffuse places where you may need it the most.
>
> • Get some help. Ask a trusted family member or friend to help you brainstorm ideas for enhancing your sense of well-being. Tell this person about well-being logs. Perhaps there could be some shared activities that would increase well-being for both of you.

Building and Sustaining Well-Being

Even if you were able to write down several experiences of well-being in the log in Exercise 7.3, you will probably find that states of well-being can be fleeting or may quickly wane as everyday concerns and worries crowd out positive emotions. Spotting and holding on to states of well-being may take practice—just like any other skill. So we recommend the ongoing, regular use of logs that help people maintain and amplify feelings of well-being.

One of the most common reasons for experiencing short-lived feelings of well-being is the tendency to have thoughts that steer us in a different direction. For example, Roberto was enjoying his daughter's softball game and trying to follow his therapist's instructions to savor a sense of well-being when he started to have interfering automatic thoughts: "I'm way behind on the work I brought home ... There's just too much to do ... I'm overwhelmed." After these thoughts ran through his head, his level of tension increased and his thinking drifted further away from the positive experience of watching his daughter's game. Soon his mind was churning as he expended large amounts of mental energy going through a list of clients whom he planned to call in the next few days. Before long, the feelings of well-being had completely dissipated.

Although we all have to devote considerable time and thought to work and other goal-related activities, a repeated tendency to interrupt even short periods of well-being with concerns and worries can steadily erode our ability to experience positive emotions. The balance can be shifted toward "all work and worry" from a healthier mixture of thinking—one that allocates adequate time to focus on tasks while leaving room to sustain positive emotions or to engage in behaviors that promote well-being.

After Roberto learned to complete the three-column log in Exercise 7.3, he began work with an expanded log that contains a column titled "Interfering Thoughts and/or Behaviors" and a column titled "Observer." The additional columns can have great value in helping people build feelings of well-being instead of letting them evaporate or drift away. His therapist explained that Roberto could write down any thoughts or activities that seemed to interrupt states of well-being and that he could use the "Observer" column to make suggestions to himself for maintaining well-being over longer periods of time or making the experiences stronger and more meaningful.

Building and Sustaining Well-Being: Roberto's Example

Event	Experiences and feelings of well-being	Interfering thoughts and/or behaviors	Observer
I was watching my daughter's softball game.	I am really fortunate to be able to sit here watching a healthy daughter who is having a great time.	"I'm way behind on the work I brought home ... There's just too much to do ... I'm overwhelmed." I start to worry about work and lots of other demands. I'm sitting in the stands, but I'm really not there. My mind is elsewhere.	Set aside time later tonight (8–9 P.M.) to make plans for contacting clients. Catch my extreme thinking (I'm overwhelmed). Tell myself that I can get the job done, and my daughter's softball game is not the best time to be doing work planning. Realize that these moments participating in my daughter's activities are "golden." Keep my mind tuned to watching all of the kids, the colors of the uniforms, their energy and vitality, and the excitement that they all feel.

Before doing your own exercise on building and sustaining well-being, some additional examples may help stir your creativity in constructing successful strategies for enhancing positive emotions.

Kate

Much like Roberto, Kate had been making good progress in reducing symptoms of depression with CBT methods. You may recall from Chapter 5 that activity schedules and the step-by-step approach gave her a real boost in overcoming her problems. As Kate moved toward full recovery, she learned methods from well-being therapy and began to apply them in daily life.

Before becoming depressed, Kate had sung with a community choir. But she hadn't been to any rehearsals and hadn't listened to the choir perform for more than 6 months. When a friend suggested that they attend one of the choir's concerts, Kate decided it was time to get out and enjoy hearing some choral music. She experienced some definite positive emotions but had to catch herself before the good feelings slipped away.

Building and Sustaining Well-Being: Kate's Example

Event	Experiences and feelings of well-being	Interfering thoughts and/or behaviors	Observer
I attended a concert of my old singing group.	It was great to see lots of people that I sang with in the past. They were in fine form. The music was thrilling. Tears came to my eyes, and they were good tears. I have loved singing with them.	I started to think "I've missed out on so much ... They all seem so happy, and I've been so miserable." Then my mind went back over all of the pain I've been through. I thought "Maybe I'll never get back to singing with them or doing other things that make life worthwhile ... maybe I'm just a loser."	Wait a minute, Kate. You've learned to spot negative thinking. Concentrate on the music. You know these pieces. Sing along with them in your mind. Feel the moods of the music and understand the message of the words. It's probably time to start singing with the group again. I'll listen to more choral music after going home to prolong the good feelings I had, and I'll call some of the people I know from the choir.

Angelina

You met Angelina when you were working on "Building Self-Esteem and Using Strengths" in Chapter 6. One of her core beliefs, "I must be in control," had been interfering with her experiencing feelings of well-being for many years. Because complete control was an elusive goal, she rarely felt satisfied or at ease. Instead she felt consistently tense and driven. When she began to use well-being therapy methods as an adjunct to CBT, she found that her perfectionistic and controlling habits often derailed attempts to feel positive emotions. However, she was able to coach herself on ways to change.

Ted

A final example of using a building and sustaining well-being log comes from the treatment of Ted, a man with depression whom you got to know in Chapters 4 and 6. Ted had made strides in modifying maladaptive core beliefs such as "All of the people in my

Building and Sustaining Well-Being: Angelina's Example

Event	Experiences and feelings of well-being	Interfering thoughts and/or behaviors	Observer
My daughter asked to talk with me about a problem she was having with her boyfriend.	It feels good that she can trust me and can open up about her problem. I treasure the close times I have with her.	I immediately want to fix the problem by telling her to drop the guy. I want to protect her and control things so everything works out perfectly in her life. Then I start thinking that she will go off to college soon. I'll really miss her. All kinds of bad things could happen to her.	Just cool It and let her talk about the problem. She wants a sounding board, not someone to rescue her from every stress in her life. Show that you understand and have compassion. It's a good thing that she wants to confront this problem. Do your best to experience all of the positives of having a "heart-to-heart" talk with your daughter. Make sure she knows that you are always there if she wants to talk. Realize that she's a strong person and she's ready to move on with life.

family have had job problems … I'm bound to fail," and he had been paying much more attention to using his considerable strengths such as his sense of humor and his ability to "remain calm in the eye of the storm." Now he was also trying to attend to experiences that could heighten his sense of well-being and help him grow as a person. One of his goals was to fully experience beautiful things in nature and to let these experiences breed feelings of contentment and satisfaction. His pattern had been to "blow off" these kinds of experiences because his mind always seemed to circle back to job concerns.

These examples show how Roberto, Kate, Angelina, and Ted were working to extract a greater sense of well-being from the ordinary experiences of everyday life. Each of them appeared to be making headway in capturing and holding on to positive emotions. But it isn't always so easy to generate feelings of well-being when you face lots of real-life problems and are being dragged down by depression. If you have lost your job, an attempt to promote well-being may seem to take energy away from the most important task—finding a new job. Or if you are in deep grief over the loss of a loved one or the breakup of a relationship, a well-being exercise could seem to be a meaningless path to take. However, even in the darkest hours, many people can find ways to experience some sense of well-being as a way of building resilience and coping with emotional pain.

If you are ready to go forward with well-being exercises, read the following Quick

Building and Sustaining Well-Being: Ted's Example

Event	Experiences and feelings of well-being	Interfering thoughts and/or behaviors	Observer
A cherry tree is in bloom in my yard.	Each of the thousands of blossoms is remarkable. They open pink and then turn to white. The effect against a blue sky is gorgeous. It is good to be alive.	I start to think of all of the projects that I have around the house that need to get done. Then I think about how the cherry trees only bloom for such a short while. I know I'm supposed to try to hang on to positive emotions, but I can't stand here forever.	Yes, you do have projects that need to be done, but it won't hurt to spend 5 or 10 minutes taking in this sight. Try to seal it in your memory so that you can bring it back to spark positive emotions when you need them. Take a photo and put it on the homepage of your computer. Use this experience to help train your senses to fully appreciate beautiful things.

Tips, then record your own building and sustaining well-being log. Photocopy the form to use it again or download it from *www.guilford.com/breakingfreeforms*.

QUICK TIPS
- If you haven't been used to searching for well-being experiences and trying to make them stick, it may take some time for you to build these capacities. So be patient and give the well-being exercises a chance to work.
- As shown in the illustrations from Roberto's, Kate's, Angelina's, and Ted's lives, well-being opportunities can often be found in the "little things" that are right in front of us if we only open our senses to experience them.
- For some people, an enduring increase in well-being can be associated with making a significant change (for example, starting and continuing a healthy relationship, becoming more involved in spiritual activities, learning something new, taking a different career path, volunteering to help others, exercising regularly and staying fit).
- However, don't be trapped by thinking you have to be a radically different person to have a deep sense of well-being. Try not to get discouraged if large changes seem to be difficult or impossible. For most people, any shift in attention that increases sensitivity to positive emotions and well-being experiences is well worth pursuing.

Although there is no set frequency for using a well-being log that works best for everybody, a general recommendation is to try to complete a log every evening for at least a week. Then you can review the logs to see what you have learned and make decisions about continuing to log well-being as part of your plan for overcoming depression.

Acceptance as a Path to Well-Being

Self-acceptance has been identified as a key feature of positive psychological functioning and well-being by Drs. Carol Ryff and Burton Singer and is a key feature of Fava's well-being therapy. The mindfulness methods from Eastern philosophical traditions (described in Chapter 13) that have been adapted by Dr. Mark Williams and associates for depression emphasize self-compassion as a part of a path to wellness. And a wave of research led by Dr. Steven Hayes has been focusing on the role of acceptance of life's twists and turns in promoting relief from a variety of mental health problems. The findings of these experts suggest that it may be very helpful to strive for increased acceptance as part of your efforts to enhance well-being and recover from depression.

To begin to understand the role of acceptance in reaching states of positive mental health, think for a moment about your answers to these questions:

1. Do you have regrets about how you have lived your life that repeatedly come back into your mind and stir up negative emotions?

Building and Sustaining Well-Being

Instructions: Use this log to record experiences of well-being. If something seems to interrupt the experience, write down the diverting thoughts or the behaviors that appeared to short-circuit the state of well-being. Then act as a thoughtful observer or coach. Write down ideas for holding on to or magnifying your feelings of well-being.

Event	Experiences and feelings of well-being	Interfering thoughts and/or behaviors	Observer

2. Do you have self-critical thoughts about perceived flaws, unmet goals, or missed opportunities? Do these thoughts interfere with your feeling positive emotions?
3. Do you have trouble accepting parts of yourself or your life that are less than ideal? Examples might be your height, physical attractiveness, athletic skill, job, marriage, childhood experiences, friends, or health.

Although we devote much of this book to methods that can help people change in positive directions and to achieve the goals they set for themselves, we also think that efforts to change must be balanced with self-compassion and acceptance. To illustrate this point, let's dig a little deeper into Ted's attempts to increase feelings of well-being. He is clearly making progress, but his mind often returns to thinking about the shame he felt when he was age 10 and 11 and his father's business was failing. He wants to do everything possible to avoid ever having to put his own children through this kind of trauma. So he has developed "workaholic" habits that far overcompensate for the problems of the past. And he dwells on any instance from his own past that raises even a little suspicion of failure.

All of the energy that Ted expends dealing with these parts of his life that he hasn't fully accepted take away from his ability to experience well-being in the here-and-now. Do you have any recommendations for Ted?

EXERCISE 7.5	**Helping Ted**

Instructions: Your role in this exercise is to be a good coach for Ted. Think of ways that he might work toward acceptance of his situation and thereby open doors to feeling more positive emotions.

What CBT methods outlined in Chapters 4 or 6 might Ted use to accept the problems of the past and stop dwelling on fears of failure?

_____

_____

_____

Write out a coping card (as explained in Chapter 4) for Ted that would help him accept the things he can't change and to stay focused on experiences of well-being.

Coping Strategy #1 _____

Coping Strategy #2 _____

Coping Strategy #3 _____

We hope you had some good ideas for Ted. From our perspective, it seemed like some of the evidence-based methods from CBT such as examining the evidence and searching for rational alternatives might help Ted gain self-acceptance. He had done previous work with these methods, but apparently not enough to put his thoughts about failure to rest. There are many coping strategies that he could use. Just a few might include reviewing a list of strengths, continuing to log well-being experiences to build up this skill while "nipping in the bud" any interfering thoughts about failure or past disappointments, and consciously telling himself to let the past go.

If you have some areas of your own life that could benefit from greater acceptance, take some time to complete Exercise 7.6.

The Thoughts–Action Path in Your Plan for Wellness

As you near the end of this chapter on well-being, you're close to completing all of the chapters from the thoughts–action path. In Chapter 4 you learned the core methods of CBT for changing negative thinking, in Chapter 5 you acquired skills for restoring energy and enjoying life, and in Chapter 6 you learned ways to build self-esteem and use your strengths. Before going ahead with the other paths to overcoming depression, we suggest you pause briefly to review what you've done and summarize some of the key steps you want to take in using the thoughts–action path. The last worksheet in this chapter should help you do this.

Before you complete the worksheet, we want to remind you of the value of using the PHQ-9 (introduced in Chapter 1) to check on your progress. If you've been working through this book for several days or weeks, this would be a good time to take the PHQ-9 again to see how you're coming along. We hope you're starting to see improvement in your symptoms and you're very encouraged about overcoming depression.

We'll show an example of a planning worksheet to give you some ideas for completing this exercise. But as you write your own plan, please remember that you don't have to do all of the things on your planning worksheet to get benefits from using the thoughts–action path. We don't want you to get down on yourself if you have difficulty putting any of the plans to work. Depression can make it hard to stay focused on making positive changes. If you have difficulties following your plans, give yourself credit for the actions you have taken and try to do some troubleshooting on ways to get the most from your plan. In the last chapter of the book, we'll offer some tips on creating a master plan for recovery from depression and giving the plan the best chance for success.

Now it's your turn to organize your ideas for using the thoughts–action path. To modify this part of your plan for recovery from depression, make photocopies of the worksheet or download it from *www.guilford.com/breakingfreeforms*.

Summary

This chapter centered on helping you cultivate and nurture feelings of well-being to help relieve depression. As an extension of the CBT methods described in Chapters 4 to 6,

Acceptance and Well-Being

Instructions: Try to identify one or more things about yourself or your life that would be difficult or impossible to change. Then write out a coping card with specific strategies that could increase acceptance and promote well-being.

Something about myself that I want to learn how to accept:

_____

_____

Coping strategies for increasing acceptance and well-being:

1. _____

2. _____

3. _____

4. _____

5. _____

Something that has happened to me that I want to learn how to accept:

_____

_____

Coping strategies for increasing acceptance and well-being:

1. _____

2. _____

3. _____

4. _____

5. _____

My Plan for Using the Thoughts–Action Path: Kate's Example

Thoughts–action methods	How much I believe that using this method(s) could benefit me (rate on 0–10 point scale where 0 = no benefit and 10 = maximum benefit)	My plan for using this method
Thought change records and related methods such as spotting automatic thoughts and cognitive errors, examining the evidence, and developing rational alternatives	9	I'll continue to complete at least one thought change record a week and keep practicing ways to change negative thinking. I'll keep a notebook with all of my thought records and similar exercises.
Coping cards	8	I'll store my coping cards in my notebook and review them at least once a week. I'll write out new coping cards whenever I think one might help me manage a situation.
Action prescriptions	5	When I'm feeling stuck, I can try to figure out an action prescription or talk with my doctor about writing down an action plan.
Activity schedules	7	The activity schedule really helped when I was more depressed than I am now and couldn't seem to get going. I can still use this method to fight procrastination and to plan how to use time effectively to enjoy life more. I'll try to check my activity schedule at least once every other week for the next month or so.
The step-by-step approach	7	This is another method that was really needed when I was deep into depression. I think I can use it when challenges arise—I probably wouldn't always need to write out the full step-by-step plan, but I could use the basic principles. When a big effort is needed, a written plan might be best.

(cont.)

My Plan for Using the Thoughts–Action Path (*cont.*)

Identifying and finding ways to use my strengths	9	*I haven't been fully recognizing or using my strengths. I'll keep a list of strengths, add to it as I can, and use the exercises from Chapter 6 to do more to put the strengths to work.*
Identifying and modifying core beliefs (schemas)	7	*My self-esteem is still pretty low. I need to work on finding some healthier core beliefs and really believing them. I'll review my list of adaptive core beliefs and design at least a couple of plans to practice using these beliefs.*
Keeping a well-being log and related methods for enhancing well-being	8	*Use a well-being log at least once a week for the next month. Work on ways to hold on to feelings of well-being. Practice the exercise on self-acceptance if I start dwelling on thoughts of being rejected and messing up relationships.*

well-being therapy can help you experience positive emotions, seek positive psychological health, and reduce the risk for return of symptoms. Because well-being is more than the simple pursuit of pleasure, you may find that working toward acceptance of yourself and others, strengthening relationships, and searching for meaning and purpose in life will add much to the methods described here. Chapters on interpersonal relationships, using spiritual strengths, and mindfulness later in this book contain strategies that can enhance your efforts to make a sense of well-being a more powerful force in your life.

The next path that we describe for breaking free from depression—the biology path—may seem to be based on a completely different set of theories and methods than the thoughts–action path covered in the last four chapters. However, research has shown that these paths (and the other paths detailed in this book) can complement one another in plans to relieve depression. For example, CBT works in part through biological pathways in the brain (see Chapter 3), while medications can reduce negative thinking and restore energy and interest. As we shift topics to describe methods for effectively using antidepressants, we suggest that you keep the lessons of the thoughts–action path in mind and continue to practice methods from this path that you have found helpful in fighting depression.

My Plan for Using the Thoughts–Action Path

Thoughts–action methods	How much I believe that using this method(s) could benefit me (rate on 0–10 point scale where 0 = no benefit and 10 = maximum benefit)	My plan for using this method
Thought change records and related methods such as spotting automatic thoughts and cognitive errors, examining the evidence, and developing rational alternatives		
Coping cards		
Action prescriptions		
Activity schedules		

(*cont.*)

Thoughts–action methods	How much I believe that using this method(s) could benefit me (rate on 0–10 point scale where 0 = no benefit and 10 = maximum benefit)	My plan for using this method
The step-by-step approach		
Identifying and finding ways to use my strengths		
Identifying and modifying core beliefs (schemas)		
Keeping a well-being log and related methods for enhancing well-being		

THE BIOLOGY PATH

8

Getting the Most from Antidepressants

Chapter Highlights

▶ How do antidepressants work?

▶ Understanding the options

▶ Choosing an antidepressant

▶ Talking with your doctor about antidepressants

▶ Dealing with side effects

▶ Maximizing chances for success

▶ What if your medication doesn't work?

▶ Biological treatments in my plan for wellness

If you've taken antidepressants or you're thinking of trying these medications, you may have some important questions. How do these drugs work? Which antidepressant might give you the best results? How can side effects be avoided or minimized? What can be done if medications don't fully relieve symptoms? This chapter is designed to help you work with your doctor to answer these questions. We'll start by looking at the evidence for effectiveness of antidepressants and exploring their potential role in your plan for wellness.

Could an Antidepressant Help?

A very large amount of research has been completed on antidepressants, but doctors are still trying to fully understand the results of all the studies. We'll try to unravel the find-

DEFINITIONS A *placebo* is a sugar pill or other nonactive substance.

A *clinical trial* is a study in which two or more similar groups of people are randomly assigned to receive different treatments. In some clinical trials people are given either a placebo or an active medication (such as an antidepressant) to see whether any improvement (for example, in depression scores) is actually due to the active medication.

A *meta-analysis* is a type of study that combines information from many clinical trials to get a more powerful idea of the true effect of a medication or other treatment. Some potential problems with meta-analyses can be whether all of the important investigations were included and whether the studies were well done.

ings for you. However, first you'll need to become familiar with a few terms.

Research on antidepressants has typically found them to be effective in reducing symptoms of depression. But there is some question about whether antidepressants are better than placebos for milder forms of depression. For example, medication has *not been shown to be superior to placebo* for a low-grade form of mood disorder called *minor depression* (defined in Chapter 1), and a meta-analysis (see Science Corner) suggested that the effects of antidepressants are strongest in people who suffer from severe depression.

SCIENCE CORNER
- A meta-analysis by Dr. Fournier and coworkers analyzed information from six clinical trials. The authors found that antidepressants were not superior to a placebo pill for minor to moderate depression. However, there was a substantial improvement in people with severe depression.
- It is important to note that people who receive placebo pills in research studies may also have a series of visits with an experienced doctor or clinician. The doctor visits may play a role in relieving depression in these studies.

Although antidepressants are not perfect treatments, many people find relief with medication. About 50 to 70% of people with depression have at least a 50% improvement when treated with one antidepressant. The response rate can be higher when one course of medication is followed by additional courses of different medications. Also, there is strong evidence that antidepressants, if taken continuously, decrease the risk of recurrence of depression. And research has shown that the combination of antidepressants plus CBT can be more effective than either treatment alone for severe depression. For these reasons, antidepressants are often a mainstay of successful treatment plans for people who have had multiple or severe episodes of depression. You can take the next quiz to find out if you might benefit from taking medication for depression.

EXERCISE 8.1	Quiz: Could You Benefit from Taking an Antidepressant?

Instructions: Circle "Yes" or "No" to answer each of the following questions. If you answered "Yes" to any, you might benefit from trying medication for depression. Please consult your doctor and keep reading for helpful tips on getting the most from antidepressants.

Do you suffer from moderate to severe depression (a score of > 10 on the PHQ-9 in Chapter 1)?	Yes/No
Have you had more than one episode of depression?	Yes/No
Have you ever had thoughts of suicide or harming yourself?*	Yes/No
Have you tried, but have had limited success with, other nonmedication treatments for depression?	Yes/No
Did you try depression medication in the past and observe some improvement in your depression?	Yes/No
If you have thoughts of hurting yourself or others, please call your doctor or get help immediately.	

From *Breaking Free from Depression.* Copyright 2012 by The Guilford Press.

How Do Antidepressants Work?

In Chapter 3 we briefly touched on how antidepressants work by increasing or enhancing the effect of certain neurotransmitters in the brain. Different types of antidepressants work on different neurotransmitters, such as serotonin, norepinephrine, and dopamine. In general, these neurotransmitters have antidepressant effects. Some also have antianxiety effects. Although there is still much we don't know about how antidepressants work, we do know that they increase the activity of neurotransmitters in the brain in a variety of ways (see the diagram on page 41 in Chapter 3 and the Science Corner here).

SCIENCE
CORNER
- Brain cells release *neurotransmitters* (NT), which are taken up by nearby cells, helping to make "connections" in important areas of the brain, such as centers for emotion. Smooth-functioning connections can promote a sense of well-being and keep us on an even keel.
- Brain cells can "reabsorb" NT for later use.
- One way that antidepressants work is by *reducing* the reabsorption (or reuptake) of NT by brain cells, causing more NT to be available for "connections" to nearby cells.

- Another way that antidepressants work is to normalize the sensitivity of nearby cells that become hypersensitive during states of depression.
- The overall effects of antidepressants are to restore functioning of neurotransmitters and related cellular activity in the brain to normal (nondepressed) functioning.

Understanding the Options

You may have heard of selective serotonin reuptake inhibitors (SSRIs), such as sertraline (Zoloft) and fluoxetine (Prozac), and serotonin/norepinephrine reuptake inhibitors (SNRIs), such as venlafaxine (Effexor). We'll give you the essentials for each of the groups (or classes) of antidepressants, including common drugs in each class, doses, side effects, and possible advantages and disadvantages of each group of antidepressants. After you read a brief section on each class of medications, you will find a table that summarizes and compares all of the key features of the antidepressants.

Selective Serotonin Reuptake Inhibitors

CAUTION If you are *pregnant or plan to become pregnant* while on antidepressants, please consult your doctor. Medication can be life-saving in severe depression during pregnancy, but the risks and benefits of medication should be considered. Paroxetine (Paxil) should *not be used* in pregnancy due to potentially serious birth defects such as congenital heart defects.

SSRIs (fluoxetine, sertraline, citalopram, escitalopram, paroxetine, fluvoxamine), which inhibit serotonin reuptake, are used for depression and several other mental health problems, such as obsessive–compulsive disorder (OCD), eating disorders, and anxiety. Immediate side effects may include stomach upset (nausea, diarrhea), restlessness or edginess, and trouble sleeping. A common long-term side effect is *sexual dysfunction* (which may include decreased libido, an inability to achieve orgasm in women, and delayed ejaculation in men). If you have side effects or limited improvement with one SSRI, you still might benefit from trying a different one.

Serotonin Norepinephrine Reuptake Inhibitors

The next class of antidepressants, SNRIs, has the added action of norepinephrine reuptake inhibition, which may help some people. Three SNRIs are currently available in the United States: venlafaxine (Effexor), desvenlafaxine (Pristiq), and duloxetine (Cymbalta). Duloxetine is also prescribed for diabetic neuropathy, chronic musculoskeletal pain, and fibromyalgia, but it should be avoided in people with liver disease or alcohol problems.

Duloxetine can cause liver damage in these situations. A common side effect is nausea, which tends to go away over time but may be worse at higher doses.

There is some evidence that venlafaxine may be more effective than some other antidepressants (see Science Corner on the next page), but it can cause high blood pressure and anxiety at higher doses in some people and can be difficult to stop abruptly (see section on discontinuation syndrome on page 203). In general, the SNRIs have similar side effects to the SSRIs because of their serotonin actions (so watch out for gastrointestinal upset early on and sexual dysfunction as a long-term side effect).

Serotonin Modulators

Three antidepressants act on serotonin a bit differently than the SSRIs. Vilazodone (Viibryd) and nefazodone (Serzone) have a variety of effects on serotonin receptors, while trazodone's exact mechanism of action on serotonin is unknown. Vilazodone is a newer antidepressant that has been reported to have a low rate of sexual side effects. Nefazodone is used infrequently because it has been associated with very rare but potentially fatal liver damage. Trazodone does not have the risk of liver failure but can infrequently cause low blood pressure, irregular heartbeat, or priapism (prolonged erection in men). One side effect of trazodone—sedation, or sleepiness—can make it a useful part of the treatment plan for people who have trouble sleeping.

Norepinephrine Serotonin Modulators

Mirtazapine (Remeron) acts on serotonin and antihistamine receptors and has sedating effects, as well as appetite-stimulating activity. Our experience shows that mirtazapine often works quickly, sometimes within one week, to improve sleep and problems with low appetite. A bonus is that mirtazapine causes minimal or no gastrointestinal upset and sexual dysfunction. One clinical trial found that mirtazapine may be more effective than some other antidepressants for moderate to severe depression. Common side effects, aside from weight gain and sedation, are dizziness, dry mouth, and constipation. People who are struggling with insomnia and weight loss from their depression, or who wish to avoid sexual side effects, might do very well with mirtazapine.

Norepinephrine Dopamine Reuptake Inhibitors

Bupropion (Wellbutrin) is a commonly prescribed antidepressant that acts on norepinephrine and dopamine. It is known for its activating (or energizing) properties and lack of sexual dysfunction or weight gain as side effects. You may have heard of bupropion (labeled as Zyban for this application) being used for smoking cessation. Bupropion should not be used in people with a history of seizures or those with active eating disorders, because it may increase the risk of seizures in people with these conditions. Common side effects (especially in the first few days) include nausea, decreased appetite, insomnia, headache, and anxiety. Bupropion might be an excellent choice in people who are overweight, are concerned about sexual side effects, are smokers, or are feeling fatigued or sleeping too much.

Older Antidepressants: Tricyclic Antidepressants and Monoamine Oxidase Inhibitors

Tricyclic antidepressants (TCAs), such as amitriptyline (Elavil) and nortriptyline (Pamelor), work by inhibiting reuptake of serotonin, norepinephrine, and (to a lesser degree) dopamine—effects that might seem great for depression. However, TCAs also affect other receptors, which can produce unpleasant side effects such as weight gain and sleepiness, dry mouth, constipation, blurry vision, and low blood pressure. Another concern is that TCAs can be fatal in overdoses. TCAs can cause a potentially dangerous irregularity in heartbeat and thus should be used with caution in the elderly and those with heart problems. Because of their sedative effects and potential for weight gain, these older antidepressants can be useful in people who have trouble sleeping or decreased appetite.

Monoamine oxidase inhibitors (MAOIs), such as tranylcypromine (Parnate) and phenelzine (Nardil), raise levels of norepinephrine and serotonin. MAOIs inhibit the enzyme that breaks down tyramine, a substance found in *aged cheese and certain other foods such as fava beans and soy sauce*. A buildup of too much tyramine can cause very high blood pressure that could lead to a stroke or heart attack. With a restricted diet, however, MAOIs can help people who have atypical depression (for example, those who sleep or eat too much) and people who have not responded to more conventional antidepressants. Great caution also is needed to avoid drug interactions. For example, MAOIs should not be taken at the same time as other antidepressants. A variety of other medications including certain cold and cough preparations also must be avoided. To manage safety concerns, MAOIs should be taken only under the close supervision of a doctor who is experienced in using this group of medications.

Choosing an Antidepressant

With so many antidepressants available, and each class having its strengths, benefits, and possible side effects, how do you and your doctor choose the medication that's right for you? In the past, studies showed that all antidepressant medications appeared to work equally well for depression. Antidepressant choice was then usually based on side effects and what may have worked well for you or a family member in the past. However, a 2009 study published in *Lancet* found that some antidepressants may be more effective (and well tolerated) than others.

SCIENCE CORNER Cipriani and colleagues performed a meta-analysis on 117 antidepressant clinical trials, including almost 26,000 patients—a very large and impressive research effort!

- They found that sertraline (Zoloft) *may be a preferred first-line medication* for moderate to severe depression.
  - Sertraline was more effective than duloxetine (Cymbalta), fluoxetine (Prozac), fluvoxamine (Luvox), and paroxetine (Paxil).

○ Sertraline was better tolerated than duloxetine and paroxetine. Escitalopram was also more tolerable than venlafaxine.

• Escitalpram (Lexapro), mirtazapine (Remeron), and venlafaxine (Effexor) were also found to be more effective than other antidepressants. However, the authors recommended sertraline as the first choice because escitalpram is more expensive (not available in generic form), and mirtazapine and venlafaxine may have more side effects in some people.

Although the Cipriani study noted in the Science Corner box showed that four antidepressants might be more effective than others, several words of caution are necessary:

• The study was so large that very small advantages were statistically significant (met scientific criteria for an advantage). A slight edge in a meta-analysis may not translate into "real-world" effectiveness.

• There are many individual differences in medication response and side effects. One medication may work beautifully for Ms. A but be ineffective for Mr. B, while Mr. B may respond nicely to a medication that didn't budge Ms. A's depression. So it's important to remember that you still have many options.

Studies show that treatment may be more successful if you and your doctor pick an antidepressant that has worked for you in the past. It's also important to remember that even if a medication did not work completely in the past, it may have a chance of working at a higher dose or in combination with another medication. Studies suggest that in some cases primary care doctors may be *undertreating* depression with doses of medication that are too low to make your depression go away completely. We'll talk more about dosing in the section on incomplete response.

Whether you have experience with taking medication for depression or not, we suggest you take a look at the table on pages 193–194 to get a sense of which medication may be right for you. We have included only the newer antidepressants in the table, but please remember that the older medications may be useful in certain circumstances. Some important things to consider when choosing a medication are dosing (is it taken once a day or twice?), side effects (are there any side effects that you could use to your advantage or that would be "deal breakers"?), and whether the medication is available in generic form (which may be more affordable). The following two examples might be helpful when looking at the table of antidepressants.

Mike

Mike is a 37-year-old auto mechanic who runs his own small repair shop. He was recently diagnosed with severe depression and, together with his doctor, decided that he would like to try medication. Aside from high blood pressure, Mike has no other medical problems and is not overweight. Since the depression set in, Mike has had trouble sleeping at night. He wakes up almost every night at 3 A.M., and his mind starts racing. He starts feeling down about a recent drop in business, and he cannot get back to sleep. He is in a long-term relationship with his partner, Julie. Although he hasn't been as active in the bedroom, he still enjoys sex and would like to avoid having sexual side effects from his medication.

Cecelia

Cecelia is a 43-year-old teacher who was recently diagnosed with a recurrence of moderate depression, triggered by the death of her sister from breast cancer. Cecelia has been sleeping until 10 or 11 A.M. on her days off (much longer than usual), but still feels fatigued much of the day. She has also noticed that she keeps "raiding the fridge" at night and has gained 5 pounds in the past few weeks. Cecelia used paroxetine in the past, which helped, but she experienced some weight gain with it and would like to try something else this time. She has been overweight for many years and says that she'll get more depressed if she gains more weight.

EXERCISE 8.2	Choosing an Antidepressant

After looking at some common antidepressants and their possible side effects in the table, can you pick out some antidepressants that Mike and Cecelia might choose with the help of their doctors?

	Antidepressant	Pros	Cons
Mike • Not sleeping • Wants to avoid sexual side effects			
Cecelia • Sleeping too much • Eating too much • Struggles with weight control			

From *Breaking Free from Depression*. Copyright 2012 by The Guilford Press.

Mike

Mike spoke with his doctor about his medication options and liked the idea that mirtazapine is usually helpful for sleep and has few sexual side effects. He also was interested to hear that mirtazapine was found to possibly be more effective than other antidepressants in a large meta-analysis. Because he was a fit guy, he and his doctor were not too concerned about potential weight gain. His doctor just encouraged him to continue exercising (which also can help with depression) and eating well. Mike's doctor gave him a prescription for 15 mg of mirtazapine each night and scheduled

Commonly Used Antidepressants

Medication	Side effects	Usual starting dose	Usual dose	Once daily?	Generic?
SSRIs	Stomach upset, sleep changes, restlessness, sexual side effects				
Citalopram (Celexa)	Arrhythmia at ≥ 60 mg	20 mg	20–40 mg	X	X
Escitalopram (Lexapro)		10 mg	10–20 mg	X	
Fluoxetine (Prozac)		20 mg	20–80 mg	X	X
Paroxetine (Paxil)		20 mg	20–50 mg	X	X
Sertraline (Zoloft)		50 mg	50–200 mg	X	X
SNRIs	Same as for SSRIs + specific side effects below				
Desvenlafaxine (Pristiq)	Similar to venlafaxine	50 mg	50–100 mg	X	
Duloxetine (Cymbalta)	Nausea (especially at higher doses)	30 mg	30–60 mg	X	
Venlafaxine ER* (Effexor XR)	High blood pressure and anxiety (at higher doses) and discontinuation syndrome	37.5 mg	75–225 mg	X	X
Serotonin modulators					
Vilazodone (Viibryd)	Diarrhea, nausea, vomiting, drowsiness, insomnia	10 mg	40 mg	X	
Nefazodone (Serzone)	Liver damage (rare), headache, drowsiness, dry mouth, nausea, heartburn	100 mg 2×/day	150–300 mg 2×/day		X
Trazodone (Desyrel)	Sedation, dry mouth, blurred vision, dizziness, sexual side effects	For depression: 50 mg 3×/day or 75 mg 2×/day For insomnia 25–50 mg at bedtime	For depression: 300–400 mg/day divided in two or three doses For insomnia: 50–150 mg at bedtime	X (for sleep)	X
Trazodone extended release (Oleptro)	Sedation, headaches, dry mouth, dizziness, nausea, sexual side effects	For depression: 150 mg at bedtime	For depression: up to 375 mg at bedtime	X	

(cont.)

Commonly Used Antidepressants (*cont.*)

Medication	Side effects	Usual starting dose	Usual dose	Once daily?	Generic?
Norepinephrine–serotonin modulators					
Mirtazapine (Remeron)	Sedation, weight gain	15 mg	15–45 mg	X	X
Norepinephrine–dopamine reuptake inhibitors					
Bupropion XL* (Wellbutrin XL)	Agitation, insomnia, decreased appetite	150 mg	150–450 mg	X	X

*Available in shorter-acting forms.

a follow-up visit for 2 weeks. Mike was asked to call his doctor if the medication seemed too sedating or had other side effects that gave him trouble.

How about Cecelia? Do any of the antidepressants in the table look like they might be worth a try?

Cecelia

When Cecelia went to see her doctor, she was at her wits' end. On top of feeling really depressed, she had gained weight and was very down about her appearance. She was nervous about trying medication again but was willing to give it a try. She and her doctor decided on bupropion because they thought it might help give her some extra energy and limit her food cravings at night. She was happy to hear that the medication was available in a generic, once-a-day form and started 150 mg XL every day in the morning. Her doctor advised her to increase the dose to 300 mg XL in the morning after 4 days if she was tolerating the medication well.

Take some time to jot down your thoughts about which medication might be the right match for you in the Exercises 8.3 and 8.4. You can take this worksheet with you to discuss options with your doctor.

Talking with Your Doctor about Antidepressants

Whether you're starting an antidepressant for the first time or have a lot of experience with taking medication for depression, communication with your doctor is often fundamental to success. It's important to let your doctor know if you're experiencing side effects, need refills, or your depression is getting worse (or better) on medication.

Your doctor might recommend frequent follow-up visits (for example, every 1–4 weeks) when starting a new medication, if your symptoms are severe, or if you are making any changes in the dose. Visits may be spaced out over time (for example, every 3

EXERCISE 8.3	Antidepressants That I Would Consider Trying		
Antidepressant	**Possible side effects**	**Expectations**	**Comments/questions**

months) if your depression is under good control, but you should expect to have periodic follow-ups in the doctor's office. Don't forget to take along (or ask for) a pen and paper to write down your questions and answers during your doctor's visit. After reading about choosing an antidepressant, can you think of some questions for your doctor?

In Exercise 8.4, check out the suggestions on the left and circle questions that you feel are important to you. Finally, list any additional questions you might have.

Most family doctors, internists, and nurse practitioners should have the medical knowledge to answer your questions and monitor your depression medication. Some primary care doctors prefer to consult a mental health professional for help with prescribing medication for depression and may refer you to a psychiatrist, a medical doctor especially trained in mental health.

EXERCISE 8.4	Questions for Your Doctor

Some suggestions	Questions for your doctor
• How does my medication work? • How often and when do I take my medication?	1.
• What side effects can I expect from my medication? • What do I do if I can't tolerate the side effects?	2.
• When should I expect the antidepressant to take full effect?	3.
• How long do I need to take the medication? • Are there any interactions with my other medications?	4.
	5.
	6.

? Who's who in depression treatment?

Primary care doctor or nurse practitioner

Your primary care physician (PCP) or Nurse Practitioner (NP) has the medical training to diagnose and treat depression, as well as other medical conditions. In Chapter 2, we reviewed how depression and medical illness can be linked. Your PCP can rule out some common medical causes that might masquerade as depression. PCPs and most NPs can prescribe medications and can manage your antidepressant therapy. In the following situations, your PCP might suggest that you see a psychiatrist to help with your depression treatment:

Possible reasons for referral to a psychiatrist:

1. Severe depression or depression with suicidal thinking.

2. Bipolar disorder (see Chapter 1 to review the symptoms of bipolar disorder).

3. Depression that is not helped by a trial(s) of medication.

4. Depression that requires multiple medications or additional treatments.

5. Interest in receiving psychotherapy.

Psychiatrist (MD)

Psychiatrists, medical doctors especially trained in mental health, are skilled in the diagnosis and treatment of all types of mental health conditions, including depression, anxiety, and bipolar disorder. In addition to prescribing and managing your medications, some psychiatrists offer talk therapy, such as CBT.

Psychologist (PhD)

Psychologists are mental health professionals who have received advanced training after college (graduate training). While psychologists cannot prescribe medications, they can provide talk therapy for depression and help guide your treatment plan.

Other mental health professionals

Many social workers, nurses, family therapists, pastoral counselors, and other health professionals are trained in mental health. Some may have certifications to provide certain types of talk therapy or group therapy. Feel free to ask providers about their credentials, background, or previous experience.

Dealing with Side Effects

Although you may experience side effects from your antidepressant medication, some people experience no side effects, and for many others the side effects are mild or go away shortly after beginning treatment. Check out some of the following strategies for managing both short-term and long-term side effects of antidepressant medications.

Short-Term Side Effects

Common side effects during initiation of treatment include nausea, stomach upset, restlessness, and insomnia. Fortunately, your body usually adjusts to the medication, and the side effects often lessen or go away within 2 weeks. One of the keys to success with antidepressant medications is knowing what side effects to expect and trying to find ways to ease them if you can. For instance, if you develop stomach upset, you might temporarily eat a bland diet without any spicy or hard-to-digest foods, take your medication with a piece of toast or crackers, or take your medication at night, right before you go to bed. You could also add an over-the-counter "stomach soother" like ranitidine (Zantac) for a few days.

If you can, try to stick with the medication for at least 4 weeks. By then, you should see some improvement in your depression, and you and your doctor can assess whether to continue, increase, or change your medicine depending on your response. But if the short-term side effects are intolerable, call your doctor to discuss the next steps. She may

CAUTION There is an FDA warning that antidepressants *may cause an increased risk of suicidal thinking* in adolescents and young adults.

- No link was found between antidepressants and actual completed suicides.
- There are no data to support an increased risk in suicidal thinking or completed suicide in adults who are middle-age or older.
- Remember, it is important to start antidepressants only under the supervision of a doctor.
- *Call your doctor or seek emergency care immediately if you feel suicidal at any point during your treatment for depression.*

suggest some additional techniques or medications to manage symptoms or try switching you to a different medication.

Long-Term Side Effects

Two long-term side effects—sexual dysfunction and insomnia—can become problems. We'll give some tips for dealing with these side effects. But first let's check in with Mike and Cecelia.

Mike

Mike has been taking mirtazapine for depression now for 2 months and has had great results. Although he has gained about 3 pounds, his slight frame could handle the extra weight. He continues to exercise, feels more energy at work, and has been sleeping well since starting the medication. Mike feels like the spark has come back in the bedroom, and his libido "is back" now that the depression is starting to lift.

Mike seems to be doing very well on mirtazapine, and he has avoided the sexual side effects (like decreased libido or delayed orgasm) commonly experienced with the SSRIs and SNRIs. These side effects can lead people to stop taking their medication (even if the depression is better). Although some people find that the benefits of taking medication outweigh the sexual side effects, others find that low sex drive or other difficulties have such a negative effect on their personal life that the side effects become intolerable over time.

? **What can you do if you have sexual side effects from your antidepressant?**

Talk to your doctor about the following options: *adding a medication, lowering your dose, or switching your medication.*

Adding a Medication

- Sildenafil (Viagra) or similar medications may help with orgasm problems due to antidepressants, even in women. But sildenafil is not FDA approved for this purpose.

Lowering Your Dose

- Your doctor may suggest lowering your dose of antidepressant. Although this has been shown to have limited benefit in studies, it may be worth a try.

Switching Your Medication

- This strategy is probably the *most likely to work*.

- You could try a medication known for its lack of sexual side effects (for example, bupropion or mirtazapine).

- Sometimes another medication in the same class as your current antidepressant (even SSRIs or SNRIs) might cause fewer sexual side effects.

Cecelia

Although Cecelia felt better on bupropion, she noticed that her sleep cycles had taken a complete 180-degree turn. Instead of sleeping too much, she found herself up at night for no reason. Her doctor had warned her about this possible side effect, and it was really starting to bother her. Cecelia thought about switching to a different medication, but she was very happy with the lack of weight gain with bupropion, and overall her mood had lifted. She was wondering what she could do to get her sleep back on track while staying on her medication.

We'll explain nondrug methods for improving sleep in Chapter 11. However, some medication options for treating insomnia are worth noting here. Similar to the strategies for managing sexual side effects, Cecelia could lower the dose of her medication or switch antidepressants (but as you recall, she would prefer to stay on her medication). If Cecelia did want to switch antidepressants, some choices commonly used for insomnia include mirtazapine, trazodone (Desryl), and the TCAs. Trazodone also can be used as an adjunct (or booster) to antidepressants to help with sleep.

Two other classes of medication used for insomnia include the hypnotics (zolpidem [Ambien], eszopiclone [Lunesta], zaleplon [Sonata], and ramelteon [Rozerem]) and benzodiazepines (such as temazepam [Restoril], flurazepam [Dalmane], lorazepam [Ativan], or clonazepam [Klonopin]). Most of the hypnotics and all of the benzodiazepines have the potential for dependency and should be used with caution (under the guidance of a physician).

Cecelia

Cecelia talked with her doctor about her options, and they decided to try adding trazodone to the bupropion. She found almost immediate relief for her insomnia but had to adjust a bit to the sedating effects of the trazodone (she learned to take it right before bedtime).

Maximizing Chances for Success

How can you get the most out of your depression medication? We've found that people have the best chance of success when they take their medication every day for the optimal length of time.

Taking Your Medication Every Day

It can be hard to remember to take medication each day, especially when you're feeling low from your depression. Some days you may feel like you can't even get out of bed, much less reach for the medicine bottle. So how do you stay motivated to take your medication each day? Here are some quick tips and a medication log to help you with taking your medication. You may want more than one copy of the log; photocopy the form or download it from *www.guilford.com/breakingfreeforms.*

QUICK TIPS   *TAKING YOUR MEDICATION EVERY DAY*

- Develop reminder systems that work for you:
  - Pill boxes
  - Cues (for example, always after brushing your teeth at bedtime)
  - Physical reminders (a sticker on the mirror, sticky note on your coffee maker, or ribbon on your keys)
- Keep a medication log like the one in Exercise 8.5 to help you track when you take your medication.
- If you have mixed feelings about taking medication, it might help to make a list of the positive reasons to give antidepressants a good try (see Exercise 8.6). Keeping these positive reasons in mind may help you stick with a daily regimen of medication for enough time to see if it works.

Does It Help to Have a Positive Attitude about Medication?

The attitudes that people have about their treatment can strongly influence results. For example, if someone is having thoughts such as "Taking an antidepressant means you're weak ... I should be able to do this on my own ... I'm always the one to get the side effects ... Nothing can help," the negative mind-set might interfere with taking the medication reliably and could undermine the chances of a good result. In contrast, a reasonably positive and hopeful view of the treatment may help a person take enough of the medication to allow it to work. Also, positive expectations could help take advantage of any good effects of medication, such as becoming more active and involved in life when energy improves.

We don't want you to sweep any questions or concerns about antidepressants "under the carpet." In fact, we have given you detailed information on possible risks of using

| EXERCISE 8.5 | **Medication Log** |

Instructions: Use this log to track your medication use over the next 4 weeks. Mark an *X* after you take your medication each day. Take note of which days on which it might be more difficult to remember (maybe Mondays or weekends are harder); use some of the Quick Tips to help keep you on track. If you take medication only once a day in the morning or evening, just use the part of the log that suits your medication schedule.

Medication(s): _____

Week	Monday	Tuesday	Wednesday	Thursday	Friday	Saturday	Sunday
1	A.M. P.M.	Λ.M. P.M.	A.M. P.M.	A.M. P.M.	A.M. P.M.	A.M. P.M.	A.M. P.M.
2	A.M. P.M.	A.M. P.M.	A.M. P.M.	A.M. P.M.	A.M. P.M.	A.M. P.M.	A.M. P.M.
3	A.M. P.M.	A.M. P.M.	A.M. P.M.	A.M. P.M.	A.M. P,M,	A.M. P,M.	A.M. P M
4	A.M. P.M.	A.M. P.M.	A.M. P.M.	A.M. P.M.	A.M. P.M.	A.M. P.M.	A.M. P.M.

these medications. However, we hope that you can keep the benefits of using antidepressants in mind if you decide to pursue this type of treatment for depression. One way to develop a positive attitude about medication is to use some of the CBT tools you learned in Chapter 4 to think as rationally as possible about the possible payoff for using medication in your path toward wellness.

Mike had a generally positive view of taking medication and what it might do for him, but he also had a few doubts. The worksheet that he completed seemed to keep him on target to take the medication consistently over the 9-month period that his doctor recommended for an adequate treatment course.

Exercise 8.6 could help you keep the positives in focus as you try to take an antidepressant daily.

Taking an Antidepressant for the Optimal Length of Time

Current studies say that if this is your first episode of depression, you should take antidepressants for a minimum of 6 months once the antidepressants take full effect. After that period, talk with your doctor about whether you should taper off your medication (with close follow-up, of course).

In people who have had previous episodes of depression (recurrent depression), studies suggest at least 12 months, and even long-term (years) of treatment may be needed. Why that long? Forty percent of people with depression will relapse after one episode of depression, and more than 70% of people who have had two episodes of depression

My List of Positive Reasons for Taking an Antidepressant: Mike's Example

1. *The medication helps me sleep.*

2. *The medication helps me get back to my old self.*

3. *I don't want to get depressed again.*

4. *My family really appreciates the improvement.*

5. *Taking a medication every day is a small price to pay for feeling well.*

EXERCISE 8.6

My List of Positive Reasons for Taking an Antidepressant

Instructions: Do some brainstorming to come up with reasons for taking an antidepressant and for taking the medication reliably for a full treatment course. Write down these reasons here.

Positive reasons to take an antidepressant:

1.

2.

3.

4.

5.

6.

7.

will relapse. Antidepressants, when taken continuously, are proven to reduce the risk of relapse in people who have recurrent depression.

Does this mean you have to take antidepressants forever? There is no simple answer to this question. The studies do suggest that discontinuing your medication increases the risk of relapse, so if your depression was severe or life-threatening, you and your doctor may decide that long-term medication is a good choice for you.

It can be frustrating to be on a medication for a long time. Yet people often take medications indefinitely for other problems such as hypertension, diabetes, or high cholesterol. Long-term medication use helps prevent potentially dangerous consequences of untreated chronic medical conditions. In the case of hypertension or high cholesterol, we are preventing heart attacks and strokes. In the case of depression, we are preventing future episodes of debilitating depression or even suicide.

Even though medication may be necessary for your health and well-being, sometimes filling the prescription can have a big impact on your psyche. It may make you feel older, or like someone who has been labeled as "ill." While taking medication may change the way you view yourself, we encourage you to challenge any negative thoughts you might be having. Try going back to the CBT techniques you learned in Chapters 4–6 to work on accepting the facts while still maintaining good self-esteem and hope for the future.

What If the Medication Doesn't Work?

There are many possible solutions when your medicine is not working, including increasing the dose, switching medication, adding another medicine (to boost the effects of the antidepressant), and using other non-medicine treatments. Before learning about these strategies, we need to talk about what happens when an antidepressant is stopped abruptly.

> **CAUTION** *Always* talk to your doctor before making changes to your medication.
>
> - Increasing or taking too much of a depression medication on your own can be dangerous.
> - Stopping a depression medication abruptly can also cause negative effects, such as a discontinuation reaction (see below).

Avoiding a Discontinuation Reaction

Stopping your medication suddenly may cause unpleasant symptoms called a "discontinuation reaction." This reaction does not mean you are addicted (in fact, antidepressant medications are not habit forming or addictive). With discontinuation syndrome, you may experience stomach upset, nausea, vomiting, fatigue, extreme anxiety or jitteriness, or worsening of depression. To avoid discontinuation syndrome, you should talk with your doctor about a slow reduction of your medication dose over several days or weeks. Or your doctor may discuss alternatives with you, such as switching antidepressants or adding a new medication.

Increasing the Dose

If you experience only a partial response to a medication or if you feel your medication isn't working as well as it did in the past, you might benefit from a dose increase. Everybody is different, and you may require a higher dose than the starting or usual dose of the medication. It can help to keep a record of medications and doses that do or don't work for you (you can use the worksheet in Exercise 8.7) so that you can show it to your doctor or refer to it in the future if needed. We are delighted when our patients bring such a record to their visits with us because it saves a great deal of time. We can quickly review the history of past attempts to treat depression with medication and then devote our energies to working on solutions. If you need additional copies of the form, photocopy it or download it from *www.guilford.com/breakingfreeforms*.

Switching Antidepressants: The Basics

There are several reasons to switch medication. First, you might experience too many side effects from the first medication you try. You could also have little or no response to a medication, even at the maximum dose. Sometimes medication that has worked for a while seems to lose its "oomph" or effectiveness. If these scenarios sound familiar, it may be time to switch medications.

SCIENCE CORNER

- Research suggests that if a first antidepressant is unsuccessful at treating depression, switching antidepressants may help.
- The *STAR*D* clinical trial, one of the largest and most influential research studies ever completed on the treatment of depression, found that only 37% of people with depression had a full remission on their first antidepressant, but 19% more got completely better when they tried a different, second medication. And even more people had full relief with additional antidepressants or combinations of medications. In all, 67% of people in the trial had a full remission on antidepressants.

Switching medications should occur only under the supervision of a doctor, because there can be some potentially dangerous side effects if you overlap certain medications. "Serotonin syndrome" is uncommon, but can occur when two medicines that strongly affect serotonin are taken together. This is a syndrome that consists of sweating, fast heart rate, diarrhea, and stomach upset. Potentially dangerous symptoms can occur when certain depression medications such as SSRIs and some of the older antidepressants, such as MAOIs, are mixed together. Other medicines are safe to switch from one day to the next, so be sure to check with your doctor about the best way to switch medications.

Let's take the example of Tabitha, who was taking venlafaxine (Effexor XR), an SNRI. Although she had some success with the medication (including more interest in

| EXERCISE 8.7 | | | | Record of Antidepressants | |

Instructions: Use this worksheet to record the antidepressants that you have tried. Rate the effectiveness and note any side effects.

Antidepressant	Dose	Length of treatment	Effectiveness rate 0–10 (10 = best response)	Side effects	Comments

things she used to enjoy), Tabitha was unhappy with the side effects of stomach upset and nausea. After discussing her concerns with her doctor, they decided to switch to bupropion XL (Wellbutrin XL), a norepinephrine and dopamine reuptake inhibitor. Because of the possibility of a discontinuation reaction with the switch from venlafaxine, her doctor suggested she cross-taper the medications.

Tabitha successfully switched medications and had better success with bupropion.

> **DEFINITION** Cross-tapering is a method of switching medication where the current medication is decreased gradually while a new medication is introduced slowly. A cross-taper with antidepressant medications can help prevent discontinuation reactions.

She eventually achieved complete remission from depression after a further dose increase of bupropion XL to 450 mg per day.

Beating Treatment Resistance: The Benefits of Augmentation

If you and your doctor have maximized the dose of your medication, but you still have not achieved full remission from depression, you might be experiencing "treatment resistance." Treatment resistance occurs when traditional antidepressant treatment (such as one of the SSRIs or SNRIs at a maximum dose) is unsuccessful. At this point you might consider adding another medication or treatment to your regimen to boost the effects of the antidepressant. Another word for this strategy is *augmentation*.

SCIENCE CORNER
- Studies have shown that 20–35% of people with depression experience persistent treatment resistance and develop chronic depression.
- Augmentation strategies have been researched extensively and offer much hope for resolving depression.

Treatment Augmentation with Medication

Several medications may be beneficial in combination with standard antidepressants. A commonly used strategy is to add another antidepressant to the current medication. Any

Tabitha's Cross-Taper between Venlafaxine and Bupropion XL

	Venlafaxine Tabitha's current dose: 150 mg XL once daily	**Bupropion XL** Goal dose: 300 mg XL once daily
Week 1	Decrease venlafaxine to 112.5 mg XL once daily	Start bupropion XL, 150 mg once daily
Week 2	Decrease further to 75 mg XL once daily	Start bupropion XL 300 mg once daily
Week 3	Decrease further to 37.5 mg XL once daily	Continue bupropion XL 300 mg once daily
Week 4	Stop venlafaxine	Continue bupropion XL 300 mg once daily

of the other antidepressants can be considered, but doctors often choose an antidepressant from a different class. For example, if you didn't have full relief from an SSRI, such as escitalopram (Lexapro), your doctor might suggest adding bupropion (Wellbutrin), venlafaxine (Effexor), mirtazapine (Remeron), or even a TCA.

Mood stabilizers such as lithium and newer antipsychotic medications (in this case used for depression instead of psychosis) such as aripiprazole (Abilify) are also used to augment traditional antidepressant therapy. These medications can be quite useful for treatment-resistant depression but should be supervised closely by a skilled physician because they have potentially serious side effects. Other options that are sometimes used include buspirone (Buspar), a nonaddictive antianxiety drug, and thyroid hormone (even if thyroid levels are normal). The use of thyroid hormone requires close medical monitoring, as do all of the augmentation methods.

QUICK Don't forget to see your PCP or psychiatrist to rule out any medical conditions
TIP   that might lead to treatment resistance, such as:

- Vitamin deficiency
- Hypothyroidism (underactive thyroid)
- Anemia

Adding Nonmedicine Treatments: A Combined Approach

As discussed in Chapter 3, antidepressant therapy can be augmented with psychotherapy, or talk therapy, with a trained therapist or counselor. In fact, for moderate to severe depression, combined medication and psychotherapy may be the evidence-based treatment of choice. Examples of other methods that could be added include CBT (detailed in Chapters 4 to 6), well-being therapy (described in Chapter 7), and making healthy lifestyle changes (see Chapter 11). Some illustrations of lifestyle changes that can help with depression are exercise and improving sleep habits.

Electroconvulsive Therapy

Electroconvulsive therapy (ECT), which takes place under the direct supervision of a psychiatrist and anesthesiologist, entails receiving small bursts of electrical energy to the brain under sedation. Although ECT has been depicted negatively in some movies and television shows, it has been tested extensively and has been found to be an effective treatment for depression. Because ECT requires anesthesia and can be associated with side effects such as headache and temporary memory loss, it is usually reserved for situations where other treatments haven't worked and symptoms are quite severe. A full medical evaluation is required before ECT to determine whether there are any physical problems that would increase the risk of this treatment or indicate that it should not be given.

Transcranial Magnetic Stimulation

Transcranial Magnetic Stimulation (TMS), a newer brain stimulation treatment, has been approved by the U.S. Food and Drug Administration (FDA) for use in persons who have failed to respond to antidepressant medication. Treatment with TMS involves having strong magnets (about the same strength as a magnetic resonance imaging test) placed on the brain to stimulate the areas that are thought to be abnormal in depression (see Chapter 3 for a figure depicting the anatomy of brain centers that have been associated with depression). Compared to ECT, the TMS method offers advantages in not requiring anesthesia and not affecting memory. Typical side effects are a tingling or mildly painful sensation in the scalp. TMS is available only at a limited number of specialty centers.

Alternative Medicine: Using Over-the-Counter Drugs to Treat Depression

You may have heard of St. John's wort, an herbal agent used for depression. It is thought to effect serotonin in a way similar to the SSRIs, but it is available over the counter in the vitamin or herbal section of pharmacies or groceries. Some people may feel that it provides a "natural" approach to treating depression. Although studies have been mixed, the consensus among researchers is that St. John's wort is not a reliably effective treatment for depression.

If you choose to try St. John's wort as an alternative treatment, please keep in mind that herbal remedies are not regulated by the FDA, and the dosage and content of different brands may not be standardized. You may find that St. John's wort has similar side effects to the SSRIs because of its serotonin effects and may have drug interactions with other medications. Women who are on oral contraception should also use backup birth control methods, because St. John's wort decreases the effectiveness of birth-control pills.

S-adenasyl methionine (SAMe) is an over-the-counter drug that is involved in the production of serotonin, norepinephrine, and dopamine. A meta-analysis found evidence that SAMe reduced depressive symptoms more than placebos, but research on SAMe has not been as rigorous or extensive as investigations into antidepressants and CBT. One research study by Dr. Papakostas and associates found that SAMe was a useful booster to standard antidepressants for treatment-resistant depression. However, these investigators concluded that there had not been enough studies to come to firm conclusions on the effectiveness and tolerability of SAMe as a stand-alone therapy.

Biological Treatments in My Plan for Wellness

In Chapter 3, you completed an exercise where you measured your level of interest in using biologically based treatments such as antidepressants in your plan for recovery. Has your interest level changed after reading this chapter? Have you developed some good ideas for using medication that you could discuss with your doctor? Before moving on with some of the other chapters, it might help to pause to organize some of your thoughts about using biological treatments to help overcome depression. Should your plan change, you'll need additional copies of the form in Exercise 8.8. Photocopy it or download it from *www.guilford.com/breakingfreeforms*.

Summary

In this chapter, we explored the principles of choosing an antidepressant, dealing with side effects, and managing treatment resistance. We hope you've gained useful tools to help you get the most from biologically oriented treatments. Remember that medication is only one option in a larger "toolbox" for relieving depressive symptoms. You've already learned about CBT and well-being therapy in Chapters 4–7, and you'll have the opportunity to explore other paths to recovery as you move ahead in breaking free from depression.

Biological Treatments in My Plan for Wellness

Instructions: Use this worksheet to record your ideas and plans for using biologically based treatments for depression. If a question does not fit your situation, skip over it and go to another question.

If you want to start an antidepressant, which choices would you like to discuss with your doctor? Are there any antidepressants that appeal to you more than others?

_____

_____

If you are currently taking an antidepressant that is effective and is well tolerated, how long do you plan to continue on this medication? What advice, if any, has your doctor given you about the length of treatment?

_____

_____

If you are currently taking an antidepressant and are having significant side effects, what ideas do you have to discuss with your doctor about reducing or coping with these side effects?

_____

_____

If you are currently taking an antidepressant, but have not had a full remission (symptoms have gone away), what options for increasing the chances of recovery would you like to discuss with your doctor?

_____

_____

If you have not had full relief from antidepressants, are there any other biologically based treatments that you would like to consider using?

_____

_____

THE RELATIONSHIP PATH

9

The People in Your Life
How Relationships Can Influence Recovery from Depression

Chapter Highlights

‣ Relationships and depression

‣ The relationship–depression cycle

‣ A relationship checkup

‣ Gaining strength from relationships

When people think about the most important things in their lives, their relationships with loved ones often stand at the top of the list. In good times and bad, our relationships can strengthen us or trouble us—take us to some of the heights of human experience or dash our hopes and dreams. In this chapter, we'll help you understand the association between relationships and depression and find ways to draw power from the positive relationships in your life. In the following chapter you'll learn about ways to cope with the problems that depression can bring to relationships, and we'll offer some strategies for managing relationship difficulties such as losses or conflicts as you work on overcoming depression.

Relationships and Depression

Research has found that interpersonal problems such as separations or divorces, conflicts with loved ones, or the death of someone close to you are very common triggers of depression. Yet people who have solid and sustaining relationships can draw on these strengths as they move from depression to wellness.

Knowledge of the close link between relationships and depression has led to the development of effective talk therapy methods to relieve depressive symptoms. For example, Drs. Gerald Klerman and Myrna Weissman pioneered the use of interpersonal psychotherapy (IPT), a specific form of psychotherapy for depression that focuses on helping people manage relationship problems. Other researchers have shown the benefits of marital and family therapy for depression. Also, CBT—an evidence-based treatment detailed in Chapters 4–6—includes methods that help people cope with relationship difficulties, enhance communication skills, and strengthen their bonds with others.

SCIENCE CORNER IPT has been shown to be an effective treatment for depression. A meta-analysis performed by Dr. Marcello de Mello and associates found that interpersonal psychotherapy (IPT) was consistently superior to placebos in treating depression in research studies.

The Relationship–Depression Cycle

There are two major ways that relationships and depression can intertwine in a downward spiral of deepening distress. One way is for a relationship difficulty, such as a breakup, an overly critical and unforgiving partner, or the death of a loved one, to set off a depression. Then the symptoms of depression can take over, and the sufferer draws inward. Before long, a vicious cycle of withdrawal from relationships and worsening depression takes the person down further. This happened to Kate, the woman with depression that you met in the first chapters of this book. Kate became depressed after a relationship with a long-term boyfriend ended. Soon she was spending most of the time after work alone in her apartment. She dropped out of most of her social activities and didn't accept her friends' invitations to go out. Kate also seemed to grow more distant from her mother and sister—two people who really cared about her. As Kate became more socially isolated, her depression intensified, and she was even less inclined to connect with others.

Another way that relationships and depression can have negative effects on one another is when a key relationship is basically strong but depression puts stress on this relationship. Mark couldn't quite figure out what was happening in his life, but he did know that his relationships with his wife and children were getting more and more strained. When he came home from a pressured day at work, the home scene often seemed to make things worse.

Mark's Story

Mark, in his early 40s, works as a manager at a cable TV company, where he is responsible for scheduling and carrying out maintenance of cable lines serving thousands of homes. He often has days when he feels overloaded and stretched to his capacity to "put out all the fires." In the last 3 to 4 months, he's noticed the return of depression that has plagued him off and on since his high school days. The depression had seemed to be in good control for a long time, but for unclear reasons it had edged its way back into his life. Maybe it was increased responsibility at work—he had had to take on supervision of cable service for another region of the city after a budget reduction and some layoffs. Or maybe it was because he was arguing more with his wife, Alice. But he knew that he didn't feel right, and something needed to be done about it.

He and Alice had been married for 15 years. They had been happy in the marriage most of the time, usually had a good sex life, and considered themselves "best friends." They had always been faithful to each other. They usually enjoyed doing things together with their kids, going to concerts, and taking hikes with their dogs on the weekends. Their two children, Abby and Luke, were 13 and 9. Both were doing well in school and had never had behavioral problems.

When Mark and Alice were dating and early in their marriage, they had played in a band together. Alice was the lead vocalist and guitarist. Mark played keyboard and also did some singing. Their band had some local gigs, but never "hit it big." Still, they had a good time being part of the group.

As they got older, the responsibilities of daily work and taking care of their two children didn't leave much room for their music. The band eventually broke up as people moved on. Alice continued to sing occasionally as a guest for several bands, but Mark seemed to have time to get the keyboard out at home only on rare occasions.

From what we have heard so far, it sounds like Mark has basically satisfying and stable family relationships. If you have had serious problems in your relationships, you may be wondering how Mark's relationships could possibly be a significant part of his depression.

Unlike Kate, who became depressed after a specific relationship event, Mark's problems had come on gradually and developed primarily due to the negative effects of depression on his relationships. Mark had experienced depression twice before—once when he was in high school before he met Alice and once in his early 30s when he had lost a job. Because he had recurrent depression, the biological factors that you learned about in Chapters 3 and 8 could have had a lot to do with the return of symptoms. Mark had decided to stop taking antidepressants about a year ago because he had been feeling well for so long. As we noted in Chapter 8, the risk for relapse in people with recurrent depression can be reduced by long-term use of antidepressants.

Mark's work stress and the demands of balancing a career and family also may have played a role in bringing the depression back into his life. But he and Alice and the kids had been getting along well before he had become depressed again.

As depression crept back into his life, Mark lost much of his usual energy and vitality. He began to start his days feeling flat instead of invigorated. It was all he could do to get his work done, let alone help out much around the house. So when he came home, he preferred to collapse in a favorite chair and be by himself instead of doing anything with Alice or the kids. He and Alice had usually shared the chores. A long-standing agreement had Alice paying the bills and doing most of the cooking and Mark doing most of the laundry and house maintenance. Now he was more irritable than happy, more withdrawn than engaging, and clearly less involved in carrying out his usual responsibilities around the house.

Alice had seen him depressed before, but she wasn't handling this depression so well. Mark's irritability and withdrawal stirred up her thoughts that it was unfair to have to go through these troubles. She had enough on her plate, with her own job managing a small retail store, helping out her mother who had rheumatoid arthritis, and what she called "a mountain" of responsibility supporting their children in after-school activities, without having to "cover" for Mark when he wasn't feeling well. And the lack of interest in sex that had come with the depression was really frustrating her. Although she knew better, she seemed to be criticizing Mark more. There were still moments of kindness and tenderness, but there was much more tension in their relationship than in the days when Mark had not been depressed.

Mark's story is a common one. It illustrates that depression can twist its way into healthy relationships and create problems that weren't there before. Then the strain in the relationship can further aggravate the depression, and it can be difficult to draw the social supports from these relationships that may be needed to foster recovery. Fortunately, there are many things that can be done to reverse this vicious cycle. We'll show you how Mark found ways to do this, but first we ask you to do a relationship checkup. Before figuring out a plan for using healthy coping strategies with the people in your life, it can help to survey the current state of your relationships.

A Relationship Checkup

In this exercise we'll ask you to make some notes about relationships that are positive forces in your life now, have been at some time in the past, or could be in the future; and about relationships that are troubling or stressing you. Try to use the brainstorming methods that you practiced in earlier chapters to open your mind up to the possibilities. Could reconnecting with some of the people in your life be a good step to take? Could you have become discouraged about a relationship problem and pulled away from a person who could become important to you again? Is there a relationship difficulty that you could address in your plan for recovery from depression? To give you some ideas, we'll take a look at two examples of relationship checkups.

Have you been thinking of your answers to these questions? Doing this next exercise should help you target some relationships that could help you in overcoming depression or may need attention as you build a plan for recovery.

Gaining Strength from Relationships

Just making a list of your some of your important relationships and answering the questions in Exercise 9.1 can give you a good start on identifying positive people in your life and recognizing how your relationships with them might give you a lift in fighting

A Relationship Checkup: Kate's Example

Instructions: Try to identify at least four family members or friends who are especially important in your life. Also, identify some other relationships with people such as coworkers, classmates, or casual acquaintances that may affect you. Then list some of the helpful or troubling features of these relationships. Finally, note any relationship that has ended that may still be causing distress.

1. **Who are the key people in your life?**

   My mother and sister. My friends Tricia, Frank, and Joanie.

2. **What are the positive things about these relationships?**

   They all have stuck with me, even though I have been so depressed I haven't paid much attention to them. They all want to help me get back into life. My sister has been especially kind. She calls almost every day and tries to set up activities for us to do together.

3. **What are the stressful or negative things about these relationships?**

   My mother always wanted me to do my best and pushed me pretty hard. I'm sure that she is disappointed because I haven't married and had children. She talks about all of the grandchildren her friends have. I can get angry at her and say things I regret later. Tricia seems to have such a wonderful life with her husband that sometimes I feel intimidated. It is hard to be around her and her husband when I'm depressed and feel down on myself.

4. **Who are some other people in your life (for example, coworkers, friends, or casual acquaintances) who may do things that affect how you feel? Try to list at least 3 of these people.**

   My boss, Samantha. Alex, the choir director. My yoga instructor. The condo superintendent.

5. **What are the positive things about these relationships?**

   Samantha has looked out for me when I've been struggling at work. She seems to understand what I'm going through. She has made good suggestions for ways for me to handle projects. Alex can be inspirational. He makes everybody feel better when they get involved with the music, and he goes out of his way to have parties and other social things with the choir that bring us together. My yoga instructor is very gentle and thoughtful. She takes an interest in everybody in the class. I can't say much positive about the condo super. He always seems angry, and you almost have to beg him to get anything done.

6. **What are the stressful or negative things about these relationships?**

   Both Samantha and I can get tense and irritable at times. Sometimes I wonder if she is upset with me and isn't telling me what she actually thinks. The condo super's attitude grates on me.

7. **What past relationships (for example, with partnerships or romances that have ended or with significant people who have died), if any, may still be troubling you or causing emotional pain? Briefly describe the difficulty you still have with the impact of this relationship on your life.**

   The breakup with Nick was really hard on me and still gets me down. I wanted to marry him, and he found somebody else. I feel like I'm always rejected, so I've given up trying.

A Relationship Checkup: Mark's Example

1. **Who are the key people in your life?**

   My wife, Alice, and my children. My dad and mother.

2. **What are the positive things about these relationships?**

   Alice is a great wife. I really love her. She's getting irritated with me, but she is still pretty supportive. She's been bailing me out by doing lots of things that I used to do around the house. I've tried to keep this depression a secret from the kids, but I think they know I've been struggling. They give us no trouble at all and are terrific kids. Being with them is one of the best things in my life when I'm feeling okay. Dad has gone through depression himself and probably understands my problem better than anyone. He and Mom look out for us; they pay for our airfare to visit them and make a big effort to visit us a couple times a year. They call me regularly to check on how I'm doing.

3. **What are the stressful or negative things about these relationships?**

   Alice has been stressed out too. She criticizes me a lot these days. Sometimes it seems like I can't do anything right. She seems to love to get away to sing with bands when she has the chance. I shouldn't be upset by this, but I can start pitying myself for having a life that seems to be too much work and not enough fun. I know she is mad at me because I haven't been interested in sex for a while. I don't really have any problems with my kids or my parents other than not doing as many activities with the kids. I can tell that they miss my being involved in their lives.

4. **Who are some other people in your life (for example, coworkers, friends, or casual acquaintances) who may do things that affect how you feel? Try to list at least three of these people.**

   Marge and Kenny, the two people that report to me at work. Dennis, one of my old friends from the band. Our neighbors, Carlie and Len.

5. **What are the positive things about these relationships?**

   Marge and Kenny are solid workers—I can really depend on them. And they both have a great sense of humor, which helps me get through some tough days at work. Dennis has kept in touch for many years. Other than Alice, he is my best friend. Sometimes we play music together just for fun. Carlie and Len are good friends. We like to have dinner with them, and sometimes we go out to a movie.

6. **What are the stressful or negative things about these relationships?**

   There really aren't any problems with these people. Maybe the only stressful thing is having to put Dennis off when he comes up with ideas for us to do something together when I'm depressed and don't feel like doing anything.

7. **What past relationships (for example, with partnerships or romances that have ended or with significant people who have died), if any, may still be troubling you or causing emotional pain? Briefly describe the difficulty you still have with the impact of this relationship on your life.**

   I've been lucky. I haven't had any breakups or anything like that. My grandparents have all died, but they lived full lives and I've gotten over losing them.

A Relationship Checkup

Instructions: Try to identify at least four family members or friends who are especially important in your life. Also, identify some other relationships with people such as coworkers, classmates, or casual acquaintances that may affect you. Then list some of the helpful or troubling features of these relationships. Finally, note any relationship that has ended that may still be causing distress.

1. **Who are the key people in your life?**

   _____

2. **What are the positive things about these relationships?**

   _____

   _____

   _____

   _____

   _____

3. **What are the stressful or negative things about these relationships?**

   _____

   _____

   _____

   _____

4. **Who are some other people in your life (for example, coworkers, friends, or casual acquaintances) who may do things that affect how you feel? Try to list at least 3 of these people.**

   _____

5. **What are the positive things about these relationships?**

   _____

   _____

(cont.)

_____

_____

_____

6. **What are the stressful or negative things about these relationships?**

_____

_____

_____

_____

_____

7. **What past relationships (for example, with partnerships or romances that have ended or with significant people who have died), if any, may still be troubling you or causing emotional pain? Briefly describe the difficulty you still have with the impact of this relationship on your life.**

_____

_____

depression. Positive people can help in many ways. You might open up to a trusted partner, family member, or friend about your problems and ask for the person's understanding, caring, and support. It can be good not to have to keep all of your painful feelings to yourself, and other people may be more understanding than you imagine.

If you're thinking negatively about yourself and the future, maybe a person who is close to you could be a voice of encouragement and hope. Depression may have taken such a strong hold on your thinking, you may not want to hear positive messages. You might be thinking that the other person couldn't possibly understand how badly you are hurting or how difficult the path ahead seems to be. However, you are probably better off hearing a message that things will get better than allowing despair to go unchecked and unchallenged. Mark's father was a very positive person in his life. His father had overcome depression and was convinced that Mark could get well and stay well. So he called Mark, wrote him notes, suggested books to read, and did many other things to convey an optimistic view of recovery. You might not have the good fortune to have a person like Mark's dad in your life, but perhaps there are other people who can give you the support you need.

Another way that positive people can help is to get you involved in activities that can energize you and bring back a sense of pleasure. In Chapter 5 you learned about CBT methods for taking action to change depressive behavioral patterns such as not engaging in stimulating and mood-lifting activities. Remember that one of the things that made Kate feel the best was doing simple things with her sister like going out for a cup of coffee or sharing vegetables she bought at a farmers' market. As Kate began to improve, another shared activity that helped a good deal was rejoining her community choir. Her friends from the choir had been calling and asking her to come to a rehearsal, and finally Kate decided to do it. She was glad she made this move. Sometimes Mark didn't feel like accepting his friend Dennis's invitations to do things like going fishing on a weekend or getting together to play music. But when he took the opportunity to spend time with Dennis, he almost always felt better.

Could you be missing out on chances to become more active with friends, family, or others and to use these activities as a way to fight depression? Some people find that walking or doing other exercise with a "buddy" helps them stick with this healthy activity. Others note that being part of a team that plays intramural sports or belonging to a group that does volunteer work keeps them active and also seems to lift their spirits. When Kate resumed attending a yoga class, she appreciated the time spent with the instructor, who was an encouraging and affirming person, and with other class members, who treated her nicely. Being more physically active also seemed to help relieve depression.

If you're already involved in mood-enhancing activities that you share with others, you might not need to make any changes. But if you are less active than before you became depressed and are feeling somewhat distanced from the positive people in your life, you might be able to combine closer connections with some of these people and getting more engaged in activities that could promote wellness.

Positive people can also help you accomplish tasks. If you are depressed and your energy is drained, you might need some help until you feel better. Many people with depression hesitate to ask others for assistance. They think that they should be able to do everything on their own and that asking for help is a sign of weakness. But if you had just had surgery and needed help with meals or household chores, would you hesitate to ask a trusted family member or friend to give you a hand? Try to remember that depression is an illness just like any other medical problem. People with depression deserve the same kindness, respect, and help as those who have other illnesses.

Kate was very reluctant to ask anyone to help, but she ultimately had a conversation with her boss, Samantha. Kate explained her illness and the treatment she was receiving and asked Samantha in a direct way to sit down with her and plan work activities so that they could accomplish them on a reasonable schedule. The decision to reveal a diagnosis of depression to an employer must be considered carefully. Of course there are some who may not understand and may react negatively to the type of discussion that Kate had with her boss. But Kate knew Samantha well. They had a very friendly and cooperative working relationship, and Kate believed Samantha would remain supportive after hearing about the problem, so their talk worked out well. They developed a schedule that made good sense to both of them, and Samantha made some welcome suggestions for ways to give Kate support.

Mark's requests for help from his wife didn't go so smoothly. Alice seemed to resent his not fulfilling his responsibilities around the house, and they got into arguments about work that was piling up. Mark hadn't talked much with Alice about how he was feeling. He just seemed to slip into a depressive behavioral pattern that was aggravating to both of them. In the next chapter we'll discuss ways to enhance communication in key relationships and to do problem solving for situations such as the one that Mark and Alice faced. You'll see that they were able to begin working together much more closely as a team for overcoming the depression.

You may be dealing with more difficult relationship problems than Mark. You could be trying to cope with a hypercritical partner or someone who has hurt you. Or maybe it seems like there is no one who could possibly help. But if depression has made it difficult for you to do the things you need to do, consider reaching out to ask someone who has had a positive influence on your life for temporary assistance until you are back to your old self.

Before doing Exercise 9.2, check over Kate's example to see how she was working on gaining strength from relationships.

As you can see from Kate's example, taking an inventory of the ways you gain strength from relationships may help you realize more fully how your connections with others affect how you feel. The exercise may also point out some problems in relationships that you may want to try to improve or resolve. We'll share some tips for working on difficulties in relationships in the next chapter. However, it's time now to focus on the positive features of relationships that can help you in your fight against depression.

Summary

Because people with depression often view themselves and the world around them through a negative lens, they can downplay, or miss entirely, the depression-fighting characteristics of their key interpersonal relationships. This chapter has detailed ways to break through the gloom of depression to tap the health-promoting features of your relationships with others. Next we'll suggest some ways to cope with relationship difficulties that may be holding you back from recovery. If you have noticed that depression has had a negative impact on one or more of your relationships, or if you have had problems such as grief, communication troubles, or a hurtful person in your life, the following chapter may help you search for answers to these challenges.

Gaining Strength from Relationships: Kate's Example

Instructions: Review the list of people in your life and the positive features of these relationships that you recorded in Exercise 9.1. Then use this worksheet to identify some specific ways to gain strength from at least two of these relationships.

A person in my life	Ways I am gaining strength from this relationship now	Ideas for gaining more strength from this relationship	Comments/possible problems/solutions
My sister	She is my biggest supporter. She almost always has time for me when I call. We enjoy being together. She gives me a bunch of encouragement.	She wants me to go out to some parties and other social activities with her and her husband. I don't want to intrude, but she wouldn't ask me if she didn't mean it. Maybe I could try to do a bit of socializing with her and Randy. I also could start to do some things for her now that I'm feeling better.	She wants me to be happy again and to meet people. I'll probably want to stay at home, but it would be good for me to go out with them sometimes.
My mother	She has a good heart and does love me. When we have family dinners on Sunday evening, I usually like being with her. She is a successful businesswoman, has weathered a tough divorce, and is a happy and independent person.	I could probably be more open to her and not try to hide so many of my problems. I've always wanted to please her so much and make her proud of me that it is hard to show vulnerability.	Mother can be critical of herself and others. I can work on this relationship in my therapy.
Tricia	Other than my sister, Tricia is my best friend. We have known each other since grade school. We sang together in an octet when we were in school, and we are in the choir together now. She's one of the main reasons I got back into the choir. Tricia always seems confident and in a good mood. She has a "can-do" attitude. She can be a bit pushy, but sometimes I need to be pushed.	There isn't too much more that I could do with this relationship. Tricia has a husband and two young kids, so she has her hands full with her own life. But I could probably make some suggestions for things to do with some of our other women friends that she would enjoy. We used to like having a night every month or so to go to the movies or a play together.	The only problem here is my getting down on myself when I see everything going so well in her life. I can try not to compare myself to others—just feel okay that she is having a good life.

Gaining Strength from Relationships

Instructions: Review the list of people in your life and the positive features of these relationships that you recorded in Exercise 9.1. Then use this worksheet to identify some specific ways to gain strength from at least two of these relationships.

A person in my life	Ways I am gaining strength from this relationship now	Ideas for gaining more strength from this relationship	Comments/possible problems/solutions

(*cont.*)

A person in my life	Ways I am gaining strength from this relationship now	Ideas for gaining more strength from this relationship	Comments/possible problems/solutions

10

Managing Relationship Problems to Improve Depression

> ## Chapter Highlights
>
> ▶ Dealing with the impact of depression on relationships
>
> ▶ Coping with loss and grief
>
> ▶ Addressing relationship conflicts
>
> ▶ Relationships in your plan for wellness

Because depression can be a cause and a consequence of relationship problems, we offer some tips in this chapter for people with three common difficulties—dealing with the impact of depression on relationships, coping with loss and grief, and addressing relationship conflicts. If you are facing one or more of these problems, we hope that the suggested strategies will be helpful. However, we typically recommend psychotherapy when relationship problems are severe, long lasting, and appear to be at the core of a depression. Interpersonal therapy (IPT) and cognitive-behavior therapy (CBT) can help individuals cope with difficult relationships or other relationship issues, even if partners or family members are unwilling or unable to attend sessions. Both of these therapies work well in couple or family formats, and other marital and family therapies also have been shown to be effective for mood disorders.

The first of the three problems discussed in this chapter is a frequent part of depressions that have lasted for more than a few weeks and have dampened one's usual ability to enjoy life, carry out tasks, and participate fully in interpersonal relationships. Even if you believe that your key relationships are still in good shape, depression may have started to erode your relations with the people you treasure the most.

Dealing with the Impact of Depression on Relationships

Both Kate and Mark had relationships that suffered when they became depressed. Although it's difficult to avoid the kinds of problems that Kate and Mark encountered, certain preventive or corrective steps may limit the impact of depression on important relationships. Three helpful actions you can take are to (1) educate and inform partners, key family members, and/or trusted friends about depression and your treatment; (2) use CBT methods and other treatments to reduce irritability, isolation, inactivity, and other symptoms that affect relationships; and (3) try to understand and cope with negative feelings about relationships.

Educate and Inform

Depression can be baffling, confusing, and upsetting to the key people in your life. They may be troubled by the changes they see in you and feel bad because they don't know what to do to stop the problem. They may want to help but not know how. Should they tell you that you look depressed or that your thinking has turned too pessimistic? Should they urge you to take medication or to get other professional treatment? Should they spend time with you or leave you alone? Sometimes family members can resent the changes when they don't fully understand them. Or they can have their own problems that interfere with giving you the support you need.

Making the effort to communicate about depression can often help keep relationships healthy when they are stressed by the symptoms of this illness. So, how should you proceed when you want to let the people in your life know about your struggle with depression?

Tips for Communicating with Others about Depression

1. *Prepare yourself.* Learn the facts about depression: its symptoms, how common it is, how it affects people, and how it is treated. Reading this book should help you understand depression and accept that it is a treatable illness that is not your fault. Be prepared to convey this understanding. Make some notes in advance of your conversation with a key person in your life. Outline the main points that you want to make. If it would help, rehearse in your mind, or to yourself aloud, how you might communicate effectively with this person.

2. *Find a good time.* It is usually not very helpful to have an important conversation about depression "off the cuff." For example, if a partner seemed irritated that you had not done a household chore and made a critical remark about it, you might be inclined to respond defensively. You might say something like "Can't you see I'm depressed? Can't you just back off and give me a break?" Trying to have a meaningful discussion about

depression at this time, when emotions may be high, may not work so well. Instead, you might do some advance planning and ask your partner if you could set aside a time to discuss your health and how the two of you could cope with the problems you've been having.

3. *Use educational resources.* You will have to do some of the educating yourself to give the key person (or people) in your life a good picture of how the depression is affecting you personally. But it also may help to suggest some resources for learning more about depression. You might recommend that the person read portions of this book, especially the first three chapters. Or you could tell her about websites, pamphlets, videos, or other books that provide information about depression and its treatment. A number of good print, video, and Internet sources are listed in the Resources section at the back of this book.

4. *Be clear and direct.* Explaining depression and how it is affecting you may create an opening to let this person know how she might be able to help. If the person is expressing an understanding of the problem and seems ready to be supportive, you can offer a few ideas for things that could be done. Examples might include becoming an exercise partner, calling periodically just to check in, reminding you to take medication, or handling a few of your routine responsibilities for a short while until you feel better. Sometimes just having this person on your side may be enough. But if specific help is needed, try to give a clear message about this need.

Use CBT and Other Treatments to Reduce Symptoms

If you're irritable, and this symptom is putting stress on relationships, you can use the methods you learned in Chapter 4 to try to calm your emotions and get along better with others. Thinking errors such as ignoring the evidence, magnifying, personalizing, and all-or-nothing thinking are often a part of irritable and angry responses to the words and actions of others. For example, when Alice came home from work and saw Mark sitting in his chair "doing nothing," and piles of laundry were all about, an anger-driven comment popped out of her mouth ("Can't you do anything to help around the house … I can't do it all!"). She regretted her words almost as soon as she uttered them because she knew Mark was depressed. But Mark had his own automatic thoughts ("All she does is complain … I can't stand her coming home and jumping on me like that … I don't know what to do … I'm letting everybody down").

If Mark had examined the evidence, he would have been able to counter the magnified and absolute quality of thoughts such as "all she does is complain." The facts were that Alice's complaints were only a small part of their life together. There was still a lot of love in the relationship, and most of Alice's actions over the past few months had been caring and supportive. However, in this situation Mark's automatic thoughts went unchecked. He sighed, gave an angry glance toward Alice, clenched his jaw, and sank deeper into his chair.

As you probably noticed, Alice had her own problem with cognitive errors. Sometimes when people are stressed, cognitive errors can be used as fighting tools. Her strong words such as "Can't you do anything to help around the house?" cut deeply into Mark

Communicating with Others about Depression

Instructions: Answer these questions to organize your ideas for communicating with others about depression.

Question	Ideas for communicating with others
Whom could you talk with about how you are feeling?	
What are the main points in the message that you want to communicate?	
What difficulties, if any, do you anticipate in communicating with this person? What ideas do you have for overcoming these difficulties?	
How would you like this person(s) to respond when you are depressed?	

and seemed to fuel his negative response. If you're using CBT to reduce irritability or other symptoms of depression, you can try to understand that other people may exaggerate or magnify their comments to make a point. This realization may help you take some of the sting out of harsh words and avoid blaming yourself excessively for behavior related to symptoms of depression.

Another valuable method from CBT that can be used to help with the negative influences of depression on relationships is activity scheduling (see Chapter 6). If you notice that inactivity, procrastination, or self-isolation is taking a toll on relationships, you can try to take some positive actions to reverse these trends by scheduling activities and rating them for mastery and pleasure. Perhaps focusing on scheduling pleasant activities with friends or family would help build up relationships that could play an important role in your recovery.

Other treatments, such as antidepressant medication, lifestyle changes, and taking care of medical problems related to depression also can assist in reversing the negative effects of depressive symptoms on relationships. Anything that reduces symptoms has the potential to help your relationships.

Try to Understand and Cope with Negative Feelings about Relationships

One basic principle of IPT is that negative emotions such as anger, resentment, disappointment, and sadness are often normal responses to social situations and tell you something about those situations. For example, anger is often a response to someone bothering you. Mark might reasonably have felt angry when Alice greeted him with an attack rather than recognizing how much his depression was paralyzing him. People who experience depression are often bursting with these types of feelings, yet they may hold them inside rather than express them. They do so for several reasons: because they find the emotions overwhelming and assume others will, too; because anger, disappointment, and other "negative" emotions feel "bad" and therefore seem shameful; and out of concern that expressing these feelings to the key people in their lives will just make things worse. They think that venting emotions such as anger will drive people away or make it more difficult to get the support they need.

If feelings are not expressed, however, other people may continue to do bothersome things, sometimes not even realizing that they're hurting the individual with depression. And not expressing a feeling like anger or disappointment means keeping it in—which can feel very uncomfortable—rather than getting it off one's chest.

When Alice came home and immediately criticized Mark for not helping around the house, he had some intensely angry thoughts but suppressed his feelings, clenched his jaw, and sank deeper into his chair. If Mark was receiving professional therapy with IPT, the therapist would probably encourage him to talk out his feelings in the treatment session and to accept the fact that depression sets people up for having lots of intense and painful emotions. The therapist would "normalize" having such feelings by explaining to Mark that it's okay to have these kinds of emotions and that expression of feelings, at least to some degree, is a healthy way to deal with them. Mark and the therapist might then practice expressing those feelings to Alice, to clear the air and improve communication in the relationship as well as the couple's understanding of each other.

Of course, it is not a good idea to vent negative emotions to others at every opportunity or in ways that seriously undermine or damage relationships. However, there may be opportunities to open up to express your sadness, anger, or other painful feelings in ways that are acceptable to the key people in your life and help you avoid the negative impact of letting intense feelings simmer for long periods of time. For example, in educating others about your depression, you might explain that it can be harmful to always hold sadness, resentments, and anger inside. Would this person understand if you sometimes let your negative feelings be known? Could this person allow you to express upsetting feelings as part of your attempts to move beyond the depression? Could you show your intense feelings occasionally and still have a good relationship with this person?

CAUTION The Guilt Trap Can Snare You

When depression makes it difficult or impossible to show the positive feelings that you would usually express to others, it can be easy to fall into the guilt trap. You can feel guilty because most of your feelings are negatively toned and you don't show as much love and concern to others as you may think they need.

So if you're having difficulties expressing positive feelings to others and you're mostly experiencing painful emotions, don't blame yourself for the problems depression is causing in your life. Try to avoid "adding insult to injury." A healthier way to look at this problem is to:

1. Recognize the effects of depression on how you show your feelings.
2. Adopt a problem-solving attitude instead of a blaming attitude.
3. Work on finding ways to express painful emotions with the people who care about you.
4. Take any small steps that you can to express positive feelings and realize that, as depression improves, your normal abilities to show affection and kindness will return.

If you're struggling with lots of negative emotions and find it difficult or impossible to express them and cope with them, your best option may be to seek professional help. IPT typically focuses on helping people handle their feelings and use them to improve relationships or cope with life crises. Other therapies such as CBT also help people express and effectively manage their painful emotions. Websites for finding therapists are listed in the Resources section at the back of the book.

We've explained three ways of dealing with the impact of depression on relationships. Do you think that any of these strategies could help you improve your key relationships and help you make progress in overcoming depression? After you review Mark's example, you can use the worksheet in Exercise 10.2 (page 233) to organize your ideas for using these strategies.

Mark had a number of ideas for putting these three strategies into action. Even if you don't see so many opportunities in your own relationships, sketching out some plans may help. Do Exercise 10.2 and, if your ideas evolve over time, photocopy the form or download it from *www.guilford.com/breakingfreeforms*.

Dealing with the Impact of Depression on Relationships: Mark's Example

Instructions: If you believe that depression has had an influence on any of your key relationships, consider the three actions noted below. Try to write down a few specific ideas for taking any of these actions that you think would be helpful.

Actions	Ideas for putting this strategy to work
Educate and inform others about depression	*I'll ask Alice to meet with me on Saturday morning at a time when we can concentrate on having a good talk. I'll prepare in advance so I can do an effective job of explaining depression and asking her for help as I'm trying to get better. One thing I'll ask her to do is to read about CBT so she'll know about what I'm trying to do to change negative thinking. Maybe some of the CBT will rub off on her, so she'll be less critical and more understanding. Another thing to do is to explain how I get all tied up with my negative feelings and how it might help sometimes to be able to have her listen to me talk about these feelings.*
Use CBT and other treatments to reduce symptoms	*This is an obvious good choice to make. Anything I can do to get back to my old way of functioning would be worthwhile. Some of the most important things to do are to take medication regularly and to use thought change records. Following an activity schedule would probably help me get back to being more involved with my family.*
Try to understand and cope with negative feelings in relationships	*No question that I try not to show my emotions, especially around Alice and the kids. It's a big jump for me to accept that talking about feelings is OK. I'll have to do this gradually, when it seems safe and wouldn't hurt anyone. An idea is for Alice and me to get a babysitter and go out for some coffee so I could open up about what I'm going through and how her criticism affects me.*

Coping with Loss and Grief

Loss and grief can strike in many different ways. Endings of relationships through either a breakup or death are well-known triggers for depression. And multiple other types of losses such as getting laid off or fired from a job, losing physical health, having an important relationship grow cold, or experiencing the death of a beloved pet can be part of the path toward depression.

The exact mechanisms by which experiences of loss and grief can lead to depression are not known. However, people who are vulnerable to depression because of genetics, previous life experiences with loss or rejection, troubled relationships, or other negative influences clearly have a higher risk of having severe or prolonged grief reactions that can evolve into despair.

When Does Grief Become Part of Depression?

Some experts suggest that grief that is still very intense after 6 months is likely to be a problem that needs treatment. However, there are so many individual differences in the extent and the meaning of loss that we don't rely on simple formulas such as the length of

---

EXERCISE 10.2	Dealing with the Impact of Depression on Relationships

Instructions: If you believe that depression has had an influence on any of your key relationships, consider the three actions noted below. Try to write down a few specific ideas for taking any of these actions that you think would be helpful.

Actions	Ideas for putting this strategy to work
Educate and inform others about depression	
Use CBT and other treatments to reduce symptoms	
Try to understand and cope with negative feelings about relationships	

grief as a primary guide for treatment decisions. Instead, we evaluate the level of depression, the person's coping skills, and the person's desire to reduce the intensity of grief in planning ways to help.

If grief is not complicated by depression and the person seems to be coping well, we listen and offer support but don't usually need to recommend any specific grief-relieving therapies. An example is the grief that Larry has had for over 3 years since the death of his teenage son in a car accident. He thinks of his son every day, still misses him terribly, and can cry easily at reminders of his presence in their family's life. Larry isn't ready to let go of these feelings. They seem completely natural to him.

When Larry visited Dr. McCray for his annual physical and took the PHQ-9, his score was 6 (mild depression). Dr. McCray had been concerned about Larry ever since his son's death, but Larry had never experienced the full symptoms of major depression, so Dr. McCray didn't suggest that he take medication or start psychotherapy. Because she knew Larry well, she was able to have a meaningful talk with him about his grief, and they discussed use of some of the positive coping strategies outlined later in this chapter.

Kate's situation was different. When her boyfriend told her he had found someone else, she was devastated. She had experienced other breakups, but Nick had seemed like the perfect match for her. They had been together for 2 years and had talked seriously about getting married and having children. There had been a few arguments, but most of the time they seemed to get along just fine.

Kate's first thoughts were "No, this can't be happening … What can I do to stop him from leaving?" But as the reality of the breakup became painfully obvious, her self-confidence plummeted and she sank into a deep depression. She was angry at Nick for deceiving her, but most of the anger was turned inward. Soon her mind was riddled with thoughts such as "I'm never good enough … I mess up everything I do … I'll never be happy … No one would ever want me" and other intense, self-critical conclusions. Her main coping strategies—keeping to herself and eating lots of "comfort food"—just seemed to add to the problem. She became increasingly lonely, found little that she could enjoy in life, and felt worse about herself as she gained weight.

When Kate first consulted Dr. Wright, her PHQ-9 score was 21 (severe depression). She clearly needed help with coping with her loss and getting her life back. Kate answered yes to all of the questions in the next exercise. What are your answers to these questions? If you answer yes to two or more of the questions, you may need to work on ways of managing your responses to a loss or losses in your plan for fighting depression.

Healthy Coping Strategies for Loss and Grief

There is no single best path for coping with loss and grief. Everyone has to find his own way to move beyond the pain. However, these commonly used strategies have helped many of our patients.

1. *Talk with others.* For most people, attempts to suppress intense feelings that have been set in motion by a loss don't have a favorable long-term outcome. It may seem easier at first to try to shut down your feelings, but the hurt, anger, and grief will probably eat

EXERCISE 10.3	Signs That Grief May Have Evolved into Depression		

Instructions: Answer the following questions about loss, grief, and depression.

Question	Yes	No
Are you experiencing prolonged, intense grief that has lasted 6 months or more?		
Do you have symptoms that suggest the diagnosis of a major depressive disorder (see Chapter 1 for criteria), with the depression occurring in the aftermath of a significant loss?		
Do you have (or have you had recently) PHQ-9 scores of 10 or above (moderate depression), with a loss apparently having triggered depressive symptoms?		
Are you preoccupied with a loss that has played a role in making you depressed?		
Do you have persistent negative thoughts about yourself that are related to a loss that you have experienced?		
Do you have intense guilt that is related to a loss?		

away at you. Well-intentioned people may offer condolences in public settings or at other times when you are not ready to talk. Others may not know what to say to you and may seem uneasy around you after you have experienced a loss. Yet there are probably positive and trusted people in your life that you can talk with openly when the time is right. A doctor, therapist, or spiritual leader can also be a very good sounding board when you are struggling with loss and grief.

2. *Stay active.* Kate was able to keep going to work, but her activity level in other areas of her life almost went into free fall after Nick left her. In Chapter 6, you learned how Kate used CBT methods to reactivate herself and climb out of the deep rut of depression. If you are suffering from loss and grief, consider using the same strategies. It's okay to keep busy and to try to experience some pleasure when grieving. These activities won't make you ignore grief that you need to work through, but they may help you better tolerate the distress.

3. *Try something new.* After a loss, there is an understandable tendency to focus on what is missing and to spend most of your energy lamenting what has been lost. To help prevent the loss from pervading every corner of your life, and to stimulate the part of you that is capable of personal growth, you might consider trying something new. Perhaps you could learn to play a musical instrument, take a class in something that intrigues

you, begin an exercise program, join a group that has a specific interest (for example, biking, hiking, playing cards, cooking, helping others, taking trips), or freshen or renovate a room in your home. Taking a step to do something creative, interesting, or productive can help serve as an antidote to feelings of loss. By taking this step, you can start to move away from loss toward a positive future.

4. *Build your support network.* Kate's contacts with family and friends began to shrivel after her loss. Then her social isolation and depression escalated in lockstep fashion. But when she reversed this trend by spending more time with her sister and her friends and rejoining a choir, her depression got better and she thought less about the breakup of her relationship with Nick. Are there things you could do to build your support network in ways that would help you cope with a loss?

5. *Think rationally about yourself.* In Chapters 4 and 5, you learned many effective methods from CBT for spotting the self-defeating thoughts that can become so pervasive in depression. These methods were just what Kate needed. After becoming involved in CBT she was able to recognize that she was taking excessive blame for the breakup, was putting herself down unnecessarily, and was falling victim to extremes in thinking (for example, "I mess up everything I do … I'll never be happy"). When Kate learned to use CBT methods to develop more rational thoughts, she gave the breakup with Nick much less power to control her sense of self and her view of what the future might hold.

6. *Use your spiritual strengths.* As we discuss in Chapter 12, depression can sometimes cause people to become distanced or disconnected from spiritual beliefs and practices. They may feel ignored by a higher power if something traumatic has happened to them, or the veil of depression may have obscured the help they could gain from their spiritual underpinnings. However, involvement in spiritual practices has been shown to decrease the risk of depression, and for many people the spiritual domain is the most important resource for coping with loss and grief. Becoming reinvolved in spiritually oriented activities offered Kate much comfort and strength as she worked to overcome her loss.

If you have suffered a loss and are grieving, take some time now to sketch out a few ideas for how you might use the coping strategies outlined here.

Addressing Relationship Conflicts

Being involved in a seriously conflicted relationship can be a principal reason for getting depressed and having difficulty finding a way out of the depression. JoAnne, a woman who came to one of us for treatment of depression, had a sad story to tell. She had been married to Frank, a salesman, for 15 years. After the first few years of their marriage, Frank became increasingly hypercritical and unforgiving. He seemed to cut her down at every turn. Frank was never physically abusive, but through the years his verbal rants escalated to the point of emotional abuse. He swore at her, called her names, and blamed all of their troubles on her. It was no wonder that JoAnne's self-esteem was at the bottom of a pit by the time she finally sought treatment.

Strategies for Coping with Loss and Grief

Instructions: Write down some plans for how you might use one or more of the healthy coping strategies for managing loss or grief. If a strategy doesn't seem to offer much promise to you right now, skip over it and try to identify another method that will give you some help.

Strategy	Plans
Talk with others	
Stay active	
Try something new	
Build your support network	
Think rationally about yourself	
Use your spiritual resources	

JoAnne's parents and her close friends all had told her that she needed to leave Frank, but it took her a long while to accept their advice. Her self-confidence had been knocked down so much by all the years of living with Frank that she was scared she wouldn't be able to manage the challenges of being a single mother. And there was a part of her that still cared for Frank and had some hope that the marriage could be salvaged.

JoAnne wasn't worried about Frank hurting her physically, but other people who are in similar situations might stick with bad relationships for much too long if they think there is a significant risk of physical retaliation for any attempts to leave. If you are in a situation like this, try to get some support and advice from a professional therapist and/or a program for people who are suffering from abuse. The National Domestic Violence Hotline (*thehotline.org*) offers help to callers 24 hours a day, 365 days a year.

After about 8 months of individual therapy and a failed attempt at marital therapy, JoAnne got to the point where she couldn't take living with Frank any longer. The marital therapy had helped her see that Frank either didn't want to change or couldn't change. And the individual therapy had helped her build back a good part of her self-esteem and to problem-solve how she could cope with going through a divorce. At the time of the writing of this book, it has been 4 years since JoAnne divorced Frank. She has continued on an antidepressant and sees Dr. Wright once every 3 months for a checkup, but she has been depression free for all of these 4 years.

Of course, ending a relationship is a radical solution to a conflict. For most people it is a last resort. In our clinical practices, we usually try to help people improve conflicted relationships, enhance their communication skills with the key people in their lives, express and effectively manage anger and other painful emotions, and learn coping strategies that can help them manage difficult interpersonal situations. Fortunately, most of our patients with depression can address their relationship conflicts and do not need to end a close relationship to recover from depression. Carl was able to make these types of adjustments in a troubled relationship with his wife, Sandy.

Carl and Sandy had been together for 8 years but had put off having children because both of them were very busy establishing their careers. In the last 2 or 3 years, increasing levels of tension made them wary about what the future might hold for their marriage. An episode of depression that Carl had experienced 2 years ago hadn't helped matters. During the depression, he quit a job that Sandy thought held a lot of promise for him. This made her angry, especially since Carl had not talked with her much about the decision. She complained that Carl didn't tell her what he was really thinking, didn't listen to her, and seemed to "be in his own world."

As Sandy began to wonder whether she could rely on Carl, she poured more energy into her own career. She often stayed at work into the evening hours and worked through weekends. It seemed to Carl that she was never available. Sometimes he wondered whether she might be having an affair, but Sandy always reassured him that she loved him and would never betray him.

In the last few months, Carl's depression had started to return. As often happened when he became depressed, his natural tendency to be quiet and to draw into himself increased. He also began to be more disturbed by Sandy's "workaholic" behavior. Carl felt that he needed tender affection from Sandy, but she seemed to grow colder and more distant as he sank further into depression. By the time Carl sought treatment for depression, he and Sandy were worrying about where their marriage was headed.

In contrast to the unsalvageable situation that JoAnne confronted, Carl's relationship with Sandy had real potential for positive change. They were still committed to each other, they had experienced some very good years in the earlier part of their relationship, and they had many shared interests such as collecting old movie posters and antiques, traveling, and caring for their dogs. They were financially stable, had a nice older house that they had restored together, and had a solid support network of family and friends.

Marital therapy was a key part of Carl's treatment for depression. He resumed taking an antidepressant, learned to use CBT methods for fighting symptoms of depression, and started an exercise regimen. But working to improve communication and resolve conflicts with Sandy offered very specific relief of the tension between them and helped restore the loving, caring, and nurturing dimensions of their life together. You'll learn about some of the steps that Carl and Sandy took as you read the rest of this chapter.

Although professional therapy is often needed when there are significant relationship conflicts, you may find the following suggestions helpful in managing troubled relationships in your own life.

Communicate Effectively

Although it can be hard to influence the communication styles of others, you can work on your own communication skills to help reduce relationship conflicts. Take a look at the communication skills table to see how your communication abilities stack up.

To change your communication style you need to become an astute observer of how you talk with others. Instead of letting your communication proceed on automatic pilot, take some time to ask yourself questions about how you might improve. For example, could you practice becoming a better listener?

QUICK Gerard Egan, author of *The Skilled Helper*, recommends that people follow the
TIP   SOLER rule:

- Squarely face the person.
- Have an Open posture (don't cross your arms or legs—it suggests anger or lack of receptivity).
- Lean slightly forward (this demonstrates your interest in what the speaker has to say).
- Make Eye contact.
- Keep your body Relaxed (a way of putting the other person at ease).

Carl and Sandy both benefited from practicing ways to enhance their listening skills. Sandy would get so consumed by her work that Carl could feel she was ignoring him. Her multitasking skills helped her be very productive in her job, but they were undermining

Communication Skills

Communication skill	Definition	Examples
Listening attentively	Focusing on the speaker without distractions	Keeping your attention on the speaker even if your phone rings, you get a text message, or there's a lot going on around you; making eye contact; thinking about what the person is saying, not how you'll respond; listening *actively*, acknowledging what the other person has said and asking for elaboration
Appropriately and honestly expressing negative feelings	Expressing emotions like anger, sadness, and disappointment in a genuine way that does not involve an attack on others; emotions are not buried or stuffed inside so that they worsen your depression, cause physical symptoms (headaches, stomach problems, back pain, etc.), or damage your relationships	Saying you're angry instead of gritting your teeth and saying nothing; admitting to feeling sad rather than trying to act as if nothing is wrong
Letting others speak for themselves	Soliciting information from others about their thoughts and feelings	Asking instead of guessing, making assumptions, or jumping to conclusions about what someone thinks or feels
Communicating with an open heart	Giving the speaker the benefit of the doubt and taking what is said at face value; assuming benevolence on the part of the speaker	Thinking before jumping in to disagree; resisting the impulse to make excuses for yourself or to justify your position; assuming the other person is *not* trying to attack you
Sticking to the subject	Following the thread of a conversation and avoiding going off on tangents or piling on old grievances	Raising problems one at a time and resolving them before bringing in past events or difficulties
Validating	Conveying that someone's ideas are valuable, understandable, and acceptable	Listening to another point of view without feeling compelled to disagree; respecting others' perspectives and right to express them; conveying empathy for a person's feelings

her marriage. So their therapist suggested that she learn to use the SOLER rule instead of trying to carry on a meaningful conversation with Carl when she was doing e-mail or rushing to an appointment with a client. Just setting aside small amounts of time when she could give undivided attention to talking with Carl made a big difference in their relationship.

When Carl sharpened his listening skills, he became more aware of Sandy's need for him to tell her what he was thinking instead of giving her the "silent treatment." He had assumed that burdening Sandy with his worries and his painful emotions would upset her, but the opposite was true. She grew more concerned and more irritated when he retreated into himself. He didn't need to unload all of his concerns all the time, yet being sensitive to her need to know and taking time to share more of his thoughts about important matters helped them grow closer.

Carl and Sandy also had a problem with "mind reading." They constantly assumed they knew what the other was thinking and feeling better than the other person did. Partners or parents and children who have known one another for years can easily fall into this trap. They jump to conclusions without giving the other person a chance to say what they mean or explain themselves. For example, when Carl was at home alone waiting for Sandy to return from a late night at work, he would have thoughts such as "She would rather be at work than spend time with me." By the time Sandy returned home he would already feel hurt and angry. Then he might jump on her and say something like "I hope you had a good day at work" in a sarcastic and disapproving tone. An alternate approach is remaining open to hearing what others have to say and even asking questions such as "What do you want to tell me?" or "What's on your mind?"

During marital therapy sessions Carl learned that he was greatly exaggerating the meaning of Sandy's late nights at work. She did admit that part of her increased emphasis on work had been out of concern that Carl's depression might interfere with his career and their financial stability. However, she still did care about him and wanted to spend time with him, especially if they could iron out their problems and get back to a happier and more enjoyable life together.

When people are depressed, it's hard to communicate with an open heart and on the assumption that others have the best intentions and are benevolent or at least neutral in their conversations. Defensiveness is very common in depression. Because people know they aren't functioning in top form, perceived criticism can set off comments such as "You just don't understand," "Give me a break," or "Why don't you do it yourself?" Other defensive reactions could include shrugging off or having difficulty accepting constructive criticism, shifting excessive blame toward others, and switching immediately into an argumentative mode whenever any hint of conflict arises. Part of Carl's plan for improving his relationship with Sandy was to reduce defensive reactions such as glaring at her or shooting back a quick retort when she complained about chores that weren't done. Do you ever find yourself communicating with a slightly hardened heart? Could you work on being less defensive and more constructive in solving relationship disputes?

Carl and Sandy's communication also got derailed by their tendency to jump around in their discussions and to pile one complaint or issue on top of another when they began to argue. For instance, Carl would occasionally complain that the level of intimacy in their marriage had deteriorated. Instead of talking directly about this problem, Sandy might bring up her concerns about their finances or start talking about some other conflicts that they had. Although these difficulties might have contributed to the emotional distancing in their marriage, the end result of dealing with multiple topics was to make Carl feel that he was to blame for everything and that there was little chance of solving any of these problems. In their marital therapy sessions they made much better progress when they stayed focused on a single topic, communicated openly about it, and tried to develop solutions.

If you notice that changing topics is interfering with your communication with an important person in your life, could you slow things down and target only one item at a time? If your partner has difficulty cooperating with this strategy, you might try to begin a conversation by being very explicit about the agenda for your conversation. You could even write down a few notes about the topic to help you stay on track if he or she suddenly changes topics or moves to another concern. Try to stay disciplined about retaining a clear focus for the conversation.

If you're depressed, you might not have a problem validating others, but you may find that they seem to have trouble validating you. Even if validation seems to be a one-way street in your relationships, being attuned to the ways that communication can be invalidating may help keep all of the hurtful comments from hitting their mark. JoAnne learned in therapy to recognize her husband's invalidating statements from "a mile away" so that she could try to let them bounce off her instead of sinking in. If you sometimes communicate with important people in your life with invalidating comments, your relationships will probably improve if you can learn to put this fighting tool aside. Practice looking for ways to express understanding of other people's feelings, even if you think they are based on false assumptions or negative thinking.

Be Assertive

When people are depressed and are involved in a conflicted or troubled relationship, they can feel rather helpless to change bad situations or to set boundaries for acceptable behavior from others. JoAnne certainly had difficulty standing up for herself until she began therapy. She felt so powerless around her husband that she didn't effectively push to have him adequately disclose their financial situation. Being in the dark about their finances made her hopelessness and helplessness worse. If you are in a difficult relationship and feel that your needs are not being respected, could you be more emphatic about these needs? If you have trouble being assertive by yourself, could you get some advice from a counselor, a spiritual leader, or a trusted family member or friend on how to proceed?

Call a Truce

If you're trying to recover from depression and a troubled relationship is standing in the way, could you ask this person to call a truce and put the conflicts aside so that you can concentrate on getting healthy again? We have seen many people who get so consumed with relationship problems that their efforts to do positive things such as exercising, following an activity schedule, or breaking patterns of procrastination fall by the wayside. Carl and Sandy called a partial truce. They agreed to try their best to stop arguing and to cooperate more effectively while Carl worked on getting better from depression. It seemed reasonable to expect that they would be more likely to solve their relationship problems if Carl's energy, interest, concentrating abilities, and self-confidence were back to normal.

Improving Communication

Instructions: Identify areas of your life in which you use the following communication skills. Then describe ways you might improve your communication by building this skill or by applying it in areas of your life where you don't currently use it.

Communication skill	Where I use this skill	How I could build this skill
Listening attentively		
Appropriately and honestly expressing negative emotions		
Letting others speak for themselves		
Communicating with an open heart		
Sticking to the subject		
Validating		

Defuse Your Anger

It's hard to make progress with relationship difficulties if you're so angry that you can't think straight. You'll need to be as rational as possible to clearly identify and resolve conflicts. One useful method for curbing excessive anger is to use the CBT skills you learned in Chapter 4. You could complete a thought change record to identify automatic thoughts that precede intense anger and then step back from the situation to see if you want to modify any of the automatic thoughts.

Often automatic thoughts that are associated with anger are very inflammatory. They almost act like a fuse to set off explosion of anger. Take, for example, Carl's anger when Sandy told him that a business meeting was lasting much longer than expected and she would need to miss a dinner he had cooked especially for her. His automatic thoughts ("She doesn't give a @@##!! … She can stay there all night for all I care") were typical of the unvarnished thoughts that people often have before a surge of anger. These weren't thoughts that he would usually express out loud to Sandy, but they still had a profound effect on how he felt.

Unfortunately, the intense anger didn't help Carl deal effectively with the situation. By the time Sandy returned home, he was seething and he had a splitting headache. Although some anger and disappointment were reasonable, the absolute and magnified quality of his automatic thoughts stoked the fires of anger that added too much heat to their conflict.

If excessive anger is a problem in any of your relationships, could you try to spot your automatic thoughts and tone them down so you can work more on solving problems than venting steam? Other well-known ways of channeling anger productively are to get involved in physical activities that can help you discharge the energy behind the anger or to find a trusted confidant to help you calm down as you talk through the difficulty. Could it be better to discharge some of the anger in these ways than allow it to fuel a counterattack on a partner or family member?

Cope by Having a Balanced Life

Too often, we've seen people slide deeper into depression when they're fixated on a relationship conflict as the core of their dilemma and can see no way to feel better unless the relationship is healed. When all of one's capacity for happiness and meaning in life is tied up in a troubled relationship, there is great potential for pain, loss, and despair. So we always encourage people with depression to cultivate multiple ways for achieving fulfillment.

One goal of this book is to help you find a variety of activities that can sustain you when times are difficult and key relationships are dysfunctional. Options might include the behavioral methods of CBT detailed in Chapter 5, the well-being therapy concepts described in Chapter 7, the spirituality resources that are discussed in Chapter 12, and, of course, the relationship building with other people in your life that we discussed in Chapter 9.

JoAnne had become so preoccupied with trying to solve the problems in her marriage that the rest of her life seemed to shrink into insignificance. While she was still trying to improve the relationship, her therapist recommended that she pay much more attention to growing the parts of her that weren't tied to Frank. At first JoAnne believed that more than 90% of her happiness was contingent on how she related with Frank. But as the therapy proceeded, she worked on developing her friendships with other women, completing a training program to be a radiology technician, and spending more time with her brother and sister, among other activities. Before long the sense that her life hinged on how Frank treated her had dissipated. And when she woke up in the morning, she could look forward to experiencing many positive things during the day.

Working on getting more balance into life can also be an effective strategy for people who are committed to staying with a less than ideal relationship. So if you find yourself troubled by a relationship that you can't seem to improve, try to think of ways that you could do more with the other parts of your life that can be changed.

Relationships in Your Plan for Wellness

Before moving on to other paths to wellness, pause briefly to make some notes on the main points you would like to remember from the two chapters on relationships. Exercise 10.6 should help you summarize your plan. If you would like to alter your plan in the future, photocopy the form or download it from *www.guilford.com/breakingfreeforms*.

Summary

Positive and supportive interpersonal relationships can be one of the most helpful resources for overcoming depression. However, relationship problems can be a primary or contributing cause of depression, escalate the downward spiral of symptoms, and undermine efforts to achieve wellness. In this chapter we coached you on ways to counter the negative effects that depression can have on important relationships. And we tried to make useful suggestions for overcoming any losses, conflicts, or relationship disappointments that may have contributed to your depression. We hope you'll be able to count on many healthy relationships as you work to reach your goals.

The next chapter, "Lifestyle Changes," opens another valuable path toward overcoming depression. You'll be able to learn how developing effective sleep, exercise, diet, and other habits can add strength to your recovery plan. You've already gained skills in using the thoughts–action, biology, and relationship paths. So you are well on your way to having an effective map for putting depression behind you.

Relationships in My Plan for Wellness

Instructions: Review the exercises in this chapter and the preceding chapter. Then fill out this worksheet to help pull together your plan for using your relationship strengths or coping with relationship problems in the fight against depression.

Relationship action	How important this relationship action is to me (0 = not important at all; 5 = moderately important; 10 = extremely important)	Specific steps I plan to take
Build quantity or quality of relationships		
More effectively use my relationship strengths		
More effectively deal with the impact of depression on my relationships		
Cope with loss and grief		
Cope with a conflicted relationship		

THE LIFESTYLE PATH

11

Lifestyle Changes

> **Chapter Highlights**
>
> ◗ Getting a good night's sleep
>
> ◗ Exercise—a natural remedy that can work
>
> ◗ Can your diet have an influence on depression?
>
> ◗ Alcohol and drugs
>
> ◗ Light therapy
>
> ◗ Lifestyle changes in your path to wellness

If you are like so many people with depression, some of your lifestyle habits, such as your sleep and your level of physical activity, could be part of the problem and part of the solution. Although modifying your lifestyle may not seem easy, small changes may produce big rewards. Think about how getting a good night's sleep or feeling more fit might help lift your mood or restore some of the energy that you have been missing.

Getting a Good Night's Sleep

How do you feel when you get a solid night's sleep and wake up in the morning feeling well rested and relaxed? Contrast this with a sleepless night filled with worrying and thoughts such as "I need to finish those reports tomorrow, and I'll never have enough time," or "What am I going to say when I have to meet with the boss next week?" Or you may wake up for no reason and lie there, wide awake in the early hours of the morning, unable to get back to sleep. You may feel down about the situation: "Here I am again, awake, when I know I need the sleep."

Whether you spend a sleepless night worrying or just lying there awake, the next day you are bound to feel depleted. You may feel groggy, irritable, or foggy, and you may not be able to focus or get the job done at work. These types of problems can make you feel bad about yourself and create a vicious cycle leading to more sleepless nights. The bottom line is that the fatigue and irritability that come with poor sleep can make depression feel even worse.

SCIENCE CORNER
- Poor sleep can affect *neurocognitive* functioning, or the way we think, make decisions, and process information.
  - Many studies show that decreased sleep leads to poorer performance on cognitive tasks, such as reading, remembering information, and performing math.
  - Negative thoughts can become worse and more frequent when you are tired (for example, feeling down about a failed relationship can feel a lot worse when you are exhausted).
- Decreased sleep also affects physical functioning and reaction time.
  - People who report fewer hours of sleep (for example, shift workers) are at higher risk for traffic accidents and falling asleep behind the wheel.
  - Mistakes on the job are more common in people who have poor sleep.

Sarah

Sarah is a 38-year-old single mother of two who works full-time as a dental hygienist. She has noticed that her sleep has been "off" for several weeks—a sign to her that depression may be creeping back into her life. Sarah has had recurring depression, which runs in her family, since her late teens. Often the first sign that depression has returned is that, just like an alarm clock, she wakes up without warning at 2 A.M. every night. She usually can't get back to sleep until 4 or 5 A.M. and then has to get up at 6 A.M. to get herself and the kids ready for the day and out the door.

The sleepless nights are really taking their toll, and Sarah has been late to work several times in the past 2 weeks—a problem that never happens when she is feeling well. Sarah also feels exhausted and tearful by the end of the day. She can barely manage to get dinner on the table and play with the kids—activities she used to enjoy. While antidepressants have worked in the past for depression-related insomnia, Sarah would like to try some natural approaches to getting her sleep back on track first.

Sarah's story is very typical of people with depression. Although it is unclear why people with depression have disordered sleep, sleeping too little or too much is one of the classic symptoms of major depression. And it is often the first symptom to appear. It's good that Sarah is tuned in to her own body and sleep–wake cycles so that she can recognize the first symptoms of her depression. This type of awareness can be a key to preventing a full-blown recurrence (see Chapter 14).

Sleep Hygiene: The Place to Start When You Can't Sleep

When Sarah went to see her doctor about the depression and sleep problems, she was a bit confused when the doctor asked, "Well, what about your sleep hygiene?" As a dental hygienist by trade, Sarah always thought of hygiene as "keeping it clean." In a way, sleep hygiene, or maintaining a set of healthy practices related to sleep, is a way to keep sleep a "polished routine" like brushing your teeth every day. By keeping a routine, your body will know what to expect, be prepared for sleep, and be situated in the most ideal environment for a good night's sleep. Although sleep hygiene may not be the answer to all of your sleep problems, it is a good place to start. We'll go over the basics of sleep hygiene, do some troubleshooting, and then discuss some alternatives to treating sleep problems related to depression.

First, let's check in with Sarah to see what her typical night looks like.

Sarah

Sarah reviewed with her doctor her typical night of sleep. She often had a beer or two after the kids went to sleep to "wind down," watched the late show in bed, then fell asleep with the TV on. When she woke at 2 A.M., she would either watch TV in bed or lie there awake until she fell back asleep (sometimes for 2 or 3 hours). Sarah sometimes sorted through bills that she had stacked on her desk next to her bed. Doing this often sent her into a tailspin of worry before she could fall back to sleep. She was so tired in the morning that she had to keep her alarm clock on the opposite side of the bed so that she wouldn't turn it off and go back to sleep.

Does Sarah's story sound familiar? Can you think of some things that might be making Sarah's sleep worse or make her bedroom a less-than-ideal environment for sleep? In the exercise on page 252, Sarah records a typical night's sleep to look for clues about what might be going wrong. After you review Sarah's entries, use the worksheet to describe the details of your own sleep routine.

Sleep Hygiene: The Basics

If you looked at Sarah's entries and thought that the TV, the stack of bills, and the cat might be big detractors from a good night's sleep, you were right. One of the key elements of sleep hygiene is to eliminate or decrease distractions in the bedroom, such as noise (the TV) or physical distractions (the cat pawing at your face or bills stacked by the bed), which might wake you from a light sleep or prevent you from getting back to sleep if you wake up. Some distractions are unavoidable (for example, a hungry infant, a scared child, or the need to urinate if you are taking a water pill for blood pressure). The key is to change those things that are modifiable to create the most ideal environment for sleep. Here are some sleep hygiene basics to try:

- Use the bed for only sleep or sex.
  - Avoid the temptation to watch TV or surf the Internet in bed. This will provide a strong psychological distraction from sleep. Also, light from a TV screen or

Describe a Typical Night's Sleep: Sarah's Example

Instructions: Think about your sleep over the past week. Describe a typical night's sleep, including your evening routine before bed, how long you slept, when you woke up, what you did when you woke up, and your typical sleep environment (for example, is your room dark or light, noisy or quiet, and are there interruptions like cats, dogs, or a snoring partner?).

Pre-bedtime routine	Time to bed	Time(s) awake during the night	What did you do when you woke up?	Time awake in the morning (what time you actually got out of bed for the day)	Sleep environment
—Drink two beers —Watch the late show on TV —Fall asleep with the TV on	11:30 P.M.	2 A.M.	Watched TV for 1 hour, then turned it off, but laid in bed awake for another hour (until 4 A.M.)	6 A.M.	—Dark room —Television often on —Bills stacked on desk next to bed —Kids sometimes wake at night with night terrors —Cat begins to beg for food at 5 A.M.

computer monitor sends a signal to your brain that it is time to be awake instead of asleep. The brain circuits for sleep are very sensitive to light.

○ Your body and brain will become used to the bed being a sanctuary for sleep and be trained to relax into slumber when you lie down. Your brain will learn: bed = sleep.

• Set a routine.

○ Train your brain to sleep by going to bed and waking up at the same time every night. Although this is not always realistic, it can reset your sleep–wake cycles to optimize the amount and quality of sleep you get each night. A good rule of thumb is to aim for 8 hours each night (for example, 10 P.M. to 6 A.M.), knowing that some people require more (or less) sleep to function well the next day.

• Create a comfortable sanctuary for sleep.

○ Make the room dark by using light-blocking shades or curtains.

○ If you can, splurge on comfortable sheets and pillows and a supportive mattress. Avoid sleeping on the couch or a futon if possible.

- Decrease distractions.

  ○ Keep pets out of the room (or use a time-activated self-feeder).

  ○ If you can, avoid physical triggers for worry, such as a stack of bills on the desk. Although it is important to address your finances, it might be better to keep bills organized in a different room like the kitchen, where they can be dealt with during the day, with a clear state of mind.

  ○ If your partner snores, have him try over-the-counter nasal strips or take a few nights a week break in the guest room if you need to catch up on sleep.

  ○ If noise is unavoidable (for example, you live next to a busy road or a train track), try a sound machine, which provides ambient noise such as ocean waves, to drown out background noise.

- Avoid alcohol, caffeine, and excessive fluid intake before bed and avoid smoking cigarettes.

EXERCISE 11.1	Describe a Typical Night's Sleep

Instructions: Think about your sleep over the past week. Describe a typical night's sleep, including your evening routine before bed, how long you slept, when you woke up, what you did when you woke up, and your typical sleep environment (for example, is your room dark or light, noisy or quiet, and are there interruptions like cats, dogs, or a snoring partner?).

Pre-bedtime routine	Time to bed	Time(s) awake during the night	What did you do when you woke up?	Time awake in the morning (what time you actually got out of bed for the day)	Sleep environment

- ○ Although alcohol might seem to help you relax, it worsens the quality of sleep.
- ○ Caffeine, found in coffee, tea, and many sodas, is a potent stimulant and can be a big barrier to getting sleep. We recommend limiting your intake to two or fewer caffeinated beverages a day (and we're talking about small portions such as 8–12 ounces, not the 30-ouncers!). Avoid caffeine after lunchtime if you can. For those who have severe insomnia, we recommend abstinence from caffeinated beverages altogether.
- ○ Excessive fluid intake or a heavy meal before bed may increase the likelihood that you will have to make a trip to the bathroom sometime during the night. Although it is important to stay hydrated, you may want to avoid eating and drinking after 8 or 9 P.M.
- ○ Avoid smoking cigarettes if possible. People who smoke heavily often wake up 3–4 hours after falling asleep due to withdrawal from nicotine.

- • When you do wake up, choose a calming activity that will help soothe your mind.

  - ○ Try some positive imagery in which you imagine yourself in a tranquil or peaceful location that could promote sleep. One example is picturing yourself on the beach under a palm tree with the cool ocean breeze and the sound of waves nearby, lulling you to sleep.
  - ○ Although there are different ways to deal with waking at night, it is widely recommended that you get out of bed if you have prolonged periods of wakefulness (for example, more than 30 minutes) in which you are worrying or getting tense about not sleeping.
  - ○ If you get out of bed, engage in a calming activity such as sitting in a comfortable chair in the dark and using positive imagery. Avoid stimulating activities such as turning on the computer or going to the kitchen for a snack.
  - ○ When you feel tired again, try getting back into bed.
  - ○ Again, you are training your brain that bed = sleep. Thus you will be more likely to fall asleep when you lie back down.

?   **Wait a second . . . what if I can't do without my coffee in the morning?**

- • It may seem as if caffeine is a necessity in the morning, especially after a poor night's sleep.

- • You may even feel "addicted" to caffeine and have withdrawal symptoms, such as headache and irritability, when you stop.

- • Remember, caffeine revs up the sympathetic nervous system, which is the body's "fight-or-flight" mechanism. It works by increasing your heart rate, blood pressure, and alertness as if you were getting ready for a fight. This is *not* what you need when you are trying to get to sleep.

- • Try some of these tips to transition off caffeine:

  - ○ Sip a half-decaf/half-caffeinated beverage in the morning.

- ○ Buy the smaller size coffee in the morning (you will save some money too).

- ○ Slowly transition to noncaffeinated sodas (or, better yet, water).

- ○ Try other ways of stimulating the brain, such as a morning walk in the fresh air or a cool shower.

After talking to her doctor about sleep hygiene, Sarah moved her TV out of the bedroom, sorted the bills in the kitchen, and got a self-feeder for her cat. Although she had a hard time changing her nighttime routine of drinking two beers, she tried to limit her alcohol intake to the weekends and an occasional glass of wine with dinner. After making these changes, Sarah saw some improvement in her sleep (especially in the early morning, because her cat was no longer bothering her before the alarm went off!), but she still had several nights a week when she woke at 2 A.M. and could not get back to sleep for about an hour. At this point Sarah's doctor encouraged her to keep a sleep log, a nightly record of sleep (a variation on Exercise 11.1). After you see the examples from Sarah's life, you can complete your own sleep log. If you need additional copies of the form, photocopy it or download it from *www.guilford.com/breakingfreeforms*.

Do you see any patterns to your sleep problems? Are any of the distractions modifiable? What seems to help you get back to sleep? Are certain nights worse than others? Keeping a sleep log can help you tease out some problem areas so that you can make necessary changes in your environment and sleep hygiene. If you tried the sleep hygiene

Sleep Log: Sarah's Example

Instructions: Log your sleep habits for the next week to see if there are any patterns or trouble spots to target. Keep the log (and a pen) by your bed, so that it is easily accessible when you wake up.

Date	Time to bed	Time(s) awake during the night	What did you do when you woke up?	How long were you awake?	Time awake in the morning	Sleep environment (any disruptions or distractions)
Monday	9 P.M.	2 A.M.	Got out of bed, read a book. Made tea.	1 hour	6 A.M.	No disruptions or distractions
Tuesday	9 P.M.	1 A.M.	Comforted son. Read a book.	2 hours	6 A.M.	Son woke up with night terror. Cat also woke up and pawed at furniture.

Sleep Log

Instructions: Each morning, log your sleep habits for the next week to see if there are any patterns or trouble spots to target. Keep the log (and a pen) by your bed so that it is easily accessible when you wake up.

Date	Time to bed	Time(s) awake during the night	What did you do when you woke up?	How long were you awake?	Time awake in the morning	Sleep environment (any disruptions or distractions)
Monday						
Tuesday						
Wednesday						
Thursday						
Friday						
Saturday						
Sunday						

techniques listed above, but still have trouble sleeping, it might be time to think about other treatment strategies. Some additional options include antidepressant medications, sleep medications, and CBT (either with a therapist or on your own, with the tips listed later in this chapter).

Using Medication for Sleep

Antidepressants specifically target depression, and sleep may improve as a result of symptom relief. As Sarah mentioned, she had used antidepressants in the past with good results. Just as sleep was the first sign of the return of depression, it was also the first to improve when she began medication. In Chapter 8 we discussed medications that can be used specifically for sleep, including antidepressants with sedating side effects (mirtazapine [Remeron], trazodone [Deseryl], and the TCAs) and hypnotics such as zolpidem [Ambien] or eszopiclone [Lunesta]).

Most sleeping pills have some potential for dependency and thus should be used with caution (and under the guidance of a skilled physician). Natural alternatives, which are not regulated by the FDA but may help with sleep, include melatonin (often used for shift work or travel-related sleep disturbances), and chamomile (often used for calming effects). Other over-the-counter sleep aids include the sedating antihistamine diphenhydramine, which is found in Benadryl, Tylenol PM, Advil PM, and Sleepinol. Diphenhydramine-containing medications are generally considered safe to use but can cause side effects such as urinary retention, dry mouth, low blood pressure, sedation, and, in rare cases, blood problems.

Remember to avoid alcohol or operating a motor vehicle when you use any medication (prescription or over the counter) for sleep. Some drug interactions may be dangerous, such as taking pain medications and sleep medications at the same time or taking an over-the-counter sleep aid with a sedating antidepressant or a prescription sleep medication. Please check with your doctor before taking any sleep aid, whether it is over the counter or prescription.

? **What if I sleep too much?**

- Do you sleep too much due to depression and have a hard time getting out of bed?

- Lying in bed may drain your energy and make you feel even more tired during your waking hours.

Try the following tips to reset your sleep–wake cycles and help devote the hours you spend in bed to quality sleep.

- Set a sleep schedule, with a limit of 10 hours in bed (for example, 10 P.M. to 8 A.M.) maximum.

- Use alarms to remind you of when to go to bed and to help wake you up.

> ○ Use what works best for you—if you need the equivalent of a bullhorn, set your alarm to a loud beep or have a friend call you.
>
> ○ If you prefer a gentler approach, set your alarm to music or buy an alarm that gradually produces light to wake you up.
>
> • Stick to the sleep hygiene tips above.
>
> ○ Remember, use the bed only for sleep or sex.
>
> ○ Resist the urge to lie there; if you lie in bed awake for more than 15 minutes, force yourself to get out of bed and do a calming activity, such as reading, drawing, or writing.
>
> • Set goals for the day to give you a reason to get out of bed (see Exercise 11.3).

If you sleep either too much or too little, you will probably feel tired in the morning, and it may be difficult to get motivated to start your day. To address this problem, try to think of some activities that could help you get out of bed. In the next exercise, list some ideas that come to mind. The activities can be as simple as taking a hot shower, sitting on the front porch, or making breakfast. Alternatively, you can schedule events outside your home to motivate you to get going, such as meeting a friend, going for a walk, or getting to exercise class.

Cognitive-Behavior Therapy for Sleep: An Evidence-Based Approach

CBT has been found to be at least as successful as medication in treating insomnia and is considered first-line treatment for sleep problems. The treatment includes all of the sleep hygiene methods described earlier plus the CBT skills that you learned earlier in the book for changing negative or anxiety-producing thoughts. For example, Sarah was able to make better progress with her sleep problem after using CBT methods to cope with some troubling automatic thoughts.

SCIENCE CORNER A National Institutes of Health consensus statement concluded that there is good evidence that CBT:

- Is *as effective* as prescription medication for the brief treatment of chronic insomnia.
- May last well beyond the end of treatment, having a more long-lasting effect than medications.

Sarah

Despite trying sleep hygiene techniques and modifying her sleep environment as much as she could, Sarah still had trouble sleeping in the early morning. When she took her

EXERCISE 11.3	**Morning Activity Schedule**

Instructions: If you have trouble getting out of bed, try scheduling morning activities to give yourself a reason to get moving.

Date	Morning activity (between 8–9 A.M.)
Monday	
Tuesday	
Wednesday	
Thursday	
Friday	
Saturday	
Sunday	

From *Breaking Free from Depression*. Copyright 2012 by The Guilford Press.

sleep log to a visit with her doctor, nothing major stood out that could be changed. However, when they delved deeper into the waking spells, Sarah and her doctor found that she had a pattern of negative thinking and worrying in the middle of the night. When something woke her from sleep (for example, the cat or her son's night terror), she began to worry. The negative "mind chatter" so common in depression started going. Sarah thought, "Why does my son keep having nightmares? Maybe I'm the cause. I'm never there for him during the day when I'm at work, when it matters most."

Sarah and her doctor put together a thought change record to explore the negative thinking that was happening at night and to create a more rational response. Sarah's nighttime thought change record is shown on page 260.

Sarah's nighttime thought change record helped her identify and change a pattern of negative thinking that often kept her up for hours at a time. She became adept at catching negative thoughts as they happened in the middle of the night, checking the thoughts for

Nighttime Thought Change Record: Sarah's Example

Event	Automatic thought(s)	Emotion(s)	Rational response	Outcome
Write down an event or situation, or a memory of an event, that triggered automatic thoughts.	1. Record the automatic thoughts that occurred while you were experiencing or thinking about this event. 2. Rate how much you believed the thought at the time it was happening. Use a 0–100 scale where 100=complete belief.	1. Identify emotions such as sadness or anger that were stimulated by the automatic thoughts. 2. Rate the intensity of the emotion on a 0–100 point scale where 100=the most extreme emotion.	1. Challenge the automatic thoughts by going off automatic pilot, examining the evidence, looking for cognitive errors, or other methods. 2. Write out some rational alternatives to the automatic thoughts. Rate your belief in the rational alternatives using a 0–100 scale.	1. Specify and rate subsequent emotions using a 0–100 scale. 2. Describe changes in behavior.
I wake up and start to worry.	I'm failing as a mom. 95 If this keeps up, my son will have a hard time in life. 75 I'm not around enough for my kids. 90 I can't do anything right. 90	Sad 95 Anxious 80 Overwhelmed 90	I'm using a lot of all-or-nothing thinking and jumping to conclusions here. It's okay to worry about my son having nightmares, but it's not all my fault. These things happen. I really do try to be a good mom. I love my kids, and I know they love me. 90 My son is doing well at school, so there really isn't any reason to believe that he will have a hard time growing up. He is surrounded by loving caregivers at home and at school. 90 I know it is tough being a single mom, but I do all right. I work hard and provide a loving home for my kids. 95 When I don't sleep, I feel more worried and sad, which makes things seem a lot worse then they really are. 90	Sad 50 Anxious 20 Overwhelmed 40 I feel like I am actually doing a good job as a mom. My kids are doing just fine, despite a few night terrors here and there. I shouldn't worry as much, especially in the middle of the night, when the exhaustion makes everything feel worse than it really is.

accuracy, and changing them to more rational alternatives. With a calm mind, she could more easily fall back to sleep. Try keeping a thought change record of your own (Exercise 11.4). You may want to keep a pen and paper at your bedside to record them as they happen or reflect back in the morning as to not keep yourself awake too long at night. Use whatever technique works best for you.

Exercise: A Natural Remedy That Can Work

As we have seen, getting a good night's sleep can help improve neurocognitive functioning and may help lift depression. There is also evidence that regular exercise may help with mild to moderate depression. You might be thinking, "How do you expect me to exercise when I don't have any energy?" or "I can't exercise because of my knee pain from osteoarthritis." We encourage you to use the CBT techniques you learned in Chapter 4 to challenge these thoughts. While emotional and physical hurdles may seem like they are insurmountable, there are many ways to make exercise work for you. Let's explore some of the options in more detail.

SCIENCE CORNER   Several randomized controlled trials have found a positive benefit of exercise for depression. Although the exact mechanism is unknown, exercise may:

- Increase the body's natural "feel-good" endorphins.
- Have positive effects on neurotransmitters.
- Decrease stress hormones.

Aerobic exercise (for example, running or walking at a fast pace) seems to have the same effect as nonaerobic exercise (for example, lifting weights or doing floor exercises).

- A small number of studies showed that higher-energy exercise had greater benefit.
- A systematic review of several studies found evidence that yoga can improve depression symptoms, adding support that even low-impact exercise can help.

Improvement in depression may or may not be related to fitness level (for example, you don't have to have a body-builder physique or run marathons to find benefit from exercise).

Alberto

Alberto, a 38-year-old self-employed carpenter, has been suffering from moderate depression for several months. He feels very sluggish, and he has been eating and sleeping much more than usual. Having gained 20 pounds in the past 6 months, Alberto feels down about his body image, and these negative thoughts have made his depression even worse. He just can't seem to get going. When a friend suggested he

Nighttime Thought Change Record

Event	Automatic thought(s)	Emotion(s)	Rational response	Outcome
Write down an event or situation, or a memory of an event, that triggered automatic thoughts.	1. *Record the automatic thoughts that occurred while you were experiencing or thinking about this event.* 2. *Rate how much you believed the thought at the time it was happening. Use a 0–100 scale where 100 = complete belief.*	1. *Identify emotions such as sadness or anger that were stimulated by the automatic thoughts.* 2. *Rate the intensity of the emotion on a 0–100 point scale where 100 = the most extreme emotion.*	1. *Challenge the automatic thoughts by going off automatic pilot, examining the evidence, looking for cognitive errors, or other methods.* 2. *Write out some rational alternatives to the automatic thoughts. Rate your belief in the rational alternatives using a 0–100 scale.*	1. *Specify and rate subsequent emotions using a 0–100 scale.* 2. *Describe changes in behavior.*

try walking in the neighborhood a few times a week, Alberto thought "How do you expect me to exercise when I can barely get dressed every day?"

Sometimes it can seem like a monumental effort to take the first steps toward feeling better. For you, it might be getting out of bed, taking a shower, or, like Alberto, getting dressed for the day. Exercise might seem like the last thing on your list. We encourage you to question this view and to consider making exercise a top priority. We're not asking you to run a race or spend hours in the gym; we simply want you to get your body moving.

The take-home point is that the overwhelming majority of research suggests that any regular exercise is good exercise. These findings suggest that even small steps toward introducing exercise may help boost your mood. Often exercise begets exercise. Once you "take the plunge" and get started, you will feel more energy and be more likely to stick to a regular exercise regimen. Can you think of some ways to get started with exercise?

Alberto's worksheet on beginning an exercise program is shown on page 265.

Alberto remembered how good he felt when he was swimming regularly in high school on the swim team. The quiet, repetitive nature of swimming helped to clear his mind and always made him feel better. Although there was some expense to joining a facility with a pool, Alberto found a good membership deal at his local "Y" and started swimming twice a week. Once he was back into the swing of things, he began to feel better physically. As he felt his energy come back, he added more sessions to the weekly routine. Now he swims three or four times a week in the mornings. Without using medications, Alberto found that his mood lifted. Along with some self-help CBT exercises, Alberto was able to pull out of the depression.

? What if I hit a plateau with exercise?

Many people find it frustrating when they hit a plateau or lose momentum with their exercise regimen. You may find your usual routine boring or stop going to the gym for a while when things get tough with depression. It's hard to get back on track, but here are a few tips that might help:

- Try to stay positive.

  - Don't get down on yourself for setbacks, but try to avoid relying on excuses to get you out of doing exercise. Remember, you don't need to set any records. Try to focus on the positive impact that exercise can have on depression.

  - Try using a fitness "mantra" (a few encouraging, calming, or inspirational words that you can say over and over) to keep you going through a workout. For example, you might say to yourself, "fit body, fit mind" or "I can do this for myself."

- Mix it up.

  - It's easy to get stuck in the same routine. If you take the same walk day after day, you might begin to lose interest, and it will be harder to maintain regular exercise. You could try doing something different, such as a new walking route or an alternate activity (for example, bike riding, jogging, or taking a dance lesson). Branch out and be creative.

- Exercise with a friend.

  ○ Ask a friend or family member to go along with you on your next jog or trip to the pool. Time can go by a lot faster with company, and you can motivate each other if you get in a slump.

- Join a team.

  ○ Some people find that exercise is easier when it doesn't feel like a "chore." Perhaps joining a team is the way to go for you. Try joining a softball team or a regular pick-up basketball game. Not only is it a good way to get exercise, but it will help get you out of the house and spend time with others.

  ○ An added bonus: When your teammates depend on you, it can make you feel good about yourself.

Martha

Martha is a 72-year-old retired social worker who has diabetes and severe knee pain from advanced osteoarthritis (wear-and-tear arthritis). She has suffered from depression for many years and lately has been feeling very down about complications from her diabetes (poor eyesight) and worsening pain from her arthritis. Martha has struggled with her weight much of her life. At her last visit with Dr. McCray, Martha expressed her frustration about exercise:

Dr. McCray: Martha, I recommend that you start some low-impact exercise to help with your medical problems. Small amounts of weight loss, even 5–10% of your current weight, can help control your diabetes and decrease the impact of extra weight on your joints. Plus, exercise can help with the depression.

Martha: No offense, doctor, but I have too much pain to do that sort of thing. How do you expect me to exercise when my knees hurt so badly? Plus, I'm scared to go walking outside because my eyesight isn't as good as it used to be, and I'm afraid I might trip and fall.

Dr. McCray: I understand it will be difficult for you, but let's try to think of some solutions. First, we need to make sure your pain is under better control …

Martha's situation is not uncommon. Many people have to deal with multiple issues that can affect their ability to make lifestyle changes such as exercising. In Martha's case, medical problems made it seem impossible for her to start an exercise regimen. Other barriers can include financial limitations (for example, access to a gym, equipment, or exercise gear), time constraints (for example, working full time, raising kids, or doing

Getting Started with Exercise: Alberto's Example

Instructions: Think of some kinds of exercise that you would like to try. Then fill in the blank spots in the table to help you get going with your exercise plan.

Exercise	Interest level (rate your interest in this type of exercise on a scale of 0–100)	Things I will need to get started	Potential obstacles to this exercise	Solutions to potential obstacles	Possible benefits to this exercise
Walking	80	Good walking shoes (I already have them)	Rough neighborhood to walk in	Walk during daylight hours with friend	Getting out of the house, getting fresh air, and spending time with an old friend. Feeling more energetic and more fit.
Swimming	90	Gym or YMCA membership to use the pool	Cost of gym membership	Try the Y first; it may be less expensive; see if there are any pool-only memberships	The rhythmic nature of swimming will help clear my mind. I may feel more energy and lose a few pounds.

shift work at night), or negative thoughts (for example, "It's just not for me," "I could never get fit," or "I've failed so many times in the past, I'm bound to fail again").

It's important to explore possible barriers to lifestyle changes with your doctor, your family or friends, or yourself. Use some of the CBT techniques you have learned to explore whether your perceived barriers are as big as you think they are. Think of ways you might be able to overcome such obstacles.

In Martha's case, she and her doctor had to be creative about finding safe ways for her to exercise (see page 267). Martha's daughter, Alice, was helpful in identifying some of the possible solutions. For instance, Alice reminded her mother that there was a gym in the senior center with support staff to help and also reassured Martha that walking with friends could be a safe way to exercise. Sometimes you have to go beyond your comfort zone or enlist family or friends to make difficult lifestyle changes such as adding exercise to your daily routine. Try Exercise 11.6 on page 268 to explore some of your barriers to exercise.

Getting Started with Exercise

Instructions: Think of some kinds of exercise that you would like to try. Then fill in the blank spots in the table to help you get going with your exercise plan.

Exercise	Interest level (rate your interest in this type of exercise on a scale of 0–100)	Things I will need to get started	Potential obstacles to this exercise	Solutions to potential obstacles	Possible benefits to this exercise

Exploring Barriers to Exercise: Martha's Example

Instructions: List some of the potential barriers to starting or maintaining an exercise regimen. Then challenge the barrier by going off automatic pilot, examining the evidence for and against the barrier, looking for cognitive errors, or other CBT methods. Then think of some possible solutions to overcoming the barrier.

Identify the barrier	Challenge the barrier	Possible ways to overcome the barrier
My knees hurt too much to exercise.	I do have knee pain, but maybe I'm on automatic pilot, so I think that everything I do will cause me pain. I haven't even tried to exercise, so I don't know if I will have pain or not. I know my daily pain is worse with stairs and bending, but I haven't tried anything like swimming or the stationary bicycle.	Talk with my doctor about better pain control for my knees. Try swimming or the stationary bicycle first. If I have too much pain, scale back and talk with my doctor.
I'm too old to exercise; I'll never be able to do it.	I'm having some all-or-nothing thinking here. I don't know if I can do it, because I haven't even tried yet. Some of my friends exercise at the senior center and walk in the neighborhood.	I'll try not to use age as an excuse. Although my vision is too bad for me to walk alone outside, maybe I can try walking with friends at the track. I can ask a volunteer at the senior center to show me how to use the stationary bicycle in the gym.

QUICK TIPS   One of the best ways to stick with exercise is to make it part of your routine.

- Pick certain days of the week when you plan to work out.
- Circle them on the calendar or mark them down in your planner to keep yourself accountable.
- Don't get down on yourself if you miss a workout.

Set healthy goals for exercise, such as:

- Join a class, walking group, or "boot camp."
- Sign up for a 5K or charity walk.
- If weight loss is a goal, shoot for ½–1 pound per week or 5–10% of your body weight over 4–6 months.

Think of reasonable "rewards" for sticking to your routine. Examples might be treating yourself to a new book or downloading some music.

Exploring Barriers to Exercise

Instructions: List some of the potential barriers to starting or maintaining an exercise regimen. Then challenge the barrier by going off automatic pilot, examining the evidence for and against the barrier, looking for cognitive errors, or other CBT methods. Then think of some possible solutions to overcoming the barrier.

Identify the barrier	Challenge the barrier	Possible ways to overcome the barrier

Can Your Diet Have an Influence on Depression?

The one-word answer to this question is *maybe*. But the story behind diet and depression is complex. If you go to a health-food store, read articles on nutrition in magazines, or search the Internet for advice on diet and depression, it is easy to get confused. There are many claims for the effectiveness of diets that are high in serotonin, carbohydrates, or other compounds, and there are suggestions that vitamin supplements can be an answer to depression. In sticking with our plan to present evidence-based recommendations in this book, we carefully reviewed research on diet and depression to help sort out the facts from the myths. Let's start with the myths about dietary intake and depression.

MYTHS ABOUT DIET AND DEPRESSION

- Foods that are high in serotonin can relieve depression.

- A diet that is heavy on carbohydrates is a good treatment for depression.

- Chocolate reduces depressive symptoms.

- Vitamin supplements help depression in people who do not have vitamin deficiencies.

Although it may seem reasonable to try to eat foods that contain serotonin-like compounds or may stimulate the production of serotonin, there is no solid evidence that you can raise serotonin or other neurotransmitter levels in the brain by altering the foods that you eat. In fact, serotonin is manufactured by the body and isn't directly available in food. There is an amino acid, L-tryptophan, that plays a role in the synthesis of the neurotransmitters serotonin, dopamine, and neurepinephrine and is available in pill form. L-tryptophan has been studied as an adjunct (or booster) for treatment with antidepressants. However, after an extensive review of this research, Dr. Jerome Sarris and colleagues from the University of Queensland in Australia concluded that there was not enough evidence to recommend use of L-tryptophan in treating depression.

Some authors have speculated that high-carbohydrate diets (for example, with lots of pasta, potatoes, and bread products) might be useful for depression, but research hasn't supported this theory. A study on chocolate and depression that was titled "Mood Food" found somewhat surprising results. While we suspect that most people would say that chocolate gives them a sense of pleasure or well-being, doctors from the University of California found that higher levels of chocolate in the diet were associated with increased symptoms of depression! People in the group with the highest depression scores ate more than double the number of servings of chocolate as those who had the lowest depression scores. This study didn't prove that chocolate caused the increased levels of depression. Perhaps people who are depressed eat more chocolate in an attempt to feel better or to soothe themselves but the chocolate doesn't do the job. We don't think that this single study should dissuade people from enjoying chocolate or justifies a recommendation to decrease chocolate intake as a treatment for depression. Yet the findings do raise questions about possible connections between chocolate consumption and mood.

Are you one of the many millions of people who take vitamin or mineral supplements daily? A survey of vitamin use in the United States found that about one-third of people reported that they regularly used one or more supplements. Although there can be many good reasons for taking vitamins and minerals, research hasn't backed up theories that supplemental vitamins help reduce depression in people who do not have a specific vitamin deficiency.

As we noted in Chapter 2, deficiencies of three vitamins—folate, vitamin D, and vitamin B_{12}—have been associated with depression in some, but not all, studies. We don't recommend routine vitamin supplements for depression unless a specific deficiency has been diagnosed with blood tests. If you have questions about possible vitamin deficiencies, you can review the section on this topic in Chapter 2 and consult with your doctor.

The Mediterranean Diet

Studies of the frequency of depression in different areas of the world have found that people who live in Mediterranean areas such as the south of Spain have lower rates of depression and suicide than those who live in northern Europe. One possible explanation for this difference is the diet of people who live in regions bordering the Mediterranean Sea. A distinguishing feature of dietary habits in the Mediterranean area is the abundant use of olive oil—a rich source of monounsaturated fatty acids. Also, people in Mediterranean regions tend to have diets that emphasize consumption of fruits and nuts, vegetables, cereal, legumes (such as beans or lentils), and fish along with moderate consumption of red wine. Northern European and American diets typically include more meat and meat products, butter, and other foods that contain saturated fatty acids.

SCIENCE CORNER

- A study conducted in Spain at the University of Navarra with more than 9,000 people found a clear link between adherence to the Mediterranean diet and lowered risk for depression.
- The risk for becoming depressed was about twice as high in people who had the lowest adherence to the Mediterranean diet compared with those who had good or strong adherence to this dietary pattern.
- Other studies have found that people who eat "Western diets" that are high in processed or "fast foods," meats, and other sources of saturated fats have higher rates of depression than those who eat healthier diets.

There isn't any research evidence that eating a Mediterranean diet can be used as an effective monotherapy (used alone, without other evidence-based treatments) for depression, but there are very strong suggestions that this type of diet may reduce the risk of depression. Also, the Mediterranean diet and similar diets that emphasize monounstaturated fats and healthy foods like vegetables, fruits, and cereals have been shown to reduce the risk of heart disease. Thus we think that this type of diet may benefit people who suffer from depression or have an increased risk of becoming depressed.

How does your diet shape up in comparison to the Mediterranean diet? The study at the University of Navarro rated the quality of diets on several key elements that we have included in the next exercise. You can use this worksheet to get a general idea of how close your diet comes to being a "Mediterranean diet." (To do the exercise again, photocopy the form or download it from *www.guilford.com/breakingfreeforms*.) We don't include alcohol consumption on this checklist because of the association between depression and substance abuse. Nevertheless, moderate consumption of red wine is a basic element of the Mediterranean diet. If you don't have a problem with excessive use of alcohol, a glass of red wine a day could be a part of a Mediterranean diet plan.

The highest score on the Mediterranean diet checklist is an 18. If your score was moderately high or at the top end of the range, you are probably eating a diet that may help reduce the risk of depression. But if your score is in the lower end of the range, there may be some diet adjustments for you to consider.

Omega-3 Polyunsaturated Fatty Acids

Omega-3 fatty acids, which are usually derived from fish oils, are popular dietary supplements because of their positive effects on blood lipids and cardiovascular health. Research has suggested that these positive benefits may extend to brain function because omega-3 fatty acids increase serotonin, norepinephrine, and dopamine levels while other fatty acids that are a common part of Western, urbanized diets may actually have a negative effect on neurotransmission (communication between brain cells).

Most of the early studies on omega-3 fatty acids found that 1–2 grams of these supplements daily were more effective for depression than placebo. But several later trials did not support their efficacy. A review of 19 studies of omega-3 fatty acid supplements for depression conducted by Dr. Rocha Araujo and associates from the Federal University of Rio de Janeiro found 13 reports of positive effects of omega-3 fatty acids and six negative studies. Other reviews and meta-analyses have also found mixed results but an overall positive trend for the usefulness of these supplements. Although the "jury is still out" on omega-3 fatty acids in the treatment of depression, these supplements are safe and have few side effects (mild gastrointestinal distress is the most common problem), can help with heart health, and may be a worthwhile adjunct to other evidence-based methods for getting depression under control.

Could Reducing Your Weight Reduce Your Depression?

Weight loss is not considered to be a treatment for depression. Yet for some people who struggle with chronic depression and being chronically overweight, a rational weight-

Mediterranean Diet Checklist

Instructions: Rate how strongly you emphasize the different food groups below in your current diet. Then you can compute a total score by adding the scores for each food group. *Note*: Positive scores are given for eating moderate or large amounts of food groups in the Mediterranean diet and negative scores for smaller amounts of foods that have lots of saturated fats.

Food or food group	I eat this food or food group infrequently. It is no more than a minor part of my diet.	I eat this food or food group a moderate amount, but it is not a major feature of my diet.	I eat this food or food group routinely. It is a major feature of my diet.	Total score for food or food group
Cereal and grains	Score: 0	Score: 1	Score: 2	
Fish	Score: 0	Score: 1	Score: 2	
Fruits and nuts	Score: 0	Score: 1	Score: 2	
Vegetables	Score: 0	Score: 1	Score: 2	
Legumes (beans, lentils)	Score: 0	Score: 1	Score: 2	
Olive oil*	Score: 0	Score: 1	Score: 2	
Meat and meat products	Score: 2	Score:1	Score: 0	
Fast foods and other convenience foods that are high in saturated fat content	Score: 2	Score: 1	Score: 0	
Total score				

*Use of olive oil is a bit hard to rate using this checklist because most people on the Mediterranean diet don't consume large amounts of it daily. The important thing is to emphasize the use of olive oil as a fat in your diet instead of butter and other saturated animal fats. So, give yourself a score of 2 on this item if you predominately use olive oil in food preparation and consumption; or give yourself a score of 0 if you rarely if ever use olive oil but consume butter and animal fats on a regular basis.

loss program can help build self-esteem and be part of a path toward full recovery. In our clinical practices, we typically don't emphasize weight-loss efforts as a major part of treating acute depression. People who are depressed have lots of other issues to face, and it can be discouraging to think that you might have to lose weight to feel less depressed. Also, research supports the effectiveness of many other approaches such as CBT and antidepressants. Thus it is usually best to tackle the depression first and then focus efforts on a weight-loss program when you are feeling better, have more energy, and your attention isn't diverted by more immediate issues and problems.

For people who seem to have depression deeply entwined with being overweight or who have had persistent depression and obesity, one of the goals of treatment can be to reduce weight. We have worked with people who have had great success at doing so and in turn have felt much better about themselves and have gained strength against depression.

When we recommend weight-loss programs to our patients, we prefer plans such as Weight Watchers, which promote healthful cooking and eating for sustainable healthy eating habits over time. If you have found the CBT approach helpful for depression, you might want to read books by Judith Beck, PhD, about CBT methods for diet control (*The Beck Diet Solution* and *The Complete Beck Diet for Life*).

Alcohol and Drugs

Many people who suffer from depression also have difficulties with drug or alcohol abuse. We've already discussed the impact that substances such as alcohol and nicotine can have on sleep. Unfortunately, people who have both depression and substance abuse are at risk for underdiagnosis and undertreatment of depression, relapse of depression, and increased rates of suicide. Check out Exercise 11.8 to see whether you might have problems with substance abuse.

If you answered "yes" to any of the questions in Exercise 11.8, you may be at risk for or are suffering from substance abuse. While it may seem difficult or impossible to break a habit like drug or alcohol use, there are many reasons to consider getting help. Despite the short-lived high from "uppers" or the numbing effect of "downers," drugs and alcohol often make people feel even worse at the end of the day and can contribute to worsening depression and suicidal thinking. People are more likely to take their own lives when under the influence, and drugs and alcohol in their own right can be fatal in overdose. Substance abuse can lead to a higher risk of trauma, including motor vehicle accidents, and medical illnesses such as liver disease and seizures.

If you or a loved one is affected by drug or alcohol abuse, please get help. Consider trying a local support group or 12-step program, such as Alcoholics Anonymous (AA). Contact your doctor to discuss treatment options, which might include intensive outpatient treatment, medication, or an inpatient (residential) stay. CBT is being used increasingly as a component of substance abuse treatment. So the lessons you are learning in this book may give you a head start on getting effective treatment. Several national resources are listed in the box on pages 274–275.

EXERCISE 11.8	The CAGE Questionnaire

Instructions: Answer the following four questions about your drinking or drug use. If you answer "yes" to one or more of them, you may be suffering from alcohol or drug abuse. Please consider talking to your doctor, therapist, or a supportive person about drinking or drug use and check out the national resources listed later in this section.

CAGE question	Answer (yes or no)
Have you ever felt the need to **C**ut down on drinking or drug use?	
Have you ever felt **A**nnoyed by criticism of your drinking or drug use?	
Have you ever had **G**uilty feelings about your drinking or drug use?	
Do you ever take a morning **E**ye opener (a drink or drug first thing in the morning to get rid of a hangover or settle your nerves)?	

From *Breaking Free from Depression*. Copyright 2012 by The Guilford Press.

QUICK TIPS   Places you can get information on substance abuse treatment:

- **U.S. Department of Health and Human Services/Substance Abuse and Mental Health Services Administration (SAMHSA):** A government agency that provides information such as a "Quick Guide to Finding Effective Alcohol and Substance Abuse Treatment."
  - *www.samhsa.gov/treatment*
  - 24-hour hotline (800) 662-HELP (4357)

- **National Institute on Drug Abuse (NIDA):** A government-sponsored institute focused on drug abuse and addiction research.
  - *www.nida.nih.gov*
  - (301) 443-1124

- **Alcoholics Anonymous (AA):** A 12-step program which holds group meetings (both in person and online)
  - *www.aa.org*
  - Check your local listings for regional phone numbers.

- **Chemically Dependent Anonymous (CDA):**
  - *www.cdaweb.org*
  - (888) CDA-HOPE

- Cocaine Anonymous (CA):
  - *www.ca.org*
  - (800) 347-8998

- Narcotics Anonymous (NA):
  - *www.na.org*
  - (818) 773-9999

- **Al-Anon and Alateen:** A support group for friends and families of problem drinkers.
  - *www.al-anon.alateen.org*
  - (888) 4AL-ANON (425-2666)

Seasonal Affective Disorder

Are you one of the people who are sensitive to the amount of light in your environment and feel more depressed when days grow shorter as the season changes? Seasonal affective disorder (SAD) is considered a "subtype" of depression in which symptoms appear during seasons of low light.

As you might expect, SAD may be more common in people who live at higher latitudes, where there is more seasonal variation and there are seasons with pronounced reductions in the amount of daylight. SAD has been linked to low levels of the neurotransmitter serotonin and shifts in circadian rhythms (the 24-hour cycle of sleeping, waking, and other activities). Light therapy (exposure to strong artificial lights from a light "box") can moderate these seasonal variations.

SCIENCE CORNER   Light Therapy for Seasonal Affective Disorder

- Experts in using light therapy typically recommend using 10,000 lux (a measure of light intensity) for 30 minutes in the morning. If a light box generates only 2,500 lux, the duration of treatment must be extended to 2 hours daily to get the same response.
- To compare light intensities, consider that indoor evening room light is usually less than 90 lux, and a brightly lit office is typically less than 500 lux.
- Common side effects of light therapy include eye strain (avoid looking directly into the light) and headache.
- If you have a disease of the retina, don't use light therapy without the approval of an eye doctor.
- People with bipolar disorder can experience overactivation from light therapy.
- *Caution*: Do not use tanning beds as a light box substitute; they have significant harmful UV rays and do not provide the same therapeutic effect.

For people who experience moderate to severe seasonal depression, depression with suicidal thinking, or SAD that doesn't improve with light therapy, antidepressants may be considered as first-line therapy before (or in addition to) light therapy. Antidepressants have been found to be effective for SAD in many studies.

CBT also has been shown to improve depression symptoms in SAD and may prevent relapse of seasonal depression. One large study by Dr. Kelly Rohan and coworkers found that adding CBT to light therapy appeared to give greater benefit than treatment with light therapy alone.

The "bottom line" on light therapy is that it is an easy-to-use, effective treatment for SAD that has few side effects. Although insurance companies usually do not pay for light boxes, there are many good online sources for light therapy devices. If you have a seasonal pattern to depression, it will probably be worth making the investment in a light box and using this helpful method when the days grow shorter. You also might look at how you spend your time in the winter. Do you tend to "hibernate" and stay indoors, or do you make a special effort to get outdoors and take in as much sunlight as possible? If you have the time and resources, could a beach trip or another vacation in the sun make a difference? On the days when you aren't working, could you make a special effort to get outdoors to take a walk or do some other exercise? Natural sunlight has a much brighter intensity than light boxes, so try to take advantage of any outdoor time that you can.

Lifestyle Changes in Your Path to Feeling Good

None of the lifestyle changes that we have outlined here should be considered "stand-alone" treatments for moderate to severe depression, but they can play significant roles in a comprehensive plan for recovery. Now that you have read about the options for lifestyle modifications and have worked through the self-help exercises, it could help to organize your plan for the future and to highlight some of the important reasons to keep focused on change. Do Exercise 11.9 (on page 277); as your plan evolves, do it again using a photocopy of the worksheet or one downloaded from *www.guilford.com/breakingfree-forms*.

Summary

If you have lifestyle issues that are affecting depression, it may be time to take action. Even if change seems difficult or impossible, there is often a way to break through long-standing habits that may be pulling you down. And there are some very practical and useful methods such as using sleep hygiene principles and getting into a steady exercise pattern that could help you reverse symptoms of depression and feel better.

In the next chapter, we'll take a look at another path toward wellness—a path that is very important for all people who are interested in the spiritual dimension of their lives and may be searching for ways to draw power from their spirituality as they work on overcoming depression.

EXERCISE 11.9	My Plan for Lifestyle Change			
Lifestyle areas	**My degree of difficulties/problems in this area** (rate on 0–10 point scale where 0 = no problems and 10 = maximum problems)	**How much I believe that change in this area could benefit me** (rate on 0–10 point scale where 0 = no benefit and 10 = maximum benefit)	**Main motivators for change (payoffs for making changes)**	**Key actions I will take to change**
Sleep				
Exercise				
Diet				
Alcohol and substance use				
Seasonal changes in depression				

From *Breaking Free from Depression*. Copyright 2012 by The Guilford Press. Additional copies of this exercise can be downloaded from *www.guilford.com/breakingfreeforms*.

THE SPIRITUAL PATH

12

Using Spiritual Resources

Chapter Highlights

◗ Defining spirituality

◗ What's the evidence? Research on the link between depression and spirituality

◗ An inventory of your spiritual resources

◗ Searching for meaning

◗ Putting your spiritual resources to work

The word "spirituality" has many meanings. For some people spirituality may be shaped largely by the beliefs and practices of a particular religious tradition. Others don't participate in a formal religion yet do consider themselves spiritual. Polls have shown that more than 95% of Americans say that they have a spiritual dimension, and more than 50% indicate that religion is a very important influence in their lives.

One of the foremost authorities on the relationship between spirituality and health, Dr. Harold Koenig, recommends that a broad concept of spirituality be used in trying to help people cope with illness "so that all patients have an opportunity to have their needs addressed (in whatever way they define those spiritual needs)." We agree with this point; and in writing this chapter we've attempted to give general suggestions that can be used by people who have a variety of spiritual backgrounds and beliefs.

Defining Spirituality

The definition of spirituality given in Chapter 2 and used here is drawn from the work of Dr. Fredrick Luskin from Stanford University and Dr. Roger Walsh, author of *Essential Spirituality.*

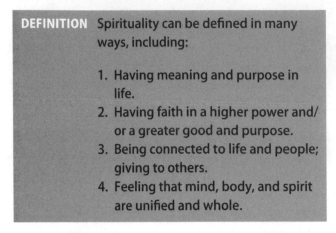

DEFINITION Spirituality can be defined in many ways, including:

1. Having meaning and purpose in life.
2. Having faith in a higher power and/or a greater good and purpose.
3. Being connected to life and people; giving to others.
4. Feeling that mind, body, and spirit are unified and whole.

The Dalai Lama has described spirituality as "being concerned with those qualities of the human spirit—such as love and compassion, patience, tolerance, forgiveness ... a sense of harmony which brings happiness to self and others." In his book *Ethics for a New Millennium*, he tells a story about how a balance between mind, body, and spirit has been so important in his life: "Having lost my country at the age of sixteen and become a refugee at twenty-four, I have faced a great many difficulties in my life. When I consider these, I see that a lot of them were insurmountable. Not only were they unavoidable, they were incapable of favorable resolutions. Nonetheless, in terms of my own peace of mind and physical health, I can claim to have coped reasonably well. As a result, I have been able to meet adversity with all my resources—mental, physical, and spiritual."

A close integration of spirituality with the mental and physical domains of life is a common theme in the teachings of many of the world's religions and philosophical traditions. For example, the YMCA, which was developed originally as a Christian-supported organization but is largely secular now and reaches out to people of all beliefs, uses the slogan "Spirit–Mind–Body" and a logo with a triangle to show the connection between these fundamental aspects of being human.

If you identify with any part of the definition of spirituality that we offer here, you may find that the following pages offer some useful suggestions for drawing from your spiritual resources in your fight against depression.

What's the Evidence? Research on the Link between Depression and Spirituality

Can spirituality be considered an "evidence-based treatment"? To get the facts straight from the beginning, it's important to note that spiritual and/or religious practices in themselves are not considered specific treatment methods for depression in the same way that antidepressants, CBT, and other evidence-based therapies are. Most religious and philosophical authorities recommend that people who have significant depression receive psychotherapy, medication, or both and have access to trained health care professionals for treatment. However, building spiritual strengths can be an important part of an overall recovery plan for many people with depression.

What about well-being therapy and mindfulness-based therapy? Are they spiritually based treatments? Earlier in this book we discussed well-being therapy, and in the next chapter we explain the basics of the mindfulness approach to treatment of depression. Both of these evidence-based therapies could be considered to have a spiritual layer among other potential mechanisms of action. Well-being therapy is concerned in part with enhancing a sense of meaning and purpose, and mindfulness practices can promote peace, calm, compassion, and other positive emotions and behaviors that are consistent with a broad definition of spirituality. However, developers of both therapies make it clear that they are not religiously based, and both therapies use a variety of methods from CBT and other approaches that do not require a spiritual orientation to life. Therefore, we discuss these two specific treatments for depression in separate chapters.

What effects does depression have on spirituality? Research on the effects of depression on spirituality has found that depression often darkens the spirit. When people become depressed they can feel empty, have trouble finding meaning in their lives, and become disconnected from people as they turn inward in their suffering. If they believe in a higher power, they may feel distant or disengaged from God, and they may drift away from attending religious services or engaging in other spiritual practices. If they feel they are spiritually oriented but wouldn't call themselves religious, they may feel a loss of connection to the natural world or other things that used to make life worthwhile. For these people, it may seem that mind, body, and spirit are not in harmony—there is no sense of wholeness and completeness.

Reduced use of spiritual resources can be part of the downward spiral of depression. As a person becomes disconnected from the things that give life meaning and purpose, a sense of despair and hopelessness can escalate. And participation in spiritually linked activities that promote positive emotional health may dwindle further or stop completely.

Can spirituality have a protective effect against depression? A large amount of research has examined the possibility that spiritually oriented practices might decrease the risk for depression or offer ways to help relieve depression; see the Science Corner for some findings.

SCIENCE CORNER   In a review of studies on spirituality and depression, Dr. Harold Koenig concluded:

1. Spiritual activities are positively related to hope, optimism, positive emotions, and life satisfaction.
2. Many people (90–95% in some studies) report that spiritual/religious practices help them cope with illnesses.
3. Most studies have shown that people who participate in religious services have lower rates of depression.
4. Spiritual/religious beliefs and activities decrease the risk for suicide.

The exact mechanisms by which spiritual involvement may serve as a protective factor against depression aren't known. But Dr. Koenig and others have concluded that social support, encouragement of positive health behaviors (for example, taking good care of your body, avoiding alcohol and drug abuse), and reaching out to help others (for example, by following the "Golden Rule" of "doing unto others what you would have them do unto you") might explain some of the reduced risk for depression.

Other studies have examined the impact of having a sense of meaning and purpose on depression. One particularly revealing study was performed by Drs. Maselko, Gilman, and Buka from Temple, Harvard, and Brown Universities. Their large investigation found that people who reported the highest levels of having meaning and purpose in life were 70% less likely to have suffered from depression than those who reported the lowest levels of meaning and purpose. In this study, people with the highest rates of religious service attendance were 30% less likely to have been depressed than those with the lowest rates of attendance. Similar findings have been reported by many other researchers. For example, in a study of people with prostate cancer and depression, Drs. Christian Nelson and coworkers found that there was a small relationship between religiosity and reduced levels of depression. However, there was a much larger effect of a more general form of spirituality on lowered depressive symptoms. They concluded that "the main component that may reduce depression is a sense of meaning and peace."

People of all beliefs and philosophical backgrounds can share the goal of finding meaning in life, so this chapter focuses largely on this important aspect of spirituality. First, however, we ask you to take an inventory of some spiritual resources that you might already have or you might want to develop further.

An Inventory of Your Spiritual Resources

If depression has seemed to weaken your spirit or you have fallen out of the habit of participating in spiritually oriented activities, the next exercise might help you identify some ways that you could use spirituality on your path to wellness. If you are already tapping significantly into your spiritual capacities, just taking stock of them now can help you plan ways to keep using them or even enhance them in the future. For some people spirituality is ingrained but rarely acknowledged, so doing the following journaling exercise can reveal resources you might be able to rely on more heavily in your quest to conquer depression. To do the exercise again in the future—or if in your journaling you need more space than the worksheet allows—photocopy the worksheet or download it from *www. guilford.com/breakingfreeforms*.

Because we intended this book for a general audience, we won't discuss details of using faith-based spiritual resources that are specific to any of the wide variety of religions practiced today. But we will ask you to think about ways of using some universally recognized spiritual resources that may help you in your efforts to overcome depression.

Searching for Meaning

Viktor Frankl, one of the most influential psychiatrists of the 20th century, was imprisoned in a Nazi concentration camp during World War II. During his time in these horrific circumstances, he was struck by how people could still find a sense of meaning and purpose, even in the face of severe deprivation and fear of imminent death. Although the ability to somehow find meaning in the darkest of hours didn't immunize people against

Taking Stock of Your Spiritual Resources

Instructions: Spend several days thinking about the following questions as you go about your daily routine. At the end of each day, note the spiritual experiences you've had. Once you feel you've recorded a good representation of your spiritual life, use the second half of the form to record any changes you might like to make.

PART I: A SPIRITUAL JOURNAL

In what ways do I find meaning in my life and the life of those around me?

_____

_____

What makes me feel as if I'm not alone but part of a larger universe?

_____

_____

How do my daily decisions take into account what's best for those beyond myself—my family, my friends, my community, the environment?

_____

_____

In times of trouble, where do I turn for solace?

_____

_____

Was I brought up in a particular religious tradition, or have I had other religious experiences? If so, what role do religious practices have in my life today?

_____

_____

How often do I attend religious services?

_____

_____

(cont.)

Do I go out of my way to commune with nature or with a deity on my own (for example, pray, meditate, go on retreats or pilgrimages)?

_____

_____

Do I read the Bible, the Koran, or other spiritual literature?

_____

_____

PART II: A SPIRITUAL ASSESSMENT

After reflecting on my answers to the preceding questions, how would I define my spirituality? Minimal? Undeveloped? Rich? Highly evolved?

_____

_____

How important is spirituality to my life?

_____

_____

Do I want to enhance my experience of spirituality or add to my spiritual resources in any way?

_____

_____

How could spiritual resources—those that I have and those that I could have—help me on my path to wellness?

_____

_____

What are three things I could do to strengthen or add to my spiritual resources should I feel the need?

1. _____

2. _____

3. _____

the terrors of the concentration camp, Dr. Frankl did observe that those with a greater sense of meaning had less despair and depression, held more hope for the future, and appeared to have a greater ability to survive.

He wrote that "one could make a victory out of those experiences, turning life into an inner triumph, or one could ignore the challenge and simply vegetate." It was obviously quite a challenge to retain a sense of meaning or find new ways of having a purpose in the concentration camp environment. But Dr. Frankl learned that the human spirit could find many ways to experience meaning—even when surrounding forces were determined to grind this spirit to dust. A core belief that kept Dr. Frankl going was that the Nazis couldn't take away a basic human freedom, "to choose one's attitude in any given set of circumstances—to choose one's own way."

Tragically, Dr. Frankl's wife, mother, father, and brother all died in concentration camps. But Dr. Frankl was liberated at the end of World War II and went on to have a distinguished career as a professor at the University of Vienna. Shortly after release from the camp, he wrote *Man's Search for Meaning*—a book that has been heralded as one of the "ten most influential books in America" by the Library of Congress. In this book he described the basic tenets of "logotherapy," a treatment method that derives its name from *logos*, the Greek word for meaning. Logotherapy hasn't been tested extensively in scientific studies, but its concepts have been integrated into many widely used, evidence-based treatments such as CBT and well-being therapy.

In his books, Dr. Frankl has given suggestions for ways to define meaning and to search for it. He considers meaning a primary motivation for life. In his framework, meaning can include these characteristics: (1) striving for a worthwhile goal, (2) acting responsibly in the world, (3) moving from a self-centered existence to loving and doing for others, and (4) experiencing and appreciating "down-to-earth" things. One of the central messages in his work is that meaning does not have to be associated with grand contributions to society or with great achievement. Meaning can be found in facing difficult experiences (as he learned so deeply during his years in a concentration camp), in doing something for others, in appreciating nature or the beauty of music, in creating a work or deed, and in the simple acts of experiencing life.

The two key lessons from logotherapy that have influenced so many people are:

1. A sense of meaning is a positive life force that can counteract despair, hopelessness, and depression.
2. It is not enough simply to identify sources of meaning; people need to commit themselves to taking actions to express that meaning.

To help stimulate your thinking about ways to find meaning, we'll share some of Dr. Frankl's suggestions with you and give you some examples of how others found meaning.

Loving and Giving

An unfortunate byproduct of depression is the tendency to pull inward and become absorbed with negative ruminations. As you do this, you may unknowingly fall into the trap of showing less loving kindness, compassion, and concern both to self and others. You may show irritability instead of empathy or self-directed condemnation instead of interest in the key people in your life. Yet finding a way to show more love, or at least friendly caring, might offer you a way to have a greater sense of meaning and happiness.

Dr. Frankl wrote that "love is the ultimate and highest goal to which man can aspire.... The salvation of man is through love and in love." A Bible passage urges us to "Love thy neighbor as yourself." Psychiatrist David Viscott noted that "to love and be loved is to feel the Sun from both sides." If your heart has been darkened by depression, could you find routes to open it back to one of the most powerful ways to find meaning?

Martina's Story

Martina is in her mid-20s and has been depressed for more than a year. Fortunately, treatment with an antidepressant and CBT helped. When she took the PHQ-9 test at her doctor's office, the scores were usually between about 7 and 10 (mild depression). Much progress had been made. Yet something wasn't quite right in her world. It often felt like she was "just going through the motions." Martina went to work every day as a veterinary assistant—a job she always thought she would love. However, the job wasn't holding her full attention. She would often find herself daydreaming about the next vacation she might take or thinking about her plans for the next weekend instead of focusing on the job at hand or finding joy in her work. After returning home she often felt empty and restless. She felt almost like she was watching life from the sidelines.

Martina also had been noticing that she had been withdrawing from her boyfriend, Al, even though she really did love him and hoped to spend the rest of her life with him. Often she would find herself telling Al that it would be best if he found things he could do by himself or with his friends. Many of the little things that she used to do for Al had fallen by the wayside. She rarely helped him with small projects around the house, suggested books he might like to read, or left him hand-written notes of affection—things that used to be a routine part of her life with Al. The same type of changes had occurred in the way she worked with the animals that she cared for in her job as a veterinary assistant. Before becoming depressed, she was very intent on giving each of the animals a very warm and caring experience when they came to the office. But now she would often realize that she had spent hours at work without really being connected to the animals or their owners. Her mind and heart had been elsewhere.

Although Martina could use many of the other methods described in this book to try to reduce symptoms of depression further and get back her old style of caring for others, there also appeared to be an opportunity for her to focus on loving and giving as a way of having more meaningful and satisfying days. She used the next worksheet to target some areas for change.

If you think that loving and giving is already a prime source of meaning in your life, you can record these thoughts in Exercise 12.2. Or you can use this worksheet to generate some thoughts about possible ways to restore or build a sense of meaning and purpose.

Loving and Giving Worksheet: Martina's Example

Instructions: Try to think of at least one place in your life in which you could tune your senses to feelings of love, caring, or concern for others. Write down some thoughts about how these feelings are meaningful to you. Then write down a few specific ideas for positive ways to show your love or kindness.

A place in my life where I have feelings of love, caring, or concern for others	Thoughts about how these feelings are meaningful to me	Specific ideas for ways to show love or kindness
My relationship with Al	He means so much to me. He is a loving, sensitive, and interesting partner. I want to be with him for my whole life.	Take time to do things with Al. Make this relationship a high priority in my life. Do little things to show kindness and caring, even if it takes a lot of effort when I feel tired.
My work with animals	Taking good care of animals is a very fine thing to do. It means a lot to the animals and to their owners. I am fortunate to have a job that can be very meaningful.	Give my full attention to my work. If I drift off, bring myself back to the reality of being with the animals. Use all my senses to appreciate them.

Facing Adversity: Coping with a Loss

In *Man's Search for Meaning* there are many good illustrations of how people have found meaning in how they deal with life problems. In Dr. Frankl's case, aching for his wife who was in another concentration camp and then ultimately coping with her death challenged him sorely. Yet he was able to find abundant meaning in his fond memories of their deeply felt moments together. Instead of becoming derailed by grief, he was able to dedicate himself to his life's work and to share his experiences with finding meaning with many thousands of people.

Depression itself offers an opportunity to find meaning in facing adversity. Could you see ways to learn from depression, to grow personally as you find out more about yourself and search for ways to overcome this illness? Could working your way through depression give you a deeper commitment to life? Thomas Moore, the author of *Care of the Soul*, suggests that we can be "instructed by melancholy." No one would suggest that somebody become depressed to find greater meaning in life. Yet if one has the misfortune to suffer from depression, an avenue may open in the search for meaning.

We all will have occasions when bad things occur and life turns sour. Perhaps it will be the death of a relative or friend, a worrisome diagnosis, or a financial blow. Can you

Loving and Giving

Instructions: Try to think of at least one place in your life in which you could tune your senses to feelings of love, caring, or concern for others. Write down some thoughts about how these feelings are meaningful to you. Then write down a few specific ideas for positive ways to show your love or kindness.

A place in my life where I have feelings of love, caring, or concern for others	Thoughts about how these feelings are meaningful to me	Specific ideas for ways to show love or kindness

think of an event in your life that may have had a negative impact or was particularly trying for you? While it might seem hard to think of how anything positive could come from such an event, there may be ways to grow spiritually from the experience. Let's take a look at how Sean, a man who was reeling from the effects of a heart attack, found a way to enrich his life and the life of others as he moved forward.

Sean's Story

Sean is a man in his early 50s who became depressed after a heart attack. Before he had to confront serious physical illness, his life seemed to be going okay. He worked steadily as a restaurant manager and enjoyed creating a pleasant dining experience and meeting customers. He went to church with his family, played some golf at public courses, and planted a vegetable garden every year. Sean's biggest problem in life before having a heart attack was coping with the death of his brother in a car accident when they were both teenagers. Grief had hit him hard then and still gnawed at him at times. Yet Sean had been able to get past the grief as he went on to complete school, begin work, and start his own family.

Sean had a good relationship with his two children; the youngest had just started college the year before, and the oldest had gotten a good job as a paralegal. He had been married for almost 30 years to his wife, Rita, and there had never been any real troubles in the marriage. He had liked his job, even though he felt like he ate too much at work and always fought a weight problem. But after the heart attack, everything seemed to have been turned upside-down. He didn't have much energy, work seemed to be a burden, and the future looked dim. Life had taken another unexpected and cruel twist, and Sean was sad, mad, and scared. Wherever he looked, it was hard to feel the same sense of being centered and knowing what to expect next. He seemed to be adrift in a sea of worry without any clear paths to safe passages or anchorages.

Dr. Wright, who was helping Sean with depression, asked him some questions to see whether he could start to see meaning in his adversity.

> *Dr. Wright:* You've told me about your fears and worries for your health and how it seems that life will never be the same after having a heart attack. I know that the heart attack was a big shock and that it's hard to adjust, but could it have opened any doors for you? Is there any way that facing this problem or learning from it could add something to your life?
>
> *Sean:* I never really thought about it that way. I don't know. How could a heart attack add anything positive?
>
> *Dr. Wright:* I didn't mean that having a heart attack was a good thing. But it did occur, and now you are left with dealing with it. So maybe we could see if there is a way to capture some sense of direction from having to go through this tough experience.
>
> *Sean:* I guess I see what you're getting at. All I've been able to think about is how my life has gotten worse. [*Pauses for a moment*] I'm the opposite of one of my good friends. He has MS [*multiple sclerosis*], but he usually seems to be happier than people who don't have such big problems.
>
> *Dr. Wright:* Sometimes people find new layers of meaning in their lives when an

> illness shakes them up. Could your friend have developed a deeper sense of what counts in life as he's struggled with MS?
>
> *Sean:* I don't know, but I guess I could ask him—we've known each other for a long time.

Sean had a searching talk with his friend and continued to consult with Dr. Wright as he worked to come to grips with having a heart attack. Although the process wasn't easy, Sean eventually came to feel that coping with his illness could be a source of meaning and purpose in his life. He could show others, especially his children, how to accept a troubling situation with grace and a sense of responsibility to make the best of it. He could work simultaneously on his physical conditioning, his mental attitude, and his spiritual life to try to bring them into harmony as he tried to focus on the joys of living each day. And he could reach out to others who had similar physical problems to offer a helping hand.

If you think you might be able to find an increased sense of meaning or purpose in coping with a problem in life, or if you have done so in the past, check over Sean's worksheet and then complete Exercise 12.3.

Finding Meaning through Faith

Dr. Frankl didn't include finding meaning through faith in his writings, but we wanted to add this route to meaning because it can be so important for people who have religious beliefs. Most religions have a central theme that belief in a higher power and following spiritual practices is a primary way of giving direction and purpose to life. Yet many people with religious backgrounds who become depressed find that their connection to God seems to weaken. In some cases it appears to be broken entirely. They may have prayed for relief from depression or some other adversity and have concluded that God isn't listening to them. They could be mad at God or simply be so weary and beaten down that they don't have the energy or interest in attending religious services or engaging in other spiritual practices.

Sean was angry at God, and his anger wasn't entirely new. From the time that his brother had been killed in a car accident at age 17, Sean had questioned how a "loving God" could let this type of painful thing happen. Although he had continued to attend church on a fairly regular basis and found comfort in the teachings and rituals, a part of his spiritual life had gone numb after his brother died. Now he was even more troubled. Having a heart attack brought back the feelings of being abandoned by God. He thought it wasn't fair to be faced with a possible shortening of life, when it seemed that he was still in the middle of it. Maybe he would never live to see grandchildren, spend more days with his wife, or have the chance to enjoy retirement.

As Sean became more depressed, he attended church less regularly, avoided volunteer activities organized by his church, and felt a growing distance from the sense of faith that had helped sustain him in the past. These changes seemed natural to Sean. A depressive mind-set had taken hold, and connectedness to all of the key elements in his life was waning.

Finding Meaning in Coping with Adversity: Sean's Example

Instructions: Identify one or more significant problems that you are facing now or have faced previously in life. Then describe how you could gain (or have gained) a greater sense of meaning through coping with the experience.

An adversity in my life	Ways that I could build (or have built) a sense of meaning in my way of coping
My heart attack	Showing my children and others that tough times can be managed.
	Listening to a "wake-up" call and getting my life into balance.
	Joining "Mended Hearts" and visiting others with similar problems to help them cope.
	Learning to appreciate the joys of each day.

EXERCISE 12.3 **Finding Meaning in Coping with Adversity**

Instructions: Identify one or more significant problems that you are facing now or have faced previously in life. Then describe how you could gain (or have gained) a greater sense of meaning through coping with the experience.

An adversity in my life	Ways that I could build (or have built) a sense of meaning in my way of coping

In the book *When Bad Things Happen to Good People*, Rabbi Harold Kushner wrote from deep personal experience. He had lost a young child to a rare disease. Through his studies and his work with others, he concluded that bad things do happen to good people. But "God does not cause our suffering. Maybe it happens for some other reason than the will of God." He tells people that it is unreasonable to expect that God will protect us from diseases, the forces of nature, or aggression from others. Instead, he suggests we look to God for love and comfort. Accepting this view can help people stop blaming God or themselves for misfortunes and thereby embrace a sense of meaning in religious beliefs and practices.

Sean seemed to need to hear Rabbi Kushner's message, and Ray, his friend with MS, knew this. Ray had been listening to Sean talk when they got together for a cup of coffee and recognized that anger, resentment, and blame were clouding Sean's ability to find meaning in his life. So he brought Sean a copy of *When Bad Things Happen to Good People* and asked him to read it. Ray also suggested that Sean make an appointment to talk with his pastor. These seemed to be good recommendations from a friend.

As the wisdom of Rabbi Kushner's book began to break down barriers to his becoming closer to God, and Sean was able to talk through his anguish with his pastor, his spiritual life began to blossom. He felt a much greater sense of peace about past losses, and his spiritual beliefs became a foundation of meaning as he looked to the future.

Finding a way to stop being angry or distant from God is just one route to building meaning through faith. If you have religious beliefs and are at the point where these beliefs are not giving you as much meaning as you wish, it might help to consult a trusted spiritual leader such as a pastor, rabbi, priest, or imam. Together you can explore some of the roadblocks that you may be encountering and work toward having your spiritual life be a fundamental source of meaning and purpose.

QUICK TIP There are good books that can help you find meaning through faith. In addition to Rabbi Kushner's book, books commonly recommended by spiritual leaders are *Finding God: Praying the Psalms in Times of Depression* by Thomas Lewis, *Essential Spirituality* by Roger Walsh, and *Dark Night of the Soul* by Gerald May.

Finding Meaning in Everyday Things

For many people a "big ticket item" such as a key relationship, an enduring commitment to a cause or purpose, or a life's work may be a cornerstone of their sense of meaning. But Dr. Frankl pointed out that there are many "small," everyday things that can also be fundamental elements of living a life of meaning. Even in the concentration camp environment, he found everyday things such as the sound of a gentle rain, the kind words of another, or the sunset that he could tune in to as sources of meaning.

If you have read Chapter 7 on well-being or have some knowledge of mindfulness concepts (discussed in the next chapter), you may recognize a common theme: becoming fully aware of the things around us that can stimulate well-being, happiness, calmness, and meaning is a prime method for adding depth to our lives. Roger Walsh, the author of *Essential Spirituality*, has written that we can miss out on the meaningful things that are right in front of us. He suggests several ways for us to increase our awareness, including (1) appreciating the beauty in our environment right now instead of putting it off until some later date; (2) becoming good listeners to what people say, to the sounds of the world around us, to music, to what you read; (3) attending to the textures, smells, and tastes of the food that we eat; and (4) becoming more attentive to your body and your physical activity.

Remember Martina, the veterinary technician who was working on enhancing her sense of loving and giving in her work and with her partner, Al? Martina wasn't finding meaning in many of the everyday things that happened in her life. She kept thinking that she would have to make some major change such as finding a new job or having children to shake her up and give her life more of a sense of meaning and purpose. Working on a major goal or having a big life change can be a way to find increased meaning. However, there seemed to be an opportunity now for her to capture more of a sense of meaning in the things that were right in front of her.

In the early part of her therapy for depression, Martina used CBT to help increase the number of pleasurable activities that she engaged in daily (see Chapter 5). The focus wasn't directly on finding meaning at this point. But as Martina began to improve, she and her therapist were able to develop an overall plan for recovery that included looking for meaning in everyday things. The next worksheet helped her do this.

In doing Exercise 12.4, you can draw on the lessons about finding well-being that you learned in Chapter 7, and you can come back to add ideas for building awareness after you read the next chapter on mindfulness.

Creating Something or Making a Contribution

When Dr. Frankl was released from the concentration camp, writing the book *Man's Search for Meaning* was high on his list of things to do. The ideas for the book had been germinating for the years that he was imprisoned, but he didn't even have a pencil or a notebook to record them. It is said that it took him only 9 days to write this book that has changed so many lives.

Dr. Frankl created something that must have given him a great sense of meaning. Although most people will never have the opportunity to write an influential book, create a world-class artwork, or make a major contribution to society, everyone has the potential to achieve meaning and purpose in creating something or making a contribution. Abundant opportunities to do this arise in everyday life but may be overlooked or underappreciated, especially when people become depressed.

The cognitive errors that you learned about in Chapter 4 can undermine efforts to find meaning through creating something or making a contribution. For example, when Martina thought about the volunteer work she used to do for the Humane Society, she minimized the impact that she could have ("The problems are so big that no one could

Finding Meaning in Everyday Things: Martina's Example

Instructions: Read the suggestions for each exercise below. Then choose at least one of the exercises and write out some ideas for how you could implement the exercise in your daily life. Write down specific things you will do.

1. Try to turn off the autopilot and really pay attention to the routine activities you do every day. Think of a few things you do without any thought or conscious enjoyment—maybe one at home, one at work, and one elsewhere—and take time to appreciate them more, to fully experience the meaning they bring to your life.

   Actions I will take: *I'll get up a bit earlier to savor time with Al instead of just rushing to get ready for work and running out the door. I'll stop to appreciate all the things that are happening in the veterinary office when it is busy and there is lots of energy in the place.*

2. Explore an activity that is not included in your usual routine but could become part of your daily (or at least weekly) life: go hiking, spend some time at the library, take a trial Pilates class at the local health club, volunteer to read to the residents at a senior citizens' center. Have fun coming up with ideas for activities that you never considered doing—get a family member or friend to help you brainstorm if you want—and then try a different one for each of the next 3 weeks.

   Actions I will take: *I'll wait to do this exercise for a couple weeks. Maybe I could take a cooking class. I always wanted to learn to cook. We get takeout food most of the time now.*

3. Concentrate on tuning in to the full glory of the earth. Pick an environment you already appreciate and find something new in it or explore a natural setting that you rarely take time to experience. If you love walking in a nearby pine forest, on your next walk pay attention to all the other trees you see besides the evergreens. If you don't ordinarily like the beach, spend a little time lying on the sand, watching the wind whip up the waves and taking in the scent of the water that wafts in the wind. Wherever you go, ask yourself what you're seeing, smelling, touching, hearing, and even tasting of the earth.

   Actions I will take: *I'll go to the lake that's only a couple of miles away. There's a quiet spot with a bench where I can sit and really pay attention to what I am seeing and hearing.*

4. Become more aware of a person in your life. Using the full power of your senses, really see and hear this person. Identify one thing about this person that you've never noticed before. Do this day after day and see how it affects your relationship.

   Actions I will take: *I am already doing this somewhat with my friend Paula. She's been going through a divorce, and we've been taking some walks together three or four times a week. I could be a better listener.*

Finding Meaning in Everyday Things

Instructions: Read the suggestions for each exercise below. Then choose at least one of the exercises and write out some ideas for how you could implement the exercise in your daily life. Write down specific things you will do.

1. Try to turn off the autopilot and really pay attention to the routine activities you do every day. Think of a few things you do without any thought or conscious enjoyment—maybe one at home, one at work, and one elsewhere—and take time to appreciate them more, to fully experience the meaning they bring to your life.

   Actions I will take:

   _____

   _____

   _____

2. Explore an acitivity that is not included in your usual routine but could become part of your daily (or at least weekly) life: go hiking, spend some time at the library, take a trial Pilates class at the local health club, volunteer to read to the residents at a senior citizens' center. Have fun coming up with ideas for activities that you never considered doing—get a family member or friend to help you brainstorm if you want—and then try a different one for each of the next 3 weeks.

   Actions I will take:

   _____

   _____

   _____

3. Concentrate on tuning in to the full glory of the earth. Pick an environment you already appreciate and find something new in it or explore a natural setting that you rarely take time to experience. If you love walking in a nearby pine forest, on your next walk pay attention to all the other trees you see besides the evergreens. If you don't ordinarily like the beach, spend a little time lying on the sand, watching the wind whip up the waves and taking in the scent of the water that wafts in the wind. Wherever you go, ask yourself what you're seeing, smelling, touching, hearing, and even tasting of the earth.

   Actions I will take:

   _____

   _____

   _____

(cont.)

4. Become more aware of a person in your life. Using the full power of your senses, really see and hear this person. Identify one thing about this person that you've never noticed before. Do this day after day and see how it affects your relationship.

Actions I will take:

_____

_____

_____

make a difference"), maximized the problems in working with this group ("Nobody is in charge ... it's a total mess), and ignored the evidence that she actually had done valuable volunteer work for an important cause ("I didn't do much of anything"). Her negative thinking seemed to be standing in the way of fully appreciating a potentially meaningful activity.

Perhaps the negative filter of depression is blocking you from seeing a creative outlet, a hobby, a skill or avocation that you want to learn, or a service or contribution to others that could be the source of greater meaning. Or maybe your daily work has more promise than you realize for enhancing your sense of purpose. Spotting cognitive errors and reducing her negative thinking helped Martina recapture the sense of meaning in her work as a veterinary assistant. And when her energy improved, a resumption of volunteer work made her feel more committed and complete as a person.

Sean also had been minimizing the meaning he could achieve through his daily work. He had been in the restaurant business for a long time, and much of his efforts seemed to be routine—ordering food, managing contracts with providers, supervising employees, greeting restaurant patrons, and so forth. The early feelings of exhilaration at opening a restaurant had faded years ago. After the heart attack, the job seemed to be more of a burden than a joy. But he needed to keep going to pay the bills and to provide for the retirement that he still hoped would take place.

Can you think of any ways in which Sean could view his job from a different perspective? If you were Ray, or another one of Sean's supportive friends, could you point out some things that he may be missing that would give him a deeper sense of purpose in his work? What might customers, employees, or family members have to say about the impact of Sean's efforts as a restaurant manager?

In a CBT session, Dr. Wright asked Sean to do the same thing we ask you to do in Exercise 12.5. After thinking for a while, Sean began to see that he had been undervaluing his work. Attitudes such as "I'm just running a restaurant; anybody could do it ... I wish I had done something important in life" gave way to more self-accepting and validat-

EXERCISE 12.5	**Helping Sean**

Instructions: From the point of view of customers, employees, family, or friends, try to identify at least two possible ways for Sean to see more meaning and purpose in his work.

1. _____

2. _____

3. _____

4. _____

5. _____

ing beliefs. For example, he wrote down these observations: "Eating out and eating good food gives a lot of people pleasure and happiness—I can help make this a great experience for lots of people ... Running a restaurant is an honest and valuable occupation—it fills a real need ... I can help provide good work for many fine employees ... I can value and enjoy my relationships with my employees and customers ... Many customers have become good friends—they come back over and over to eat at our restaurant ... I can still enjoy the creativity of planning new menus and exploring new ways to prepare food."

Have you been thinking about ways that you could create something or make a contribution that you may not have recognized previously, fully appreciated, or plumbed to their full potential? A brief list of some possible avenues for building meaning in this way is given here to help get you started. Read over this list and then complete Exercise 12.6.

Possible Avenues for Creating Something or Making a Contribution

- Reexamine your daily work or other daily responsibilities—focus on the meaningful parts of these activities, keep them in top-of-the mind awareness, and let them guide your attitudes about your work.
- Find meaning through artistic or musical expression, a hobby or interest that can stimulate your passion, a sport or athletic pursuit, or a skill that you want to learn.
- Commit time and energy to helping others—do this in your everyday life with your relatives, friends, and coworkers and/or consider reaching out through volunteer work or other community activities. Give to others in need.
- Try to model to others the values that you would want them to follow in their own lives.

Finding Meaning through Creating Something or Making a Contribution

Instructions: List at least two ways that you are already finding meaning through creating something or making a contribution or could do so in the future. Note specific actions you are taking or could take to put this idea into action.

A way to create something or make a contribution	What I am doing now to put this idea into action	What I could do to put this idea into action

Putting Spiritual Resources to Work

A fundamental part of all religions, the logotherapy principles of Dr. Frankl, and most other spiritual orientations to life is making a commitment to putting one's beliefs and spiritual practices into action. Depression often makes it hard to do this, but the spiritual path toward recovery includes finding ways to act in the world that are consistent with your spiritual underpinnings and the things that give your life meaning and purpose. In this last section of the chapter we want you to build an overall plan for using your spiritual resources. To do this, we recommend you start by reviewing Exercise 12.1, where you completed an inventory of spiritual resources. Next you can scan through the other exercises in the chapter to remind yourself of the ideas you have already sketched out. Then you can write out a plan similar to the examples shown here for Sean and Martina.

? **Are you having difficulty getting connected to your spiritual domain and bringing your mind, body, and spirit into harmony? Try these ideas:**

1. Take a mini-break from daily concerns—schedule a weekend trip to a quiet and potentially inspiring place. Or if you can't get away for a few days, set aside an hour or two when you can free yourself up to get in closer touch with your spiritual side.

2. Sign up for a retreat where leaders will stimulate you to think about your spiritual life.

3. Take a class on a spiritually oriented topic and/or study spiritually oriented books or videos.

4. Spend time meditating (see Chapter 13) and/or obtain training in meditation.

5. Engage in therapy with a clinician who can encourage you on building your spiritual connections.

Sean

As you've learned so far, Sean was able to work through his anger and blame to become more accepting of the tragedy of the past and to find strength in his religious beliefs as he faced his heart condition. And he was able to find meaning in how he coped with adversity and in his daily work. But his love for his family counted the most. So when he completed the next exercise, he put "my wife and children" in the first position.

In the second part of the exercise ("Other spiritual resources that I could use now or develop in the future"), Sean wrote down two items: "mindfulness meditation" and "taking better care of my body." Although experts in mindfulness meditation (see Chapter 13) note that this approach is not based on religious beliefs, it does have a spiritual dimension for many people. Mindfulness can enhance awareness of meaningful things in life and promote loving kindness and acceptance. Dr. Wright had recommended that Sean develop mindfulness skills as part of his plan for recovery.

The other entry ("taking better care of my body") in the second part of the exercise also seemed to have a spiritual flavor to Sean. While many people who exercise may not see physical activity as a spiritual pursuit, Sean was in touch with the need to connect his mind, body, and spirit as he moved toward wellness.

Martina

Martina felt like she was a spiritual person and believed in God. But unlike Sean, she was not involved in an organized religion. So she didn't identify the comforts of religious experiences as a key part of her spirituality. However, when Martina did the exercises earlier in this chapter, she realized that her relationship with her boyfriend was an area of her life that was full of meaning. She also found a sense of purpose in her work and felt that she could find more meaning in everyday things. Yet Martina was still searching for meaning. She had more questions about her spirituality than Sean, but Martina was putting some of her spiritual resources into action now and was thinking about where she would go in the future.

Are you ready to work on your own plan for putting spiritual resources to work? We hope that the exercises and the examples in this chapter have stimulated you to think of ways to tap your spiritual resources in the struggle against depression. Do Exercise 12.7 (on page 306), and if you want to modify your plan in the future, photocopy the form or download it from *www.guilford.com/breakingfreeforms*.

Summary

The spiritual path can add a rich element of meaning and purpose to plans for recovery from depression. Although spiritually oriented practices are not evidence-based treatments for depression, many studies have found a decreased risk for depression in people who have a significant spiritual dimension. And many people have found that their spiritual strengths help them cope with depression and other adversities in their lives. As you move ahead to the next chapter of this book, on using mindfulness as a path to recovery, we encourage you to work on uniting your mind, body, and spirit in your search for wellness.

My Plan for Putting Spiritual Resources to Work: Sean's Example

Instructions: Use this worksheet to organize your ideas for using spiritual resources. You can also use the worksheet to make notes on spiritual resources or connections that you want to explore further.

I. FINDING MEANING

Key things that give my life meaning and purpose	Specific plans/commitments/actions related to this source of meaning	Comments/notes/questions related to this source of meaning
My wife and children	Show my love and appreciation every day. Be fully mindful of the blessing of having them in my life. Be "in the moment" with them as much as possible.	I need to watch out for the worries of the day interfering with my fully living my life with my family. I need to truly savor each day with them.
My faith and my church activities	Look to God for love and comfort—not to directly intervene to stop natural forces that can harm me or others. Pray for grace to accept my life and to live it fully and lovingly. Attend services regularly. Volunteer to work with the food bank program.	It would help to keep reading and studying about my spiritual beliefs and to have some more visits with my pastor.
My work	Keep my positive attitudes about my work in mind every day. Remind myself that I am doing honest work that fills a real need for my customers, employees, and family.	I realized that making a contribution through work is extremely important to me. If my heart condition makes it impossible for me to work, I'll need to figure out another way to feel like my days have purpose.
Facing the troubles in my life	Be an example to my family and others of how to cope with an illness in a healthy way. Volunteer work through "Mended Hearts."	The possibility of having complications or another heart attack still worries me. But using my spiritual connections is a big help.

(cont.)

Sean's Example (*cont.*)

II. OTHER SPIRITUAL RESOURCES THAT I COULD USE NOW OR DEVELOP IN THE FUTURE

Other spiritual resources	Ways I could put them into action	Comments/notes/questions
Mindfulness meditation	Practice meditations daily. Work on being fully aware of the things that give my life depth and meaning.	Mindfulness adds to the work I am doing in finding meaning and purpose. It also calms and centers me.
Taking better care of my body	Continuing with exercise (walking for 30 minutes or more 4–5 times a week and strength training at the Y).	I neglected my physical side for too many years. It feels good to get my whole life in better balance.

My Plan for Putting Spiritual Resources to Work: Martina's Example

Instructions: Use this worksheet to organize your ideas for using spiritual resources. You can also use the worksheet to make notes on spiritual resources or connections that you want to explore further.

I. FINDING MEANING

Key things that give my life meaning and purpose	Specific plans/commitments/actions related to this source of meaning	Comments/notes/questions related to this source of meaning
My love for Al	Make this relationship my top priority. Do things like helping with projects around the house, writing him affectionate notes, and asking about his day that show that I am loving, kind, and attentive. Affirm my commitment to being with him for life.	I need to keep showing my love even when I am tired or stressed out. I can work on forgiving his little quirks that have irritated me in the past—they count for nothing in comparison to the love we have.
My work with animals	Put myself in their place. Think about how they'd like to be treated. If my attention drifts, bring myself back to the connection I am making with the animals and their owners. Continue to learn more about how to take care of animals. Commit to weekly volunteer work with the Humane Society.	I think as I become less depressed it will be easier to get back to my old self at work. I really do love my job. I need to treasure it.

(*cont.*)

Martina's Example (*cont.*)

Key things that give my life meaning and purpose	Specific plans/commitments/actions related to this source of meaning	Comments/notes/questions related to this source of meaning
Everyday things	I'll pay better attention to some of the everyday things at home and at work that are meaningful—for example, watching Al enjoy reading the morning paper, just sitting with Al and listening to good music, the kindness and good humor of the people at work.	Depression really interfered with my finding meaning in daily life. I'm making progress in reconnecting to the little things that can mean so much.
Having a family	I think I'm still a bit too young for this, and Al and I are just getting settled financially. But I think having children would be hugely meaningful for me. I've always thought that loving and caring for children is one of the most important things to do in life.	This is a dream for the future.

II. OTHER SPIRITUAL RESOURCES THAT I COULD USE NOW OR DEVELOP IN THE FUTURE

Other spiritual resources	Ways I could put them into action	Comments/notes/questions
Getting in touch with nature	I always feel better when I am around lakes, the mountains, or the woods. I get inspired and feel like I'm experiencing something very special. I've talked with Al about making regular plans to get away from the pressures of our city life. We may start to do some hiking.	Too many days fighting city traffic, being cooped up inside, and not seeing the beauty of nature depresses my spirit. We really need to get away on a routine basis, and we need to find things that we could do any day that don't require a lot of travel (walk in parks or go to the zoo).
Learning more about spirituality and what it means to different people	I haven't had any education in spirituality. I could read some of the books that my therapist recommended.	I think I'll give this idea a try. It wouldn't hurt to learn more about spirituality.

Instructions: Use this worksheet to organize your ideas for using spiritual resources. You can also use the worksheet to make notes on spiritual resources or connections that you want to explore further.

I. FINDING MEANING

Key things that give my life meaning and purpose	Specific plans/commitments/actions related to this source of meaning	Comments/notes/questions related to this source of meaning

(cont.)

II. OTHER SPIRITUAL RESOURCES THAT I COULD USE NOW OR DEVELOP IN THE FUTURE

Other spiritual resources	Ways I could put them into action	Comments/notes/questions

THE MINDFULNESS PATH

13

Mindfulness

In Western cultures, mindfulness is a relatively new addition to the treatments available for depression, but the basic practices of mindfulness have their origins in Buddhist teachings that have been refined for more than 2,500 years. Modern application of mindfulness principles for relieving symptoms of physical and emotional diseases was pioneered by Dr. Jon Kabat-Zinn, who developed a mindfulness-based stress reduction (MBSR) program in 1979. His ground-breaking research has shown that meditative exercises that build mindful awareness of ourselves and the things around us can have a highly positive impact on chronic illnesses, pain, and psychological health.

If you're wondering whether you will have to adopt Buddhist religious principles or spend large amounts of time in meditation to benefit from mindfulness practices, the answer is no. In their book *The Mindful Way through Depression: Freeing Yourself from Chronic Unhappiness*, Dr. Mark Williams, John Teasdale, Zindel Segal, and Jon Kabat-Zinn show people ways to tap the strength of mindfulness in everyday activities and to integrate mindfulness with the CBT methods described earlier in this book. In this chapter we introduce you to the mindfulness practices recommended by Dr. Williams and other experts in this approach and suggest exercises that can help you build mindfulness skills as part of your plan for overcoming depression.

What Is Mindfulness?

When you're depressed, your mind may be "full," but it is full of the kinds of thoughts that cause distress instead of calm. You may be thinking of all of the things that you need to do, the things you forgot to do, or the things you didn't do right. Your mind may get mired in loops of unproductive negative thinking that seem to lead nowhere but down. In a cruel twist, this type of thinking robs you of the experiences you need most—experiences of the richness and beauty of life. Because mindfulness is the opposite of the negative, ruminative thinking of depression, it can offer an uplifting path toward wellness.

> **DEFINITION** According to Dr. Mark Williams and his associates, *mindfulness* is "the awareness that emerges through paying attention, in the present moment, and nonjudgmentally to things as they are."

The phrase "staying in the moment" captures the spirit of the mindful approach to living. When people stay in the moment, they attempt to fully experience the things that are occurring *right now* instead of allowing reflections about the past to take over their mind or to get caught up with looking ahead to what must be done to achieve happiness. Dr. Ronald Siegel, author of *The Mindfulness Solution*, notes that we can often miss out on the moments that enrich life because we are rushing forward to reach some goal or achievement that we believe may be essential to arrive at some distant, imagined better moment.

Wouldn't it be a shame to wake up at some later point in your life to realize that many of your days were so fully occupied with regrets, strivings, and preoccupations that vast swaths of moments with potential meaning had slipped away unnoticed and undervalued? Dr. Siegel explains that an alternative to "mindlessness" is to "actually experience what is happening in the moment: to be attentive to what we are doing rather than operating on automatic, to appreciate the present moment rather than wishing it away."

The fundamental philosophy of the mindful approach includes more than the cultivation of full awareness of present experiences. Another equally important layer of mindfulness is the nonjudgmental *acceptance* of these experiences. Experts in mindfulness recommend that people learn to accept experiences in the moments of their lives with kindness, warmth, and compassion. If you are continually judging your experiences and rehashing all the details to see whether you could have done a better job or could have spent your time more profitably, you will short-circuit your mind's ability to have healing moments of awareness.

Benefits of Mindfulness

Experts in mindfulness such as Drs. Jon Kabat-Zinn, author of *Wherever You Go, There You Are*, Christopher Germer, author of *The Mindful Path to Self-Compassion*, and Mark Williams, coauthor of *The Mindful Way through Depression*, describe numerous benefits, such as:

- *Shifting from the "doing mode" to the "being mode."* With the pressures of modern life, most of us spend the majority of our time in the "doing mode"—performing tasks, thinking about tasks, evaluating ourselves, trying to reach goals, and so forth. Often our "being mode" (being fully aware and living life in each present moment) is underdeveloped. People who practice mindfulness can cultivate the being mode and in doing so be more at peace with their emotions and more open to experiences of happiness and self-acceptance.

• *Learning to experience the world directly with full awareness while disengaging from the restless torrent of our thoughts.* Jon Kabat-Zinn notes that mindfulness practices help us "get out of this current [of thoughts, worries, and concerns], sit by its bank and listen to it, learn from it, and then use its energies to guide us rather than to tyrannize us." This capacity is especially useful for calming the storm of negative thinking that is so common in depression.

• *Viewing our thoughts as "mental events that can come and go in the mind like clouds across the sky instead of taking them literally."* According to Dr. Mark Williams and his associates, thoughts that people have when they are depressed (such as "I'm no good ... I'll never get anywhere ... What's the use?") can be viewed simply as ideas, not an accurate accounting of the truth. A mindful attitude can help people disregard or dispel these types of thoughts.

• *Turning off the autopilot in our minds.* We can act like robots as we plod through our days, moving from task to task, crossing out yet another item on our "to-do" lists. However, we are not really in touch with our senses, our emotions, and our thoughts. Mindfulness can help us live our lives fully and make healthy choices about where we really want to go.

• *Spotting and avoiding the downward spiral into depression.* By building awareness, we can learn to recognize the types of thoughts and emotions that can pull us down into depression. Mindfulness practices can be blended with CBT methods (described in Chapters 4–6) to stop the downward spiral and maintain wellness.

SCIENCE CORNER

• A study by Dr. John Teasdale and associates found that an 8-week program of MBCT reduced the risk of relapse by about half in people who had had three or more previous episodes of depression.

• Dr. Willem Kuyken and his coworkers showed relapse prevention effects for MBCT that were comparable to long-term treatment with antidepressants. MBCT was more effective than ongoing antidepressant treatment in:

  ○ Reducing residual symptoms (the symptoms that remained after previous treatment for depression).

  ○ Improving quality of life.

• An investigation by Dr. Mark Allen and others found that people who had completed MBCT reported that the program helped them:

  ○ Gain better control over depression.

  ○ Accept that depressed thoughts were part of the illness and not an accurate representation of themselves.

  ○ Improve the quality of their interpersonal relationships.

Where to Begin?

Before going further, we want you to know that there are two different types of mindfulness practices that you might read about elsewhere as well as here. They are referred to as "informal" and "formal" practices. Informal mindfulness practices don't require extensive training in meditation or a set schedule for meditation experiences, but they can help you sharpen your awareness of everyday things in your life and explore some of the basics of meditation principles. Formal mindfulness practices typically involve a significant commitment to participating in meditation experiences. For example, the MBCT program for depression developed by Dr. Mark Williams and his colleagues requires fairly intensive meditation and other mindfulness exercises over an 8-week period.

It's important to know the difference when you are dealing with depression. We want you to understand why we primarily emphasize informal mindfulness exercises in this chapter:

1. Formal, intensive mindfulness training is usually not recommended for people who have acute depression or severe symptoms of depression. It is designed primarily as a relapse prevention method for people who have already recovered from depression or who have low-grade symptoms.
2. Formal mindfulness training can require levels of concentration and effort that may be difficult for people with acute depression.
3. However, informal mindfulness training can be empowering for people with all degrees of depression. And informal training can give people a sample of what might be involved in more extensive training if they decide to pursue this opportunity at a later date.

> *CAUTION* If you suffer from acute or severe depression, don't rely on mindfulness methods as a primary treatment approach. Use CBT, antidepressants, and/or other evidence-based approaches for acute depression.

Our intent with this chapter is to expand your ability to experience a sense of mindfulness in your daily life and to show you what further mindfulness training might have to offer.

Cultivating Mindfulness

To understand and cultivate a greater sense of mindfulness, it might help to take an inventory of some of the places in your life where your mind is functioning on autopilot. Have any of the situations listed in Exercise 13.1 occurred to you? This exercise could stimulate you to think of specific examples in your life in which you are not fully mindful of your experiences. When Angelina, one of the people with depression whom you met earlier in this book, started to learn about mindfulness practices, she wrote out a list of examples of mindlessness (see page 316). Each of these examples offered Angelina opportunities to become more mindful in her daily life. When you do Exercise 13.2, try to spot some examples of depressive or anxious thoughts that take you away from being

EXERCISE 13.1   **A Mindlessness Inventory**

Instructions: Using a scale of 0–5, rate how often each of the following happens to you.

0 = Never, 1 = Rarely, 2 = Sometimes, 3 = Often, 4 = Very often, 5 = Most of the time

Occurrence	Rating of how often this occurs
I run on automatic without much awareness of what I am doing.	
I get so focused on goals that I lose touch with what I'm doing right now.	
I listen to someone with one ear, doing something else at the same time.	
I find myself ruminating or worrying about the past or future without having much awareness of the present moment.	
I snack or eat meals without being really aware of what I am eating.	
I get lost in my thoughts or feelings.	
I drive my car on automatic pilot without paying attention to what I am doing.	
I daydream or my mind drifts when I could be appreciating good things that are "right in front of my nose."	

The mindlessness inventory is adapted with permission from *The Mindfulness Solution* (2010) by Dr. Ronald Siegel.

"in the moment" and also some examples of everyday activities in which you might learn to be more mindful.

Now that we have recognized some of the ways that mindlessness can creep into our lives, it's time to try some exercises to cultivate a sense of mindfulness. As mentioned above, our focus here will be on mindfulness practices that can be blended into everyday life and don't require large investments of time or effort. The first exercise suggested by Jon Kabat-Zinn in his book *Wherever You Go, There You Are* is *stopping*. He notes that the essence of meditative practices is "stopping and being present, that is all." Because we spend most of our lives running around and doing, it can be very revealing and refreshing to stop for a moment and become attuned to watching the moment without trying to change it at all.

Situations in Which I Am Not Very Mindful: Angelina's Example

Instructions: Try to identify at least three specific situations in your life in which you are not very aware of being in the moment, you are ruminating, or you are "mindless."

1. *I am sitting watching TV with a diet soda and a bowl of chips. Before I know it, half of the bowl of chips is gone and I can hardly remember eating any of them.*

2. *My mind gets filled with worry about having an anxiety attack, and I can't think of anything else.*

3. *I start thinking about problems that I had in my job months ago. My mind goes over and over the situation. I am trying to second-guess what I should have done. I am paying little or no attention to what is going on in the present.*

4. *I am trying to practice the piano, but my mind doesn't stay on this experience. It drifts all over the place—often to all of the things I think I should be doing instead of playing the piano.*

QUICK TIPS
- It's normal and natural for your mind to jump back into the "doing" mode when you try to build awareness through mindfulness exercises.
- If you're practicing mindfulness and your mind wanders off or starts to ruminate, gently bring it back to the moment that you're in right now.
- With practice, you'll probably be able to increase the amount of time that you can "stay in the moment," and you'll be able to let these experiences of awareness suffuse your everyday life.

EXERCISE 13.2 ## Situations in Which I Am Not Very Mindful

Instructions: Try to identify at least three specific situations in your life in which you are not very aware of being in the moment, you are ruminating, or you are "mindless."

1. _____

2. _____

3. _____

4. _____

5. _____

EXERCISE 13.3	**Stopping**

Instructions:

1. Stop what you are doing for a brief while (5 seconds to 5 minutes) several times a day.

2. Sit down if possible.

3. Become fully aware of what is happening in this moment. Don't try to change anything at all. Just breathe and become aware of your sensations—what you are hearing, what you are seeing, what you are smelling, what you are feeling.

4. When you are ready, end the exercise and move ahead where you want to go.

Try the stopping exercise now. Read the instructions and gently put your book down for a few seconds or minutes to experience the moment. When you're ready, come back to the book.

After you do the stopping meditation, jot down a few observations on what you experienced. Were your sensations sharpened in any way? Did you see, hear, smell, or feel things that would have been missed if you continued to be fully in the doing mode? Were any emotions more or less apparent? Did you have any stirrings of a sense of peace or calm?

When Angelina practiced one of the brief stopping meditations, she was at her desk and had been doing e-mail for about an hour. The doing mode was in top gear. Her mind and body were on full alert to get everything "just right" in how she answered messages. Her neck and shoulder muscles were "tight as a drum." A large part of her mental effort was focused on writing effective responses, but her mind was also jumping back and forth between self-condemning thoughts about work-related e-mails from the past that she believed she could have done better and worrying about an upcoming dinner engagement she had with her boss.

Although it was difficult at first for Angelina to exit the doing mode for even a few seconds, the stopping exercises seemed to open doors to a deepened awareness and appreciation of what was happening in the moments of her life. She wrote down these observations in her notebook about the stopping meditation she tried when taking a break from doing a flurry of e-mails: "I was working at home, and the windows were open. I tuned in to the sounds around me. They were very vivid when I paid attention. I could hear cars passing on a street two blocks away; there were creaks in the floor from my boyfriend walking in the room above my head. There was a very slight but pleasing sound coming from my nostrils as I focused on my breath. I would have never heard this if I wasn't trying to be really aware of all of the sensations. There were birds singing in the yard. Again, I didn't even hear them when I was immersed in the e-mails. The rhythms of my breath were calming as I tuned in to them. I looked at the lamp beside my desk. The sunlight was dancing in patterns on the glass as I just slightly moved my head to look at the lamp from different angles. I stopped for just about a minute, but I did learn that I could become more aware. It was a good feeling."

Angelina was just starting to practice mindfulness, but she had already seemed to grasp one of the main points of mindfulness training: shifting from the doing to the being mode can help us step away from worries, concerns, deadlines, and other pressures for at least brief intervals and to allow awareness to calm our emotions and enrich our lives.

QUICK TIPS   Are you wondering whether spending time in mindfulness practices might take away from your efficiency or your ability to complete tasks? Could it be that taking moments for full awareness could derail you from goal-oriented activities such as meeting work deadlines, getting your house chores completed, or doing things to help others?

- Mindfulness practices typically don't make people less efficient. In fact, mindfulness may improve your ability to function if you can learn ways of being in the moment while reducing fruitless ruminations or worries.

- The being mode and the doing mode can be close partners in leading a fulfilling life. We all need to spend considerable time in the doing mode to get things done. But expanding our ability to experience the being mode can give life balance and depth. Also, gaining mindfulness capacities can help us be happier and more effective while we are in the doing mode.

Another commonly used exercise in mindfulness training focuses on the experience of eating. The "raisin" exercise could help you build your mindfulness sensitivities for eating and also teach lessons for expanding the role of mindfulness in other areas of your life.

After you do Exercise 13.4, try to answer these questions. How did the eating exercise make you feel? Were you more aware of the texture and flavor of the food? Did you tune in to the process of eating and how your mouth and tongue processed the food? Notice how long it took you to eat one raisin. Was this different from your usual method of eating? Do you think you can use parts of this exercise in your everyday life to bring more awareness or pleasure to your eating?

Eating mindfully is just one of myriad ways that people can bring greater awareness of the present moment into their lives. Can you think of some other everyday experiences that might be good targets for practicing mindfulness? Angelina did a little brainstorming and came up with a list (shown on page 320) of routine activities that she wanted to experience more fully just as they were happening.

Angelina had lots of good ideas for increasing her mindfulness in her daily routine. It was tempting to try to make all of these changes at once. As with so many other people, the "lightbulb" went off in Angelina's mind as she realized the potential power of mindfulness in moving away from depressive thinking and infusing her days with more aware-

EXERCISE 13.4	**Eating One Raisin**

Instructions: Select one raisin or another food item such as one cracker or a section of an orange. Choose something that is an ordinary food item, something you like, and something you would ordinarily eat in a bite or two. Then go through the following steps to build your sense of awareness. The steps are based on eating a raisin; please adapt them if you pick another food item.

1. Sit in a comfortable position (in a chair or cross-legged on the floor) in an area without distractions. Turn off the TV, radio, or computer, and begin to bring your awareness to your own body and the raisin in front of you.

2. Pick up the raisin and put it in your hand. Feel the soft, mushy texture and the smooth ridges on the raisin. Roll it between your fingers to feel its size and borders. Focus on the sensation of touching the raisin. (approximately 1 minute)

3. Now bring the raisin to your nose. Smell the raisin and notice any feelings or memories this might bring. (approximately 1 minute)

4. Put the raisin on your tongue and leave it there for a minute. Experience the full taste of the raisin without biting into it. Feel the texture of the raisin now on your tongue, instead of your hand. How does it feel different? How does it taste? (approximately 1 minute)

5. Roll the raisin around in your mouth, experiencing how it feels against your cheek and behind your lips. Has the flavor changed or intensified? (approximately 1 minute)

6. Now slowly begin to chew the raisin. How does this feel against your teeth? Notice the chewiness and the changes in flavor. Feel how the raisin breaks apart in your mouth. (approximately 1–2 minutes)

7. Finally, swallow the raisin. As you swallow, pay attention to the act of swallowing and the sensation of the raisin going to the back of your tongue, your throat, then down your esophagus and on to your stomach.

ness. Yet she accepted her doctor's recommendation to go slowly and to begin practicing mindfulness with only a few daily activities.

One of the activities she targeted was taking a walk. Most days she walked for about a mile and a half in her neighborhood. She knew that the exercise was good for her physical health and also could help with depression, so she kept at it even though she rarely enjoyed the experience. Most days that she walked, her thoughts focused on getting done with the walk so that she could do something else ("I can't wait for this to be over ... I need to get that project done for work"), the unpleasantness of having to push herself to exercise or being unhappy with the conditions ("This is too much effort ... I hate to sweat and get messy when it is hot outside ... I'm cold, I wish I were home now taking a hot shower"), or ruminations about her past life, present problems, or future challenges ("I could have handled that meeting better ... I need to get the bills paid today ... I just have too much to do to ever get my life in control"). Before bringing a mindful

Being More Mindful in Activities of Everyday Life: Angelina's Example

Instructions:

1. Think of some routine activities that you do every day or most days.

2. Make a list of at least five of these activities that you typically do without being very attentive to what is happening in the moment.

3. Then circle two or more of these activities as initial targets for spreading mindfulness more fully into your life.

4. Try to be attentive to mindfulness principles in performing at least one routine activity every day.

Routine Activities in Which I Could Become More Mindful:

1. (Eating meals or snacks)
2. Brushing my teeth
3. (Taking a walk)
4. Doing the dishes
5. Talking on the phone with my mother
6. Getting dressed in the morning
7. Looking at my house plants
8. (Listening to music)
9. Sitting in my favorite chair after coming home from work
10. (Taking a shower)

---

attitude to her walking, Angelina was essentially avoiding the experience. Even though she was grinding out a walk most days, she was rarely if ever in the moment—she was somewhere else.

Here's what Angelina reported to her doctor after she was able to bring mindfulness to her daily walks:

"I used to dread the walks. I just wanted to get them over with as fast as possible. But now things are different. I open my eyes and my ears. One thing that is really calming is watching the play of the light on the trees and seeing the wind move through the leaves. I never paid much attention to that before. There are millions of different angles of light, and the colors are really beautiful if you tune in to them. I listen for the sounds around me as I walk—things like some kids playing in a yard or a plane going overhead. I try to take in these sounds as deeply as possible so that I fully experience them. Sometimes I just focus on the feeling of my feet touching the ground, the sounds of my legs moving forward and rustling my clothes, and my breathing as I walk."

In Angelina's example, an activity that previously had been mostly onerous became something to appreciate and savor. By becoming more mindful, she was fully engaged in living her life in the moment of her walking instead of letting this time slip by or allowing it to be dominated by troubling thoughts and unpleasant feelings.

When you work on the next exercise, be sure to choose at least a few ordinary activities that don't take too long to complete and are not likely to stir up lots of negative emotions or conflicts. For example, you might become more attentive to the actions you take in making a cup of tea or a pot of coffee. Becoming more mindful in these types of activities can help you build skills for increasing awareness in more complex areas of your daily routine.

? What if I have trouble staying "in the moment"?

The old phrase "easier said than done" often applies to attempts to become more mindful in activities of everyday life. You've probably had years of solid practice in functioning in the doing mode, and considerably less experience in intentionally practicing mindfulness. So try to have reasonable expectations.

At first you may not be able to stay as tuned in to your experiences as Angelina was in the example. Your mind may quickly skip back into the doing mode. Or you may wonder whether the mindfulness exercises could possibly be worthwhile. So try to:

- Give mindfulness a chance by practicing it in everyday activities at least once a day for at least 2 weeks.

- Remind yourself that everyone has difficulties staying completely in the moment. Even people who are highly experienced in mindfulness meditation note that their minds can wander away when they are trying to experience full awareness.

- View each episode of inattentiveness to the sensations of the moment as an opportunity to practice mindfulness. There will be plenty of opportunities!

- Don't judge yourself. Just gently direct your attention back to the moment.

- Imbue your efforts to become more mindful with kindness. Be tolerant and accepting of yourself.

The exercises that we recommend here for increasing awareness in routine, everyday activities do not require formal meditation skills, but they do fit the definition of meditative experiences given by Jon Kabat-Zinn ("stopping and being present, that is all"). We

Being More Mindful in Activities of Everyday Life

Instructions:

1. Think of some routine activities that you do every day or most days.

2. Make a list of at least five of these activities that you typically do without being very attentive to what is happening in the moment.

3. Then circle two or more of these activities as initial targets for spreading mindfulness more fully into your life.

4. Try to be attentive to mindfulness principles in performing at least one routine activity every day.

Routine activities in which I could become more mindful:

1. _____

2. _____

3. _____

4. _____

5. _____

6. _____

7. _____

8. _____

9. _____

10. _____

use these everyday mindfulness methods in our own lives and believe they offer much to people who suffer from depression. Full awareness of the richness of everyday experiences can give respite from the repetitive chatter of negative thinking and the painful emotions that people experience so often in depression.

Before going ahead to help you learn additional mindfulness skills, some tips on bringing increased awareness to everyday activities may be helpful.

Tips for Becoming More Mindful in Routine Activities

- *Be more mindful of eating and drinking.* Many facets of your daily experiences with eating and drinking could be ripe for increased attention and awareness. For example, could you be more mindful of food preparation? Even if it's peeling an orange or pouring milk on your cereal, you may find delights in becoming more attentive. Instead of performing these activities in an automatic manner, open yourself up to the sights, sounds, and smells of the activity. When you have a meal, put the lessons of the raisin exercise to work. Fully appreciate the textures and tastes of the food. Develop a finely grained picture of the food in your mind.

- *Be more attentive of times when you are starting or ending your day.* When you wake up, take a few moments to tune in your senses before you rush headlong into the day's activities. You could observe your breathing for 5 or 10 breaths. You could stretch your muscles and fully experience the sensations in your hands, arms, neck, back, legs, and feet. Or you could pause for a moment to kindly appreciate a partner who is still asleep next to you. When you prepare to go to sleep at night, you could also attend to your breathing and stretch your muscles. You could pay attention to the physical feelings of removing your clothes and freeing your body from its daily covering. Or you could focus full attention on looking at some photos in a magazine you're reading.

- *Be more mindful when listening to others.* Could you build your ability to be mindful by being more attentive when others are speaking to you? Angelina put "talking on the telephone with my mother" on her list. Even though she loved her mother deeply and did want to talk with her, she knew that a sense of obligation had been washing over the daily calls. Often she found herself just "going through the motions" when she called her mother to check in. As her mother was talking, Angelina could be thinking of a host of other things. So working to stay in the moment during these phone calls was a very meaningful goal for Angelina.

Perhaps you could practice mindfulness in your own listening skills. When your mind wanders away from the experience, gently direct your attention back to the person who is talking with you. Listen with sensitivity and appreciation to the textures of the voice and the content of the message.

- *Practice mindfulness when you see everyday objects.* Ice in a glass of water, the look and feel of a smartphone, a book cover, a house plant, the design on a pillow—all of these objects and many more can be appreciated more mindfully. Just stop for a moment and look fully at an object. Then go on your way.

- *Really listen to the music you hear.* Many of us "listen" to music as we drive to work, do chores around the house, work out at the gym, or participate in other everyday activities. But how often do we really listen with full attentiveness, soaking in the sound, appreciating the expressiveness of the voice or the musical instrument, hearing the nuances of the sounds and rhythms? Set aside a brief time to intentionally choose music that you want to hear. Then try your best to stay in the moment of the musical experience. Keep nudging yourself back into the moment for at least 5 minutes.

- *Become more aware of tension in your body.* Several times a day, take a brief break to attend to body sensations of tension, soreness, or tightness. Most of us have such areas. Maybe it's stiffness or pain in your neck, a tightness in your jaw, or sore muscles in your back. Stretch these areas and gently massage them if needed. Then focus on your breathing and try to let excess tension escape from your body. As you pay attention to your breathing, let tense or worrisome thoughts fade into the background.

SCIENCE CORNER **What effects does mindfulness have on the brain and on the body?**

- Studies by Dr. Richard Davidson and colleagues at the University of Wisconsin have suggested that meditation can have positive effects on brain wave activity and the development of new connections between brain cells in people with depression.

- Research by Dr. Antoine Lutz and associates has shown that meditation can enhance the activity of brain centers that are linked to positive emotions and empathy.

- Dr. Sara Lazar at Massachusetts General Hospital, who performed magnetic resonance imaging on meditators, found that meditation on a regular basis thickened (enlarged) several areas in the cerebral cortex of the brain. Presumably building the thickness of the cortex is a good thing because that part of the brain is responsible for conscious thought. Some studies have shown a loss of cerebral cortical functioning in depression.

Being Mindful toward Your Body

In a way, mindfulness is like using a camera lens that allows us to focus our attention very intently on a single object or process. Dr. Ronald Siegel notes that mindfulness is "focusing the mind's lens." This focusing can instill calmness and peace. It steadies your mind by activating brain circuits needed to attend to the focus, while it turns down activity in circuits involved in processing competing thoughts, worries, or negative emotions. In this section of the chapter we introduce you to two mindfulness exercises—breathing and body scan meditations—that are key parts of the MBCT program developed by

• The breathing and body scan meditations described here can be part of formal meditative practices if performed repeatedly over 8 weeks or more.

• If you're acutely or severely depressed, it might be best to delay routine use of these meditations until you have reduced symptoms and can fully concentrate on mindfulness exercises.

• However, anyone with depression can at least try out the exercises in this section to see what they are like and to consider using them in the future.

Dr. Mark Williams and associates. They recommend regular practice with these meditations to build the mindfulness skills that can help reduce the risk of relapse into depression.

Mindfulness of Breathing

Focus on the breath has been used as a meditative exercise for more than 2,500 years and is recommended by mindfulness experts as one of the pillars of the meditative experience. Because the breath is always with us, it's an ever-present resource for mindful attentiveness. And the strong calming and centering effect of mindful breathing has made it a foundation for many other mindfulness practices.

Mindfulness of breathing can be as simple as paying attention to 5–10 breaths while allowing your mind to be fully absorbed by these few moments of breathing. You may recall that we suggested attention to a few breaths as one way to experience mindfulness in everyday activities (for example, when arising from sleep and preparing for sleep). Mindful attention to a few breaths can also be part of the stopping exercise described earlier. Just stop and be mindful of your breathing for a short while. Let this moment of peaceful contemplation soak in. Then move on.

The seated mindfulness of breathing exercise described next requires more effort, time, and practice. But it could help you reach some of the deeper states of peace that mindfulness can instill. An audio recording of Jon Kabat-Zinn leading this mindfulness practice is contained in a CD in the book *The Mindful Way through Depression*.

Angelina really liked the mindfulness breathing exercise and thought it helped her cope with depression and anxiety by reducing the power that worrisome thoughts seemed to have over her. She used the CD prepared by Dr. Kabat-Zinn to help her stay in the moment of mindful breathing. But sometimes she did fall into the trap of trying to control her breathing—either slowing it down or taking a deep breath. She needed to keep reminding herself that her breathing would function just fine on its own without her regulating it. The breathing meditation was not about modifying her breathing; it was about becoming fully aware and accepting of what is happening right now in each breath.

When her mind wandered, Angelina tried her best to bring it back to the moment of the breath. Yet plenty of distractions got in the way. They were mostly the concerns or distractions of everyday life—thinking of what she might prepare for dinner, wondering when her partner might come home, feeling hot and sticky because it was a very warm day. Or her attention could waver if she began to think of some of her problems—financial

EXERCISE 13.6	Mindfulness of Breathing

Instructions: To get in touch with your breath moving in the body right now, sit in a comfortable position or lie down on your back and place one hand over your belly (in the region of the navel). You may notice that in this position the abdominal wall rises with the in-breath and falls with the out-breath. See if you can pick up on and feel this movement, first with your hand, then without your hand, just by "putting your mind in your belly." There is no need to control the flow of the breath. Allow it to come and go as it will, sensing as best you can the changing pattern of physical sensations. Rest here in awareness, with the feeling of the breath moving in the body in this way or however you find the movement of the belly to be with your own breathing.

Adapted with permission from Williams, M., Teasdale, J., Segal, Z. V., & Kabat-Zinn, J. (2007), *The Mindful Way through Depression.*

From *Breaking Free from Depression.* Copyright 2012 by The Guilford Press.

worries, job concerns, chronic pain in her back. A host of other potential trouble spots were lurking there waiting to absorb her energies and take her away from the moment of the breath.

These types of doing-mode thoughts were exactly why Angelina persisted with her mindful breathing exercises. By bringing herself back time and time again to the mindful breathing experience, she knew she was gaining a capacity that would help her be less troubled by the daily travails that were certain to come her way.

The Body Scan

In the full 8-week MBCT program described in the *The Mindful Way through Depression*, the body scan meditation is used for about 45 minutes a day throughout the first 2 weeks of the program and continues to be a routine meditation for the remaining 6 weeks, making it a cornerstone of the formal mindfulness training in MBCT. We include the body scan meditation here to give you another example of a formal meditative experience that you can try if you want to explore more extensive mindfulness experiences.

Some people find that an abbreviated version of the body scan in which attention is focused for a brief time on one of the body areas can be beneficial. So take a look at the body scan meditation to see whether any or all of it might help build your capacity for mindful awareness.

Many people note that the body scan mediation can lead to states of deep relaxation and inner peace. In fact, you might find yourself drifting off to sleep during a body scan mediation. Sometimes we have noticed this tendency ourselves when we use the body scan exercise. Because awareness—not relaxation—is the main goal of meditation, you might want to make a few adjustments if you find yourself falling asleep when you try body scanning methods. For example, you might do the body scan in a seated position with your eyes open. Or you could choose a time of day when you may be more alert.

Dr. Mark Williams and his colleagues emphasize the body scan in their MBCT program because they believe it helps us connect with our bodies, which "play a key role in

The Body Scan

Instructions:

1. Make yourself comfortable lying down on your back, in a place where you will feel comfortable and undisturbed. You may choose to sit in a chair if that will work better for you. Allow your eyes to close gently.

2. Take a few moments to get in touch with the movement of your breath and the sensations in your body. When you're ready, bring your awareness to the physical sensations in your body, especially to the sensations of touch or pressure where your body makes contact with the floor or chair. On each out-breath, allow yourself to sink a little deeper into the surface you're lying or sitting on.

3. If you're feeling pain, or having difficulty attending to one area of your body, try not to pass judgment; just be aware of the sensation you're feeling. Continue to focus on bringing the breath and attention to that area. The intention of this practice is to bring awareness to any and all sensations you are able to be aware of (or lack of sensation) as you focus your attention systematically on each part of the body in turn.

4. Now bring your awareness to the sensations in the belly, becoming aware of the breath as it moves into the body and as it moves out of the body. Take a few minutes to feel the sensations as the belly rises on the in-breath and falls on the out-breath.

5. Having connected with the sensations in the belly, now bring the focus of your attention into the left foot and all the way to the toes. Focus on each of the toes in turn, bringing a gentle attention to the sensations you find, perhaps noticing the sense of contact between the toes, a sense of tingling, warmth, or perhaps numbness. Whatever you are experiencing is okay. It is what is here right now.

6. Now, when you are ready, on an out-breath, let go of the toes and bring your awareness to the sensations in the bottom of your left foot—bringing a gentle, investigative awareness to the sole of the foot, the instep, the heel (noticing, for example, the sensations where the heel makes contact with the mat or bed). Experiment with "breathing with" any and all sensations—being aware of the breath in the background as, in the foreground, you explore the sensations in the bottom of the foot.

7. Now expand your awareness into the rest of the foot—to the ankle, the top of the foot, right into the bones and joints. Then take a deeper and more intentional breath in, directing it down into the whole of the left foot, and, as you breathe out, let go of the left foot completely, allowing the focus of awareness to move into the lower left leg—the calf, shin, knee, and so forth, in turn.

8. Continue to scan the body, lingering for a time with each part of the body: the left shin, the left knee, the left thigh. Then move over to the right toes and then foot and ankle, the right lower leg, the right knee, the right thigh; the pelvic area—groin, genitals, buttocks, and hips; the lower back and the abdomen, the upper back and the chest and shoulders. Then we move to hands, usually doing both at the same time. We rest first with the sensations in the fingers and thumbs, the palms and the backs of both hands, the wrists, the lower arms and elbows, the upper arms; the shoulders again and the armpits; the neck; the face (jaw, mouth, lips, nose, cheeks, ears, eyes, forehead); and then the entirety of the head.

9. When you become aware of tension or of other intense sensations, you can use the in-breath to gently bring awareness right into the sensations, and, as best you can, have a sense of what happens in that region as each breath lets go.

10. The mind will inevitably wander away from the breath and the body from time to time. That is entirely normal. It is what minds do. When you notice it, gently acknowledge it, noticing where the mind has gone off to, and then gently return your attention to the part of the body you intended to focus on.

11. After you have scanned the whole body in this way, spend a few minutes being aware of a sense of the body as a whole and of the breath flowing freely in and out of the body.

Adapted with permission from Williams, M., Teasdale, J. D., Segal, Z., & Kabat-Zinn, J. (2007), *The Mindful Way through Depression*.

the experience and expression of emotion," and it helps us "uncouple the links between body sensations and thinking that keep the cycle of rumination and unhappiness going." Simply put, mindful awareness of the body offers a wonderful opportunity to focus our attention in a way that can calm distressing thoughts and feelings. So try to come back to the body scan meditation if you aren't ready to fully engage in it now. Or take a brief break (just 1–5 minutes could be worthwhile) each day to practice some of the awareness methods taught in the body scanning exercise.

The Mindful Path toward Overcoming Depression

If the mindfulness practices described in this chapter have struck a chord with you, and you want to find a way to implement an MBCT program, we highly recommend the book *The Mindful Way through Depression*. This book with the companion CD gives detailed guidance on learning to use mindfulness to reduce the risk of relapse from depression. It's listed in the Resources section at the back of the book along with other recommended readings for building mindfulness skills.

Even if you don't pursue a path of formal meditation, you can be like so many other people who have learned to spend more of their lives "in the moment" and use informal mindfulness practices to help them cope with depression and anxiety. The key steps you can take to do this are (1) learning to allow painful emotions and negative thoughts to pass by, (2) taking mindful action, and (3) practicing the basic mindfulness skills outlined in this chapter. Each of these steps can be integrated into an overall plan for overcoming depression that includes methods from CBT, pharmacotherapy, and/or other useful approaches.

Allow Negative Thoughts and Distressing Emotions to Pass By

When depression produces negative, self-condemning thoughts and distressing emotions (such as sadness, anxiety, and anger), there is a natural tendency to try to do anything possible to get rid of these thoughts and feelings. A common response is to get into the doing mode to try to solve a problem or make some positive changes. There is nothing wrong with taking such actions in the doing mode. In fact, we explained valuable methods from standard CBT in earlier chapters that help people change their thinking and their behavior in ways that can reduce upsetting emotions, and we explained how lifestyle modifications such as exercise can make people feel better. But findings of MBCT research suggest that there is another way to manage negative thoughts and painful emotions—getting into the being mode.

So far we've described mindfulness exercises that would typically be expected to generate positive or neutral emotional experiences and produce calm. But people with depression who work to become more mindful may at times have a heightened awareness of negative internal states. Although it's certainly not a goal of mindfulness to make people feel worse, Dr. Mark Williams and his associates observe that "bringing a gentle openness and interest to something troublesome is, in itself, an enormously important part of acceptance.... Intentionally holding something in awareness is already an affirmation that it can be faced, named, and worked with."

> **?** **How could it possibly help to become more mindful of negative thoughts and distressing emotions?**
>
> - The key to using mindfulness to cope directly with negative thoughts and painful emotions is *gentle acceptance*. If you can be aware of the thoughts and emotions and then use mindful breathing and/or attention to the body to induce a sense of calm and peace, then the negative thoughts and emotions may lose some of their hold on you.
>
> - If you try to become more mindful of internal states that are painful and you *feel worse*, don't proceed unless you have professional guidance in how to use this technique. The full 8-week MBCT program teaches people advanced methods for managing negative thoughts and emotions.

To illustrate a mindful way to let negative thoughts and distressing emotions pass by, we'll look in once more on Angelina. Using the basic mindfulness philosophy of just trying to experience things as they are, right now, without trying to change them, she practiced ways of getting into the being mode when she began to dwell on a work problem that had occurred 3 years ago but still tormented her. She had a habit of going over and over an incident where she sent an e-mail without checking it for accuracy and was later reprimanded by her boss. She still felt shame at having made "such a stupid mistake" and really "fouling up." As a result, her beliefs about "needing to be in control" had grown stronger and stronger, and she was always tense when doing e-mails or sending any other communications at work.

With coaching from her doctor, Angelina began to try these mindfulness approaches to the problem:

1. When I begin to worry about the e-mail incident, I'll pause to breathe into my negative thoughts and my tension and shame. I'll focus on the calming sensation of the breath in my belly and then through my nostrils.
2. As I focus on the breath, I'll gently accept the thoughts and emotions as they are right now without trying to get rid of them. I'll accept myself in a kind and gentle way.
3. I'll give the thoughts a name: "The unforgiving judge."
4. I'll view the thoughts and emotions as passing clouds in the sky. I can choose to be aware of them but let them pass by without letting them upset me.

If you think you're ready to try this type of mindfulness exercise, choose for Exercise 13.8 a troubling thought or emotion that seems to come back at you frequently. Then you can use some of the methods that Angelina found helpful. If you're acutely or severely depressed, you may want to skip over this exercise until your symptoms are improved.

Allowing Negative Thoughts
and Distressing Emotions to Pass By

Instructions: If you have a recurring thought or emotion that troubles you, try this mindfulness method:

1. Use mindfulness of breathing to calm and center you.

2. Experience the thoughts and emotions as they are right now without trying to immediately fix or eliminate them.

3. Name the thoughts and/or emotions to help you accept that you can face and work with these negative internal experiences.

4. View the thoughts and emotions as phenomena that you can decide to let pass by. You can use an image of clouds passing in the sky, bubbles in a pool of water that rise to the surface and pop, or any other image that will help you.

My plan for letting the thoughts and emotions pass by:

1. The thoughts/emotions I will focus on are:

_____

_____

2. The mindfulness breathing method I will use is:

_____

_____

3. Some of the words I'll use to gently accept myself are:

_____

_____

4. The image I'll choose to help me let thoughts and emotions pass by is:

_____

_____

Take Mindful Action

In some ways, the principles of mindfulness seem to take a 180-degree turn from the standard CBT methods described in Chapters 4–6. Instead of trying to directly change negative automatic thoughts, mindful awareness seeks to defuse their power by another route. The mindfulness method is drawn more from an Eastern philosophical tradition, whereas the direct route to change, as in classic CBT, is derived primarily from Western ways of thinking and acting. Although the approaches seem to be different, their methods can complement and enhance one another.

The MBCT designed by Dr. Mark Williams and associates fuses the attentive and accepting awareness of mindfulness with many of the action-oriented methods of CBT. So MBCT involves not only doing mindfulness practices but also making mindful choices about actions you can take to help you pull out of depression and lead a happier life. If, for example, your experience with depression included reduced interest and ability to experience pleasure, you might review a pleasant events checklist (described in Chapter 5) with mindful awareness and choose several activities to do in the next week. If you mindfully considered options for solving a problem, you might then elect to use the step-by-step method from CBT (also described in Chapter 5). The key addition of MBCT to traditional CBT is the heightened awareness and acceptance of the being mode.

MBCT is not an "armchair philosophy." It actually embraces and heavily uses the doing mode, but it does so in a way that balances taking action with an ability to be in the moment. As Dr. Williams and associates have observed, mindfulness is "very much about wise doing, a doing that emerges and flows out of the domain of being—'mindful doing,' if you will."

An example of mindful doing is the next step that Angelina took after she used the mindful approach to her recurrent thoughts about the e-mail incident from several years ago. As noted earlier in the chapter, she had a repetitive pattern of worrying about making a mistake. So her behavior when she was doing her e-mail, especially when it was related to her job, was very tense and driven. After labeling her self-condemning and punitive thoughts "The Unforgiving Judge," and using mindfulness methods to gently accept herself, she made the following behavioral plan:

1. When doing e-mail, stretch muscles and feel areas of tension at least every 15 minutes. Pause for a moment to be aware of the breath. Then breathe into the tension and let it go.
2. Review e-mails that I need to send for my work only once before hitting the send button. Once is enough.
3. Remind myself that I don't have to get everything perfect all the time and that trying to never make a mistake takes its toll on me. Let the thoughts about the past e-mail mistake that got me in trouble pass by. Realize that I am doing well at work and the one mistake from years ago means very little, if anything, now.
4. Practice sending some e-mails that aren't fully groomed for punctuation and phrasing to family or friends.
5. After I do some work activities online from home, treat myself to a relaxing activity to wind down.

EXERCISE 13.9	**Taking Mindful Action**

Instructions: Select a problem, concern, or worry that you might like to approach by taking mindful action. Then follow these steps:

1. First, allow yourself to enter the being mode. Pause for a few mindful breaths and stay in the moment. Be mindful of an everyday thing. Or, if you can, engage in the mindfulness of breathing meditation in Exercise 13.6.

2. Gently accept your thoughts and feelings in a nonjudgmental way. Be kind and friendly to yourself.

3. When you are ready, try to make a wise choice about an action you will take.

Angelina's plan contained elements from mindfulness but also included "wise choices" for how she would begin to change her behavior when she spent time communicating by e-mail. If you recall the core methods of CBT from earlier in this book, you probably spotted some action items that could spring from use of the CBT approach.

For Exercise 13.9, try to identify an area of your life in which you want to take action and can do so with the support of self-accepting, mindful awareness.

Practice Basic Mindfulness Skills

We've explained how to use simple mindfulness exercises such as stopping, being more mindful in the routines of everyday life, and pausing briefly to become fully aware of the breath. And we've introduced you to some commonly used meditation experiences. A value of practicing these skills is that increased experiences of mindfulness, even in brief moments, have the capacity for inducing calm and peace in the face of tension and inner strife. And a growing sense of mindfulness could help you experience more happiness and less despair.

To continue building your efforts to use mindfulness in overcoming depression, it might be helpful to sketch out a plan with some specific ideas. Angelina's plan for ways to increase mindfulness experiences in her life is shown on page 333.

We hope Angelina's examples will stimulate some ideas for increased mindfulness in your own life that you can jot down now, in Exercise 13.10. If you want to modify your plan in the future, make photocopies of the form or download it from *www.guilford. com/breakingfreeforms*.

Summary

Mindfulness practices offer an alternate way to cope with the negative thoughts and painful emotions of depression. Although mindfulness methods are rooted in Buddhist traditions that had their origins over two millennia ago, modern scientists have adapted

My Plan for Using the Mindfulness Path: Angelina's Example

Instructions: Review the exercises you have completed in this chapter. Then note specific ways you will practice mindfulness.

Mindfulness activity	How important or valuable I think this mindfulness practice could be for me (rate on 0–10 point scale where 0 = no benefit and 10 = maximum benefit)	Actions I will take to practice this mindfulness activity
Be more mindful in activities of everyday life	9	Use my list of "Being More Mindful in Activities of Everyday Life" to stay focused on things I can do to stay "in the moment." Continue to use my daily walks as opportunities to become more mindful. Be more mindful in my daily phone calls to my mother.
Use simple mindfulness meditations such as the "stopping" meditation or a brief meditation on the breath	7	Practice mindful breathing at least once a day and more if possible. At a minimum, try mindful breathing for 2–5 minutes after I wake up and before I get out of bed.
Use the body scan meditation	4	I'm not sure I'm ready to put a lot of effort into daily body scan meditations, but I'll try at least a part of the body scan (especially around my shoulders and neck, which get very tight) a couple of times a week.
Practice mindfulness methods of letting negative thoughts and distressing emotions "pass by"	7	I'll write a coping card to remind myself to use mindfulness to let some of my thoughts pass by.
Take mindful action	6	I'll try adding a mindfulness layer to the CBT methods I learned for taking action.

My Plan for Using the Mindfulness Path

Instructions: Review the exercises you have completed in this chapter. Then note specific ways you will practice mindfulness.

Mindfulness activity	How important or valuable I think this mindfulness practice could be for me (rate on 0–10 point scale where 0 = no benefit and 10 = maximum benefit)	Actions I will take to practice this mindfulness activity
Be more mindful in activities of everyday life		
Use simple mindfulness meditations such as the "stopping" meditation or a brief meditation on the breath		
Use the body scan meditation		
Practice mindfulness methods of letting negative thoughts and distressing emotions "pass by"		
Take mindful action		

the practices for today's world and have found that mindful awareness can enhance both physical and psychological health.

Mindfulness is not recommended as a stand-alone treatment for acute or severe depression, but basic practices such as trying to be in the moment and being mindful of everyday things offer ways to experience more of the richness and depth of positive life experiences. Mindfulness methods have been shown to be effective in reducing the risk of relapse, and they can be used in combination with other evidence-based treatments in comprehensive efforts to overcome depression. In the next chapter of this book you'll have the opportunity to pull together your ideas for using all of the paths to recovery in an overall plan for getting well and staying well.

14

Getting Well
Staying Well

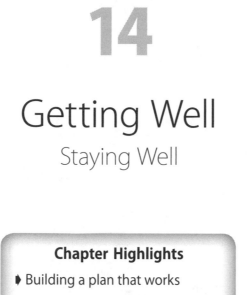

Chapter Highlights

▶ Building a plan that works

▶ Overcoming obstacles to success

▶ Staying well

As you've traveled the paths to recovery, you've explored a wealth of opportunities for overcoming depression. If you already have come up with specific plans for using one or more of the paths, and these strategies are working for you, just keep at it. However, if you haven't recovered fully yet, or want to reduce your risk for relapse, you may want to read on. The first section of this final chapter will help you pull together your ideas for using the paths to recovery to create an overall strategy for getting well. The middle part of the chapter gives tips for surmounting common obstacles that can stand in the way of success in overcoming depression. The concluding section covers the important topic of how to increase your chances of staying well.

Building a Plan That Works

One of the advantages of developing a multifaceted, comprehensive plan for recovery is that it gives you plenty of options. You can work on several fronts with the hope that following more than one path will give you a better chance of achieving wellness. Or if you want to try just one approach at a time, you can have a backup plan in case the first strategy doesn't provide full relief.

When you were introduced to the paths to wellness in Chapter 3, you rated your degree of interest in using each one. Now that you've learned more, it could be very helpful to reevaluate your interest in the paths and make some notes about the actions you want to emphasize in your overall plan for recovery. To help you build a comprehensive plan, we'll give you examples of how some of the people from this book organized their plans. And we'll provide a worksheet for sharpening your major ideas for overcoming depression.

Kate read about all six of the paths to wellness and tried out a number of the strategies that appealed to her. After several weeks she was feeling much better but still had symptoms of mild depression. Recognizing the distance she had already traveled along the paths to recovery, and armed with the extra energy that some relief from depression afforded her, she decided the time was right to see how much further she could go toward wellness. Her first step was to complete the worksheet on page 339.

Kate's example shows an encouraging amount of progress. In 6 weeks, her PHQ-9 score had dropped by almost two-thirds, and she had been able to use at least a small part of each path to recovery. You might recall from Chapter 1 that Kate's PHQ-9 scores eventually fell to a very low level after 12 weeks of following a comprehensive plan and getting professional help. The graph on page 16 shows her PHQ-9 scores dropping to 4 by week 10 and 2 by week 12.

Kate considered the thoughts–action path the most important part of her recovery plan, so she used the self-help exercises from this path routinely in daily life and participated in professional therapy that emphasized CBT methods. Although she credited medication with helping reduce symptoms, Kate liked the idea of learning skills to cope with problems and felt empowered by her work in using the paths to wellness. The relationship path was also quite important to her. A relationship breakup had triggered her depression, and working through the pain of this loss and the negative effects on her self-esteem were important steps in restoring positive feelings and hope for the future. Relationships with helpful and supportive people were an excellent resource for breaking out of the rut of depression and getting back to a happier, more socially stimulating life.

Efforts to use the other paths also had a place in Kate's overall plan, but she thought the lifestyle, spirituality, and mindfulness paths were not quite as important. As you can see in looking at her plan, she decided to try a strategy or two from these paths and also to consider investigating a deeper experience with mindfulness in the future to reduce the risk for return of severe depression.

Before you use the worksheet in Exercise 14.1 to write out your own comprehensive plan, we'll show the priority scores from three of the other people you've met in this book. And we'll briefly describe some of the reasons they emphasized certain paths over others. These scores illustrate the diversity of approaches that people have found helpful in overcoming depression. Although Mark, Angelina, and Sean took their own paths, they all were able to find ways to put depression behind them.

Mark

Thoughts–action path	Biology path	Relation-ship path	Lifestyle path	Spirituality path	Mindful-ness path
2	1	2	4	4	3

My Plan for Using the Paths to Wellness: Kate's Example

Instructions:

1. Record PHQ-9 ratings to check on your progress.

2. Review Exercise 3.13 (page 56), where you first rated your interest in the paths. Then review the plans you've written for using each of the paths to wellness. You can find these plans at the end of Chapters 7, 8, 10, 11, 12, and 13.

3. The next step is to decide on the weight you want to give each path in your overall plan for recovery. Use a 1–5 priority rating, where 1 = the highest priority. These ratings will give you an idea of the relative importance of the different paths in your comprehensive plan.

4. Then record some of the principal steps you have taken or would like to take to put plans into action.

5. Finally, you can make some notes about your experiences in using the paths and/or write down ideas you have for future plans.

Beginning PHQ-9 score (from Chapter 1): ____21____   Number of days (weeks) since completion of first PHQ-9 rating: ____6 weeks____

PHQ-9 score now: ____8____   My goal PHQ-9 score: ____4 or less____

Path to recovery	Priority	Key actions I have taken or am taking to use this path	Key actions I haven't taken yet but would like to take to use this path	Notes/comments
Thoughts–action path	1	—I'm recognizing negative thinking and using thought change records to change automatic thoughts. —I have five coping cards that I carry with me in my purse. Also, I try to follow action prescriptions that I write out with my doctor. —I am using an activity schedule to increase the numbers of interesting and stimulating events (especially doing things with people) in my life.	—Do more step-by-step plans to manage things like joining a club or starting some other activity that would help me meet some new people. —Do more well-being logs. I did only one, but it seemed to lift my mood.	The CBT methods are really helping. My self-confidence is getting back to where it was before the breakup. But I still have a way to go.

(cont.)

339

My Plan for Using the Paths to Wellness: Kate's Example (cont.)

Path to recovery	Priority	Key actions I have taken or am taking to use this path	Key actions I haven't taken yet but would like to take to use this path	Notes/comments
		—I used a step-by-step exercise to get going with cleaning out my garage. —I have a list of positive and negative schemas and am trying to practice using some revised schemas in daily life.		
Biology path	2	—I'm taking sertraline, and I've definitely improved.		—I don't think I need to do anything else with medication now. But I'll stay on the medication for at least 6 months as my doctor recommended.
Relationship path	2	—I'm following the plans to draw strength from my important relationships (especially with my sister and my friend Tricia). —I'm working with my doctor on handling the grief over the breakup with Nick.	—I could try to communicate better with my mother. —I'll eventually want to get out to meet new people and possibly date again.	—I'm doing much better with getting out with the friends I do have. But I'm not ready to date anyone now.

Lifestyle path	3	—I'm attending yoga classes three times a week. —Sleep is okay. I've cut back on coffee to only one cup in the morning, and I've moved files from work that I had stored in my bedroom.	—I could follow a Mediterranean diet more closely.	—Yoga is good for me. I get some exercise, and I feel more relaxed after classes.
Spirituality path	3	—I'm attending church services again. —I did the worksheet on ways to find meaning, and I am paying more attention to looking for meaning in everyday things like spending time with my sister.	—I'm planning to get more involved with church activities. The whole idea of finding meaning and purpose appeals to me. Now that I am feeling better, I think I can focus more on developing this sense of being connected.	—Spirituality is very important to me. But I gave it a 3 on the priority scale because I think some of the other paths are giving me more specific help for depression.
Mindfulness path	4	—I haven't done much with this path except to practice a few of the exercises for mindfulness in everyday life and to do some breathing meditations.	—I might read the book by Dr. Williams on mindfulness and depression to see if it could help me avoid getting so depressed again.	—This is probably a good idea for the future. I have enough to do right now with the other paths I'm using.

341

Mark is a man with a history of recurrent depression who stopped taking an antidepressant before depression returned to his life and began to put a strain on his marriage. In Chapters 9 and 10, you learned how he used the relationship path to deal with the impact of depression on his family life and tap his support system to help him move toward wellness. Mark also found methods from the thoughts–action path to be very helpful. But he ranked the biology path as the most important part of his recovery plan. He realized that medication needed to be the cornerstone of his attempt to pull out of the depression. An antidepressant had worked before, and he regretted that he had decided to go off it.

Mark had never had much interest in athletic activities or exercise, so initially he gave the lifestyle path a lower priority score. Later, when his depression was in better control, he decided it would be a good idea to try to exercise regularly and lose some weight. His efforts to overcome procrastination and get involved in exercise are described later in this chapter.

The spirituality path also seemed somewhat less important to Mark. He considered himself a spiritual person and clearly wanted to have a sense of meaning in his life, but he hadn't noticed any significant erosion of his spiritual connectedness. The mindfulness path seemed to have somewhat greater appeal because of studies that showed a reduced risk for relapse. Also, Mark had enjoyed doing the exercises to enhance mindfulness in Chapter 13. So he gave this path a middle priority score and concluded that it might be worth exploring more thoroughly in the future.

Angelina

Thoughts–action path	Biology path	Relation-ship path	Lifestyle path	Spirituality path	Mindful-ness path
1	5	4	3	3	1

Angelina's story was featured in Chapters 6, 7, and 13. Her plan gives an example of someone who didn't want to take medication and instead decided to rely on psychotherapy methods to achieve wellness. She primarily used CBT strategies. For example, she worked on changing schemas to help build her self-acceptance and self-esteem. But Angelina also became very interested in mindfulness as a method for calming her worries and helping her avoid the return of depression. Angelina didn't have significant relationship problems or issues. However, she thought the advice in the relationship path helped her better manage the impact of depression on her communication with family members and get support for her recovery. She decided to participate more regularly in exercise at her local Y and found the section of the book on finding meaning to be helpful. Nevertheless, she continued to put most of her effort into CBT and mindfulness strategies.

Sean

Thoughts–action path	Biology path	Relation-ship path	Lifestyle path	Spirituality path	Mindful-ness path
2	2	3	3	1	4

Sean took a somewhat different path toward wellness. Although he was able to draw strength from all of the paths, spirituality was especially important to him. You may recall from Chapter 12 that Sean developed depression after suffering a heart attack and that a sense of feeling spiritually disconnected was a core part of his problem. Therefore, working to resolve his spiritual dilemma and to use his spiritual resources became a fundamental part of his plan for overcoming depression. He also relied heavily on CBT methods and accepted his doctor's recommendation to use an antidepressant.

Sean used the tips from Chapters 9 and 10 to help get support from the positive people in his life, to educate these people about depression, and to limit the potential negative effects of depression on relationships. On the lifestyle front, Sean's plan included eating a low-fat diet and following a cardiac rehab schedule for aerobic exercise. He found that becoming more mindful of activities of everyday life was helpful. But he decided not to pursue more extensive experiences in mindfulness meditation.

We hope these examples have illustrated that the paths to wellness are extremely flexible and can be blended together in myriad ways to overcome depression. After you sketch out your own customized plan, we'll help you troubleshoot difficulties that can be encountered in putting plans to work. As with all the other individual plans in this book, you may find yourself wanting to modify your overall plan, in which case you can photocopy the worksheet in Exercise 14.1 or download it from *www.guilford.com/breakingfreeforms*.

Overcoming Obstacles to Success

We hope your plan for wellness goes very smoothly and you make steady progress toward your goals. But if you encounter obstacles along the way, some of the tips we give here may help you stay on track toward recovery.

Lack of Previous Success in Following Plans

Are you a person who has tried several diets or exercise programs but hasn't been able to stick with the program long enough to achieve success? Have you had other experiences where well-intended plans fizzled out? Many of our patients tell us they've had so many experiences with not being able to follow through with the specifics of plans that they don't have great optimism for trying again.

If you're plagued with memories about plans that haven't worked, and part of you remains somewhat discouraged about following a plan for recovery from depression, you can try using some of the skills you've learned from CBT. For example, you might be able to spot cognitive errors or other distortions in thinking in automatic thoughts or schemas like "I can never stick with anything long enough … What's the use of trying? My plans all end up the same way—going nowhere." Is there any evidence that you have followed a plan and had it work out, even to a partial extent? Have you learned ways to improve your chances of following a plan? Angelina changed some of her negative thoughts using the exercise on page 346.

If you've had some negative thoughts about your ability to follow a plan for wellness, use Exercise 14.2 to try to develop a mind-set that can send you on your way to recovery.

My Plan for Using the Paths to Wellness

Instructions:

1. Record PHQ-9 ratings to check on your progress.

2. Review Exercise 3.13 (page 56), where you first rated your interest in the paths. Then review the plans you've written for using each of the paths to wellness. You can find these plans at the end of Chapters 7, 8, 10, 11, 12, and 13.

3. The next step is to decide on the weight you want to give each path in your overall plan for recovery. Use a 1–5 priority rating, where 1 = the highest priority. These ratings will give you an idea of the relative importance of the different paths in your comprehensive plan.

4. Then record some of the principal steps you have taken or would like to take to put plans into action.

5. Finally, you can make some notes about your experiences in using the paths and/or write down ideas you have for future plans.

Beginning PHQ-9 score (from Chapter 1): _____   Number of days (weeks) since completion of first PHQ-9 rating: _____

PHQ-9 score now: _____   My goal PHQ-9 score: _____

Path to recovery	Priority	Key actions I have taken or am taking to use this path	Key actions I haven't taken yet but would like to take to use this path	Notes/comments
Thoughts–action path				
Biology path				

Relationship path	**Lifestyle path**	**Spirituality path**	**Mindfulness path**

Modifying Negative Cognitions about Sticking with a Plan: Angelina's Example

Instructions: Write down negative cognitions you might have about your ability to follow a plan for personal change. Then examine the evidence, spot cognitive errors, and write down a rational alternative that will increase your ability to make the plan work.

Automatic thought or schema: *I can never stick with diets or other plans to change.*

Evidence for:

It is true that I have tried lots of diets, but always quit.

Many times I have tried to teach myself to relax and to not get so stressed out, but I always return to my "workaholic" lifestyle.

I had a plan to get another job, but didn't follow through with all of the things I'd need to do.

Cognitive errors in evidence for this thought:

There is an all-or-nothing quality to all of this evidence.

It also magnifies the problem and ignores the evidence that I actually have followed some plans.

Evidence against:

Although I've quit many diets, my current eating pattern isn't too bad.

I'm trying to cut down on fast food and to eat more fruits and vegetables.

I'm using mindfulness and am finding it very helpful.

I did follow my plan to complete my education.

I'm actually fairly well organized, and I have made many plans that I have completed (for example, planning holiday dinners with family, planning a vacation with friends, planning with my daughter for managing after-school activities).

Rational alternatives:

I've quit some plans, especially diets, but I've also had some positive outcomes for other plans.

This plan for getting over depression is a challenge. However, I have had enough experience with carrying out plans that I can keep going and try to make it work out.

I have some skills in following plans. I'd like to get better at following plans—I can work on learning ways to do this.

Stressful Events Set You Back

One of the most common problems our patients encounter is that just as they seem to get going with putting their plans into action, some trouble pops up or a new crisis looms. Whether the problem is a child who's having difficulties at school, a downturn in physical health, a financial worry, job concerns, or something else, it seems to commandeer their energy and attention at the expense of their plan for recovery from depression. If you find yourself failing to make headway against depression because you end up jumping from crisis to crisis, you can do these two things:

1. *Narrow the focus.* For at least a short while, reduce the number of actions you're taking in your plan for wellness. Choose a few methods that you think will give the highest yield. Perhaps it will be as simple as taking a medication and using strategies from the thoughts–action path. Or maybe there are other stress-management methods or spiritually oriented activities that you find helpful and want to be sure to include. After the level of stress is reduced, or you have moved beyond the crisis, you can get back to a more comprehensive plan. The most important thing is to try to keep moving forward in your journey to overcome depression.

2. *Expend most of your efforts on mending yourself.* When important people in your life face big problems, it seems natural to put your own concerns aside to help them. But we've seen innumerable people in our clinical practices who get so consumed with helping relatives or friends that they begin to drift away from using the paths to their own recovery. Before long, their depression takes a turn for the worse. If you're responding to crises in the lives of others, try to keep a reasonable balance between the energies you devote to their problems and the energies you devote to your own health. A good reason for expending most of your efforts on mending yourself is that you might be able to be a more effective mother, father, partner, or friend if you take care of yourself first.

Procrastination

Has procrastination been a limiting factor in your life? Have you noticed that you put things off and then feel bad when they languish? Breaking through procrastination isn't easy, but many of our patients have been able to do it. The following tips have worked for them—and for us.

1. *Change your thinking.* The lessons you learned in the thoughts–action path can really pay off if you decide to tackle procrastination. Use the same strategies recommended earlier in the chapter for coping with "lack of success in following a plan." In this case, though, you will target automatic thoughts and schemas that keep you from getting started. A particularly useful strategy is to complete a thought change record when you realize you're procrastinating.

When Mark wrote his initial plan for wellness (described earlier in this chapter), he played down the importance of making any lifestyle changes, especially exercising. Over time he reconsidered as he heard more and more about the benefits of exercise and

Modifying Negative Cognitions
about Sticking with a Plan

Instructions: Write down negative cognitions you might have about your ability to follow a plan for personal change. Then examine the evidence, spot cognitive errors, and write down a rational alternative that will increase your ability to make the plan work.

Automatic thought or schema: _____

_____

Evidence for: _____

_____

Cognitive errors in evidence for this thought: _____

_____

Evidence against: _____

_____

_____

_____

Rational alternatives: _____

_____

_____

_____

admitted to himself that he had gained a lot of weight through the years. But every time he thought of joining a health club or starting a walking program, procrastination would get in the way.

We won't show you Mark's entire thought change record, but we'll give some highlights to demonstrate how this method helped him cope with procrastination.

Event: I told my doctor I would walk three times a week. It's Sunday, and I haven't gone out walking this entire week. There's always something else to do—activities with the kids, work I've brought home, cleaning up the kitchen, etc.

Automatic thoughts: I'm too busy; there's never enough time. (100% belief) I hate exercising—I've never been athletic. (90%) What's the use? I'll always be fat and out of shape. (90%)

Emotions: Anger at self (45%), sadness (50%)

Rational thoughts: There are plenty of cognitive errors here—magnifying the problem, thinking in absolutes, jumping to conclusions, and so forth. Actually, there would be enough time if I got organized. (95%) It's true that I never participated in sports, but I don't know if I could enjoy certain types of exercise unless I give it a fair chance. (95%) I've seen other people get into an exercise routine and have it work for them. Maybe I have it in me to do the same. (40%)

Outcome: Reduced anger (15%) and sadness (20%). I went on a walk Sunday afternoon with my wife. I think I can walk at least twice a week (Saturdays and Sundays), and I'll try to find another day to meet the goal of three walks per week.

Did Mark's example give you any ideas for self-defeating cognitions that you may have that are promoting procrastination? Some of the procrastination-stimulating cognitions that our patients have reported are "I can do it tomorrow … I'll mess it up (or fail) anyway, so why try? … It will be too hard … Everybody else has their life in order—mine's a total mess … If I do succeed, then there would be pressure on me to do even more." If you have these types of thoughts, you can examine the evidence and try to develop more rational cognitions that will help you make positive changes.

People who have had significant problems with procrastination often find some degree of truth in their automatic thoughts. Perhaps there have been problems with putting tasks off repeatedly because you think you can "do it tomorrow." Or maybe you've had a pattern of viewing tasks as being too hard and beyond your capacities. If this is the case, then you may need to admit the problem and use some of the other tips given here to have some positive experiences in getting things done.

2. Build your motivation. In Chapter 5 you learned how to use motivational enhancement strategies to increase your chances of following behavioral plans such as activity schedules and the step-by-step approach. You can use the same methods to help you stay the course in following an overall plan for wellness. Do you remember doing the motivational enhancement exercise? To use this method you set a specific goal for change, list some key motivators that will encourage you to work on reaching the goal, and then identify some demotivators that might get in your way. You then try to keep the motivators in top-of-the-mind awareness while you figure out ways to cope with the demotivators.

If you have trouble with motivation to follow a plan for wellness, the worksheet on page 123 (in Exercise 5.8) could give you a boost.

3. *Get organized.* A common mistake of procrastinators is lack of organization. If you don't structure adequate time to carry out the plan, you may find that other responsibilities take over and a plan that once seemed so reasonable will fall by the wayside.

A strategy that might be helpful is to:

- Review your plan for wellness to see if you're carving out specific time to follow important parts of the plan.
- Prioritize actions so that you can decide how much time should be devoted to each of these key parts of the plan.
- Be practical in making choices. Don't overload yourself, but try to organize your days to do the things that you think will help most.
- Use an activity schedule or other planner to make specific commitments of time to follow plans.

When Mark used these principles, he decided that exercise was an important priority and that procrastination would get in the way unless he set aside defined times to take walks. After talking with his wife, Alice, he wrote on his schedule that he would walk for at least 30 minutes every Saturday and Sunday starting at about 4:30 in the afternoon and he would walk after work at about 6 P.M. on Tuesday or Wednesday.

4. *Reach out for support.* People who have problems with procrastination often fall into the trap of believing that they have to do it alone. If procrastination has been a chronic issue, one might feel shame at not being able to accomplish tasks and thus hesitate to let others know about the difficulty. However, a helping hand can sometimes lead to a breakthrough in overcoming procrastination. Alice became an "exercise buddy" for Mark and helped him stick with his commitment to walk three times a week. She also had open discussions with him about his entire plan for wellness and gave him lots of support in carrying it out. Are there positive people in your life who could give you encouragement and support in making your plan for wellness a success?

Hitting a Plateau

Finding that you've reached a plateau in a path to recovery is both good and bad. It means you've made progress and aren't as depressed as before, but it also leaves you frustrated to be stalled. The fact is, hitting a plateau is common in treatment for depression, especially among those who are receiving only one form of treatment.

SCIENCE CORNER

- Most studies have found that 60% or more of people who are treated with a single antidepressant, or a single course of evidence-based psychotherapy without any other treatments (monotherapy), do not reach full remission.
- Residual symptoms are very common, but research has shown that further improvement can occur with additional treatment.

• If you seem to be stuck in depression and are not receiving professional treatment, don't wait any longer. Find a doctor or therapist to help you in your path to recovery.

• If you're receiving professional treatment, be sure to discuss all of your ideas for getting past a plateau with your doctor and/or therapist.

One of the reasons that we have gone to lengths in this book to explain multiple paths to recovery and to encourage you to learn a variety of methods is to provide tools that you can use to reach full remission. Although methods from any of the paths might be considered as ways to move toward recovery, we'll highlight several especially promising ideas here.

1. *Reconsider the diagnosis.* If depressive symptoms are lingering, it's often a good idea to take a step back to be sure the diagnosis and treatment plan are on target. If you haven't had a recent visit to your primary care doctor, make the effort to do so. Because many physical problems and medications used to treat medical illnesses can trigger or aggravate depression, be sure your physical health is not part of the reason your depression hasn't resolved completely. Also, you can ask your doctor to take another look at the diagnosis of depression. When patients are referred to us for a second opinion, we often find that they still have symptoms because they were misdiagnosed—for example, having bipolar disorder but being treated for unipolar major depression or having an unrecognized anxiety disorder or substance abuse problem.

2. *Use aggressive pharmacotherapy or other biological treatments.* In Chapter 8 we described how antidepressants and other biologically based therapies can be used to overcome treatment resistance (lack of effectiveness). The same strategies can be used to move beyond a plateau. There are many helpful methods for switching antidepressants or combining them with other medications or for using more than one antidepressant at a time. Transcranial magnetic stimulation is another example of a biological treatment that can increase the possibility of a full recovery.

3. *Start an evidence-based psychotherapy if you have not already done so.* Several studies and meta-analyses have shown that adding an evidence-based psychotherapy such as CBT to a treatment plan can lead to greater levels of improvement. If you've been using CBT self-help only and haven't had the opportunity to try professional therapy, ask your doctor for a referral or go online to look for therapists in your area who have received training in this approach. Websites that list cognitive-behavioral therapists are listed in the Resources section at the end of this book. If you have been participating in CBT but haven't fully immersed yourself in this approach, try increasing the frequency of visits.

4. *Use well-being therapy methods.* Research by Dr. Giovanni Fava and others has found that adaptations of CBT that focus on building a sense of well-being are useful strategies for treating depressive symptoms that aren't been fully relieved by other treatments. These methods are featured in Chapter 7.

5. *Address an interpersonal issue or other nagging problem that may be holding you back from full recovery.* Sometimes an ongoing stress such as a troubled marriage, a difficult relationship with a child, or unemployment can interfere with progress toward wellness. Can you get help from a therapist in solving this problem? Or can you make some decisions that will help you meet this challenge? We gave examples of ways that people have dealt with relationship problems in Chapter 10.

6. *Add light therapy if you have a pattern of seasonal depression.* As noted in Chapter 11, light therapy with a 10,000 lux intensity light source for 30 minutes in the morning is an effective treatment for people who have a seasonal pattern to their depression.

7. *Examine your lifestyle to see if further changes may be helpful.* If you haven't done much with the lifestyle path yet or believe you haven't used this path to its full potential, you might consider going back over this chapter to see if any of the strategies might help relieve symptoms. If sleep remains a problem, use the methods described in Chapter 11 to improve your sleep habits. If you aren't exercising or think more exercise might be helpful, organize a plan to make exercise a core part of your weekly routine. And consider looking at your diet to see whether there are any changes that might give you a lift as you work toward recovery.

If you've hit a plateau, or may hit a plateau in the future, the next worksheet (Exercise 14.3) could help you focus your ideas for making renewed progress. You might find it useful again in the future as well; photocopy the form or download it from *www.guilford. com/breakingfreeforms*.

Staying Well

Because depression has the unpleasant tendency to reappear in people's lives, we always try to work out plans with our patients that will reduce the risk of recurrence. The best-case scenario is to treat depression to full remission (no significant symptoms) the first time it occurs and put a plan into action so it never returns. But we know that people who have had two or more previous depressions are at especially high risk for having another episode. Thus people with a history of multiple episodes will probably need a long-term plan to keep depression away.

The strongest scientific evidence for methods that can sustain recovery is for CBT, antidepressant medication, and mindfulness meditation. Although there is no therapy that guarantees a depression-free future, many studies have shown that these treatments are highly useful in reducing the risk of relapse.

SCIENCE CORNER A review by Hollon and colleagues of major studies of depression found the lowest relapse rate (about 20%) in people treated with CBT. A considerably higher relapse rate (about 50–80%) was observed in people who received acute treatment with antidepressants but *did not* continue them long term.

However, the review by Hollon and colleagues also found that continuing antidepressants for long-term therapy reduced the relapse rate about to the level achieved by CBT.

Other studies, such as a large investigation conducted by Dr. Martin Keller and associates, have found that ongoing treatment with antidepressants is much more effective than placebos in reducing the risk for relapse.

Mindfulness meditation has been found to be an effective method of reducing the risk of relapse in studies by Drs. Teasdale, Segal, and others.

Instructions: Consider each of the strategies on this worksheet and make specific notes on ideas you would like to use to get past a plateau. Take this worksheet with you to discuss these ideas with a doctor or therapist.

Strategy	Specific ideas I have for using this strategy	Comments/notes
See a doctor to reconsider the diagnosis		
Use more aggressive pharmacotherapy or other biological treatments		
Start an evidence-based therapy or increase level of participation in therapy		
Use well-being therapy methods		
Address an interpersonal issue or other nagging problem		
Use light therapy		
Examine lifestyle to see if changes would help		
Use other strategies derived from the paths to wellness		

Research has also shown some benefit of booster sessions for people who have responded to interpersonal psychotherapy (IPT).

~~~~~~

Although an ideal program that works every time for relapse prevention hasn't been discovered yet, these recommendations may help you maximize the chances of staying well.

1. *Develop a long-term relationship with a health care professional who can help you stay well.* Even if you've finished treatment and are completely recovered, it's a good idea to have an ongoing arrangement with a doctor or therapist who can assist you if symptoms start to return. And if some form of maintenance therapy such as continued use of medication or booster psychotherapy sessions is part of your plan, you'll need to have a trusted health care professional on your team.

2. *If a single episode of depression is treated with an antidepressant, the medication should be continued for at least 6–9 months after symptoms have been resolved.* Research has shown that early discontinuation of medication greatly increases the rate of relapse.

3. *If you have a history of three or more episodes of depression, long-term treatment with an antidepressant should be considered.* People who have had multiple bouts of depression have a very high risk of relapse if antidepressants are withdrawn and thus should strongly consider ongoing use of medication. We have many patients in our practices with histories of multiple episodes who are in full remission and are committed to indefinite therapy with antidepressants. They don't want to be depressed again and know that continuing an antidepressant is an integral part of their plan to maintain wellness.

4. *CBT should be considered if you have not yet received this treatment.* Although this book has featured self-help methods from CBT, professional treatment could be needed to help you reach full recovery and sustain these gains. Whether you have been treated professionally with CBT or not, the exercises in this book are designed to help you draw strength from this treatment approach and to use self-help methods over the long haul.

5. *Mindfulness meditation can offer a unique and effective way to maintain wellness.* The discipline and practice required to fully utilize mindfulness meditation may not be for everyone, but research has clearly supported the usefulness of this method of preventing recurrence of depression. If you've suffered from one or more episodes of depression, mindfulness deserves careful consideration as a part of your plan to stay well.

6. *Key strategies that were helpful for treatment of acute depression should be continued.* Although research has not yet looked at the value of continuing to use a comprehensive plan that includes strategies from many paths to wellness, we think it makes good sense to follow plans that promote psychological health over the long term. For example, if exercise has been beneficial, it probably wouldn't be wise to drop out of your exercise routine as soon as your depression eases. If you've found that a focus on well-being has

been helpful, why not sustain your efforts to look for ways to enhance your feelings of well-being? If you realized that a greater sense of meaning is very important to you, could you go further in your efforts to live a purposeful and meaningful life? If a relationship problem has been a part of your depression, could you work on maintaining gains that have been made, or could you target relationship issues that you want to resolve in the future?

Our last exercise in *Breaking Free from Depression* will help you organize your ideas for staying well. If you are still trying to resolve an acute depression or are contending with chronic symptoms, this exercise can be delayed until you feel that your depression is in good control. However, we hope that you've made good progress and that you're ready to start planning ways to make your recovery last.

Kate completed this worksheet after she had been using her plan for wellness for about 12 weeks and her PHQ-9 score had fallen to 2. Scores of 4 or less are generally considered to be in the range of remission.

Kate was able to write out some great plans for staying well. She included evidence-based methods such as medication and CBT and added some depth to the plan by making commitments to use yoga, move on after her relationship breakup, and use her spiritual resources. Now it's your turn to complete this final exercise. To modify your plan for staying well down the road, photocopy the form in Exercise 14.4 or download it from *www.guilford.com/breakingfreeforms.*

Summary

In this book you've been able to develop a plan for using six paths to wellness in your journey to overcome depression. You've had the opportunity to build skills for using methods from evidence-based treatments, and you've learned many ways to cope with symptoms and move toward recovery. Starting in Chapter 1 and continuing through this last chapter, we've encouraged you to monitor progress and to refine your plan until you achieve lasting success. We hope that you're breaking free from depression and that the path ahead looks bright with promise.

My Plan for Staying Well: Kate's Example

Instructions: Review each of the strategies for staying well and write out specific things you will do to use these strategies. You can check over your comprehensive plan for wellness (Exercise 14.1) to get ideas for maintaining wellness.

Strategy	My specific plan for using this strategy	Comments/notes
Develop a long-term relationship with a health care professional	*I have a good relationship with my doctor and will see him at least once every 3 months to check on progress and do any troubleshooting needed.*	*I can make more frequent appointments if needed.*
If medications have been used, develop a plan for how long they should be continued.	*I've been on sertraline for about 3 months. My doctor recommends I take it for at least 6 more months. This plan is okay with me.*	
Consider use of CBT. Or if you have already had treatment with CBT, note your plans for continuing to use these skills.	*I don't need to use activity schedules any longer because I'm back to my old self. But trying to spot and change automatic thoughts is definitely worthwhile. Coping cards and well-being logs are also high on my list of useful things to keep doing.*	*I can get a tune-up on using CBT when I see my doctor every few months. Reviewing my notebook from CBT can help me remember to use these methods.*
Consider use of mindfulness meditation.	*I enjoyed doing some of the mindfulness exercises, especially being mindful of everyday things. But I am doing well now and have other plans in place to stay well. So I don't think I'll get more involved with mindfulness exercises.*	*I can save this approach for later if I need it.*
Continue to use other strategies from the paths to wellness.	*I will keep going to yoga classes—they are a big help in putting me in a good mood.* *I'm pretty much over the breakup with Nick. It's time to start meeting some other people.* *Spirituality remains very important to me, and I'll put effort into this part of my life.*	*My life is going well now. I need to keep up the balance I've achieved.*

My Plan for Staying Well

Instructions: Review each of the strategies for staying well and write out specific things you will do to use these strategies. You can check over your comprehensive plan for wellness (Exercise 14.1) to get ideas for maintaining wellness.

Strategy	My specific plan for using this strategy	Comments/notes
Develop a long-term relationship with a health care professional.		
If medications have been used, develop a plan for how long they should be continued.		
Consider use of CBT. Or if you have already had treatment with CBT, note your plans for continuing to use these skills.		
Consider use of mindfulness meditation.		
Continue to use other strategies from the paths to wellness.		

Resources

Books

Addis ME, & Martell CR. (2004). *Overcoming Depression One Step at a Time: The New Behavioral Activation Approach to Getting Your Life Back*. Oakland, CA: New Harbinger.

Antony MM, & Norton PJ. (2009). *The Anti-Anxiety Workbook*. New York: Guilford Press.

Barlow DH, & Craske MG. (2000). *Mastery of Your Anxiety and Panic: Client Workbook for Agoraphobia*. Burlington, MA: Academic Press.

Basco, MR. (2009). *The Procrastinator's Guide to Getting Things Done*. New York: Guilford Press.

Basco, MR. (2006). *The Bipolar Workbook*. New York: Guilford Press.

Bonanno, G. (2009). *The Other Side of Sadness: What the New Science of Bereavement Tells Us about Life After Loss*. New York: Basic Books.

Greenberger D & Padesky C. (1995). *Mind over Mood: Change How You Feel by Changing the Way You Think*. New York: Guilford Press.

Henry AD, Clayfield JC, Phillips SM, & Nicholson J. (2001). *Parenting Well When You're Depressed: A Complete Resource for Maintaining a Healthy Family*. Oakland, CA: New Harbinger.

Miklowitz, DJ. (2002). *The Bipolar Survival Guide: What You and Your Family Need to Know*. New York: Guilford Press.

Real, T. (1998). *I Don't Want to Talk about It: Overcoming the Secret Legacy of Male Depression*. New York: Scribner.

Rosenquist, S. (2010). *After the Stork: The Couple's Guide to Preventing and Overcoming Postpartum Depression*. Oakland, CA: New Harbinger.

Wright JH, & Basco MR. (2002). *Getting Your Life Back: The Complete Guide to Recovery from Depression*. New York: Touchstone.

Personal Accounts of Depression and Bipolar Disorder

Duke, P. (1992). *Brilliant Madness: Living with Manic Depressive Illness*. New York: Bantam Books.

Jamison, KR. (1995). *An Unquiet Mind*. New York: Knopf.

Shields, B. (2005). *Down Came the Rain*. New York: Hyperion.

Styron, W. (1990). *Darkness Visible: A Memoir of Madness*. New York: Random House.

CBT and IPT

Burns, D. (1999). *Feeling Good: The New Mood Therapy*. New York: Harper.

Greenberger D, & Padesky CA. (1995). *Mind Over Mood*. New York: Guilford Press.

Weissman, MW. (2005). *Mastering Depression through Interpersonal Psychotherapy: Patient Workbook*. Oxford, UK: Oxford University Press.

Wright JH, Basco MR, & Thase ME. (2005). *Learning Cognitive-Behavior Therapy: An Illustrated Guide*. Arlington, VA: American Psychiatric Publishing.

Medications

Chew RH, Hales RE, & Yudofsky SC. (2009). *What Your Patients Need to Know about Psychiatric Medications*. Arlington, VA: American Psychiatric Publishing.

Preston JD, O'Neal JH, & Talaga MC. (2009). *Consumer's Guide to Psychiatric Drugs: Straight Talk for Patients and Their Families*. New York: Simon & Schuster.

Stahl, SM. (2008). *Essential Psychopharmacology* (3rd ed.). Cambridge, UK: Cambridge University Press.

Relationships

McKay M, Fanning P, & Paleg K. (1994). *Couple Skills: Making Your Relationship Work*. Oakland, CA: New Harbinger.

Gottman J, Notarius C, Gonso J, & Markham H. (1979). *A Couple's Guide to Communication*. Champaign, IL: Research Press.

Sleep

Hauri P, & Linde S. (1996). *No More Sleepless Nights*. Hoboken, NJ: Wiley.

Jacobs, GD. (1998). *Say Goodnight to Insomnia*. New York: Holt.

Morin, CM. (1996). *Relief from Insomnia: Getting the Sleep of Your Dreams*. New York: Doubleday.

Diet and Exercise

Beck, JS. (2007). *The Beck Diet Solution: Train Your Brain to Think Like a Thin Person*. Birmingham, AL: Oxmoor House.

Ornish, D. (2000). *Eat More, Weigh Less: Dr. Dean Ornish's Life Choice Program for Losing Weight Safely While Eating Abundantly*. New York: Harper.

Weight Watchers. (2010). *Weight Watchers New Complete Cookbook*. Hoboken, NJ: Wiley.

Light Therapy/SAD

Rosenthal, N. (2006). *Winter Blues: Everything You Need to Know to Beat Seasonal Affective Disorder*. New York: Guilford Press.

Subtance Abuse

AAWS. (2002). *Alcoholics Anonymous: The Story of How Many Thousands of Men and Women Have Recovered from Alcoholism*. New York: Alcoholics Anonymous World Services.

Miller WR, & Munoz RF. (2005). *Controlling Your Drinking: Tools to Make Moderation Work for You*. New York: Guilford Press.

Spirituality

Dalai Lama. (1999). *Ethics for the New Millennium*. New York: Penguin Putnam.

Frankl, VE. (1959). *Man's Search for Meaning*. New York: Simon & Schuster.

Kushner, HS. (1981). *When Bad Things Happen to Good People*. New York: Schocken Books.

Moore, T. (1992). *Care of the Soul: A Guide for Cultivating Depth and Sacredness in Everyday Life*. New York: HarperCollins.

Lewis, TG. (2002). *Finding God: Praying the Psalms in Times of Depression*. Louisville, KY: Westminster John Knox Press.

Walsh, R. (2000). *Essential Spirituality: The Seven Central Practices to Awaken Heart and Mind*. New York: Wiley.

May, GG. (2004). *The Dark Night of the Soul: A Psychiatrist Explores the Connection between Darkness and Spiritual Growth*. New York: HarperCollins.

Mindfulness

Kabat-Zinn, J. (1990). *Full Catastrophe Living: Using the Wisdom of Your Body to Fight Stress, Pain, and Illness*. New York: Hyperion.

Kabat-Zinn, J. (2005). *Wherever You Go There You Are*. New York: Hyperion.

Salzberg, S. (2010). *Real Happiness: The Power of Meditation*. New York: Workman.

Siegel, RD. (2010). *The Mindfulness Solution: Everyday Practices for Everyday Problems*. New York: Guilford Press.

Williams M, Teasdale J, Segal Z, & Kabat-Zinn J. (2007). *The Mindful Way through Depression*. New York: Guilford Press.

Organizations

Information, Support, and Help with Depression

United States

Academy of Cognitive Therapy
Website lists certified cognitive therapists by location.
www.academyofct.org
267-350-7683

Association for Behavioral and Cognitive Therapies
Website lists therapists trained in cognitive and behavioral techniques, by location.
www.abct.org
212-647-1890

National Institute of Mental Health
www.nimh.nih.gov
301-443-4513 (local)
866-615-6464 (toll-free)
301-443-8431 (TTY)
866-415-8051 (TTY toll-free)

Depression and Bipolar Support Alliance
www.dbsalliance.org
800-826-3632

Depression and Related Affective Disorders Association
www.drada.org

National Network of Depression Centers
www.nndc.org
734-332-3914

Massachusetts General Hospital Mood and Anxiety Disorders Institute
www.moodandanxiety.org
617-724-7792

University of Louisville Depression
Center
www.louisville.edu/depression
800-334-UofL (8635)
502-813-6606

University of Michigan Depression
Center
www.depressioncenter.org
800-475-MICH (6424)
734-936-4400

Canada

Mood Disorders Society of Canada
www.mooddisorderscanada.ca
519-824-5565

The Organization for Bipolar Affective
Disorder
www.obad.ca
403-263-7408
866-263-7408

United Kingdom

Depression Alliance
www.depressionalliance.org
0845 123 23 20 (for an information
pack)

Depression UK
www.depressionuk.org

Mood Swings Network
www.moodswings.org.uk
0845 123 60 50 (help line)

Ireland

Aware
www.aware.ie
01 661 7211

Australia/New Zealand

Balance NZ: Bipolar and Depression
Network
www.everybody.co.nz
0800 111 757 (depression helpline)

Black Dog Institute
www.blackdoginstitute.org.au
02 9382 4523 (community/consumer
inquiries)

Substance Abuse

United States

Substance Abuse and Mental
Health Services Administration
(SAMHSA)
www.samhsa.gov/treatment
800-662-HELP (4357)

National Institute on Drug Abuse
(NIDA)
A government-sponsored institute
focused on drug abuse and
addiction research.
www.nida.nih.gov
301-443-1124

Alcoholics Anonymous (AA)
Check your local listings for regional
 phone numbers.
www.aa.org

**Chemically Dependent Anonymous
 (CDA)**
www.cdaweb.org
888-CDA-HOPE

Cocaine Anonymous (CA)
www.ca.org
800-347-8998

Narcotics Anonymous (NA)
www.na.org
818-773-9999

Al-Anon and Alateen
www.al-anon.alateen.org
888-4AL-ANON (425-2666)

Canada

Canadian Centre on Substance Abuse
www.ccsa.ca
613-235-4048

United Kingdom

**National Treatment Agency for
 Substance Misuse**
www.nta.nhs.uk
020 7972 1999

Ireland

**National Drug Advisory and Treatment
 Centre**
www.addictionireland.ie
353 1 6488600

Australia/New Zealand

**Australian Centre for Addiction
 Research**
www.acar.net.au
61 (0) 411 286 109

**Alcohol Drug Association New
 Zealand**
www.adanz.org.nz
03 379 8626

Computer-Assisted CBT Programs for Depression

"Good Days Ahead"
www.empower-interactive.com

"Beating the Blues"
www.beatingtheblues.co.uk

Hotlines

National Suicide Prevention Hotline
800-273-TALK
www.suicidepreventionlifeline.org

National Domestic Violence Hotline
800-799-SAFE
thehotline.org

References

Allen M, Bromley A, Kuyken W, & Sonnenberg SJ. (2009). Participants' experiences of mindfulness-based cognitive therapy: "It changed me in just about every way possible." *Behavioural and Cognitive Psychotherapy, 37*(4), 413–430.

America A, & Milling LS. (2008). The efficacy of vitamins for reducing or preventing depression symptoms in healthy individuals: natural remedy or placebo? *Journal of Behavioral Medicine, 31*(2), 157–167.

Araujo DMR, Vilarim M, & Nardi AE. (2001). What is the effectiveness of the use of polyunsaturated fatty acid omega-3 in the treatment of depression? *Expert Review of Neurotherapeutics, 10*(7), 1117–1129.

Bertone-Johnson, ER. (2009). Vitamin D and the occurrence of depression: Causal association or circumstantial evidence? *Nutrition Reviews, 67*(8), 481–492.

Cipriani A, Furukawa TA, Salanti G, Geddes JR, Higgins JP, Churchill R, et al. (2009). Comparative efficacy and acceptability of 12 new-generation antidepressants: a multiple-treatments meta-analysis. *Lancet, 373*(9665), 746–758.

Cuijpers P, Dekker J, Hollon SD, & Andersson G. (2009). Adding psychotherapy to pharmacotherapy in the treatment of depression disorders in adults: A meta-analysis. *Journal of Clinical Psychiatry, 70*(9), 1219–1229.

Dalai Lama. (1999). *Ethics for a New Millenium.* New York: Penguin Putnam.

Davidson RJ, & Lutz A. (2007, September). Buddha's brain: Neuroplasticity and Meditation. *In the Spotlight Magazine,* 171–174.

Dimidjian S, Hollon SD, Dobson KS, Schmaling KB, Kohlenberg RJ, Addis ME, et al. (2006). Randomized trial of behavioral activation, cognitive therapy, and antidepressant medication in the acute treatment of adults with major depression. *Journal of Consulting and Clinical Psychology, 74*(4), 658–670.

de Mello MF, de Jesus MJ, Bacaltchuk J, Verdeli H, & Neugebauer R. (2005). A systematic review of research findings on the efficacy of interpersonal therapy for depressive disorders. *European Archives of Psychiatry and Clinical Neuroscience, 255*(2), 75–82.

Eccleston C, Williams AC, & Morley S. (2009). Psychological therapies for the management of chronic pain (excluding headache) in adults. *Cochrane Review.* Retrieved from *onlinelibrary.wiley.com/o/cochrane/clsysrev/articles/CD007407/frame.htm.*

Egan G. (1986). *The Skilled Helper: A Systematic Approach to Effective Helping.* Washington DC: Thompson Brooks/Cole Publishing.

Fava GA, Rafanelli C, Cazzaro M, Conti S, & Grandi S. (1998). Well-being therapy: A novel psychotherapeutic approach for residual symptoms of affective disorders. *Psychological Medicine, 28,* 475–480.

Fava GA, & Ruini C. (2003). Development and characteristics of a well-being enhancing psychotherapeutic strategy: Well-being therapy. *Journal of Behavior Therapy and Experimental Psychiatry, 34*(1), 45–63.

Fava GA, Ruini C, Rafanelli C, Finos L, Conti S, & Grandi S. (2004). Six-year outcome of cognitive behavior therapy for prevention of recurrent depression. *American Journal of Psychiatry, 161*(10), 1872–1876.

Fava GA, Ruini C, Rafanelli C, & Grandi S. (2002). Cognitive behavior approach to loss of clinical effect druing long-term antidepressant treatment: A pilot study. *American Journal of Psychiatry, 159*(12), 2094–2095.

Fava M, & Mischoulon D. (2009). Folate in depression: Efficacy, safety, differences in formulations, and clinical issues. *Journal of Clinical Psychiatry, 70*(Suppl 5), 12–17.

Fountoulakis KN, & Moller HJ. (2010). Efficacy of antidepressants: A re-analysis and reinterpretation of the kirsch data. *International Journal of Neuropsychopharmacology, 27*, 1–8.

Fournier JC, DeRubeis RJ, Hollon SD, Dimidjian S, Amsterdam JD, Shelton RC, et al. (2010). Antidepressant drug effects and depression severity: A patient-level meta-analysis. *Journal of the American Medical Association, 303*(1), 47–53.

Frank E, Kupfer DJ, Buysse DJ, Swartz HA, Pilkonis PA, Houck PR, et al. (2007). Randomized trial of weekly, twice-monthly, and monthly interpersonal psychotherapy as maintenance treatment for women with recurrent depression. *American Journal of Psychiatry, 164*(5), 761–767.

Frankl, VE. (1959). *Man's Search for Meaning.* New York: Simon & Schuster.

Friedman ES, Wright JH, Jarrett RB, Thase ME. (2006). Combining cognitive therapy and medication for mood disorders. *Psychiatric Annals, 36*(5), 320–328.

Gaynes BN, Warden D, Trivedi MH, Wisniewski SR, Fava M, & Rush AJ. (2009). What did STAR*D teach us? Results from a large-scale, practical, clinical trial for patients with depression. *Psychiatric Services, 60*(11), 1439–1445.

Gelenberg AJ. (2009). And a one, and a two … exercise for depression. *Biological Therapies in Psychiatry, 32*(11).

Gelenberg AJ. (2009). Folate and depression. *Biologic Therapies in Psychiatry, 32*(8), 29–30.

Gelenberg AJ. (2010). Diet and depression. *Biological Therapies in Psychiatry, 33*(3), 12–13.

Gelenberg AJ. (2010). Treating persistent insomnia: Therapy, meds, or both? *Biological Therapies in Psychiatry, 33*(3), 11–12.

Germer CK. (2009). *The Mindful Path to Self-Compassion.* New York: Guilford Press.

Goering PN, Lancee WJ, & Freeman SJ. (1992). Marital support and recovery from depression. *British Journal of Psychiatry, 160*, 76–82.

Hayes SC, Strosahl K, & Wilson KG. (1999). *Acceptance and Commitment Therapy: An Experiential Approach to Behavior Change.* New York: Guilford Press.

Hollon SD, DeRubeis RJ, Evans MD, Wiemer MJ, Garvey MJ, Grove WM, & Tuason VB. (1992). Cognitive therapy and pharmacotherapy for depression: Singly and in combination. *Archives of General Psychiatry, 49*, 774–781.

Hollon SD, DeRubeis RJ, & Seligman MEP. (1992). Cognitive therapy and the prevention of depression. *Applied and Preventive Psychology, 1*, 89–95.

Hollon SD, Jarrett RB, Nierenberg AA, Thase ME, Trivedi M, & Rush AJ. (2005, April). Psychotherapy and medication in the treatment of adult and geriatric depression: Which monotherapy or combined treatment? *Journal of Clinical Psychiatry, 66*(4), 455–468.

Jacka FN, Pasco JA, Mykletun A, Williams LJ, Hodge AM, O'Reilly SL, et al. (2010). Association of Western and traditional diets with depression and anxiety in women. *American Journal of Psychiatry, 167*(3), 305–311.

Jacobson NS, Dobson KS, Truax PA, Addis ME, Koerner K, Gollan JK, et al. (1996). A component analysis of cognitive-behavioral treatment for depression. *Journal of Consulting and Clinical Psychology, 64*(2), 295–304.

Kabat-Zinn J. (1990). *Full Catastrophe Living: Using the Wisdom of Your Body to Fight Stress, Pain, and Illness*. New York: Hyperion.

Kabat-Zinn J. (2005). *Wherever You Go, There You Are: Mindfulness, Meditation in Everyday Life*. New York: Hyperion.

Keller MB, Kocsis JH, Thase ME, Gelenberg AJ, Rush AJ, Koran L, et al. (1998). Maintenance phase efficacy of sertraline for chronic depression. *Journal of American Medical Association, 280*(19), 1665–1672.

Kingston T, Dooley B, Bates A, Lawlor E, & Malone K. (2007). Mindfulness-based cognitive therapy for residual depressive symptoms. *The British Psychological Society, 80*, 193–203.

Kirsch, I. (2009). Antidepressants and the placebo response. *Epidemiologia e Psichiatria Sociale, 18*(4), 318–322.

Koenig HG. (2007). Spirituality and depression: A look at the evidence. *Southern Medical Journal, 100*(7), 737–739.

Koenig HG. (2008). *Medicine, Religion and Health: Where Science and Spirituality Meet*. West Conshohocken, PA: Templeton Foundation Press.

Kushner HS. (1981). *When Bad Things Happen to Good People*. New York: Schocken Books.

Kuyken W, Byford S, Taylor RS, Watkins E, Holden E, White K, et al. (2008). Mindfulness-based cognitive therapy to prevent relapse in recurrent depression. *Journal of Consulting and Clinical Psychology, 76*(6), 966–978.

Lazar SW, Kerr C, Wasserman RJ, Gray JR, Greve D, Treadway MT, et al. (2005). Meditation experience is associated with increased cortical thickness. *NeuroReport, 16*(17), 1893–1897.

Lewis TG. (2002). *Finding God: Praying the Psalms in Times of Depression*. Louisville, KY: Westminster John Knox Press.

Lin PY, & Su KP. (2007). A meta-analytic review of double-blind, placebo-controlled trials of antidepressant efficacy of omega-3 fatty acids. *Journal of Clinical Psychiatry, 68*(7), 1056–1061.

Lutz A, Brefczynski-Lewis J, Johnstone T, & Davidson RJ. (2008). Regulation of the neural circuitry of emotion by compassion meditation: Effects of meditative expertise. *PLoS ONE, 3*(3), e1897.

Martinez M, Marangell LB, & Martinez JM. (2011). Psychopharmacology. In RF Hales, SC Yudofsky, & GO Gabbard (Eds.), *Essentials of Psychiatry* (3rd ed., pp. 455–524). Washington, DC: American Psychiatric Publishing.

Maselko J, Gilman SE, & Buka S. (2009). Religious service attendance and spiritual well-being are differentially associated with risk of major depression. *Psychological Medicine, 39*(6), 1009–1017.

May GG. (2004). *The Dark Night of the Soul: A Psychiatrist Explores the Connection between Darkness and Spiritual Growth*. New York: HarperCollins.

Moore T. (1992). *Care of the Soul: A Guide for Cultivating Depth and Sacredness in Everyday Life*. New York: HarperCollins.

National Institutes of Health. (2005, June 13–15). Consensus and State-of-the-Science Statements. *NIH State-of-the-Science Conference Statement on Manifestations and Management of Chronic Insomnia in Adults, 22*(2), 1–30.

Nelson CJ, Jacobson CM, Weinberger MI, Bhaskaran V, Rosenfeld B, Breitbart W, et al. (2009, October). The role of spirituality in the relationship between religiosity and depression in prostate cancer patients. *Annals of Behavioral Medicine, 38*(2), 105–114.

Nemeroff CB. (2008). Recent findings in the pathophysiology of depression. *Focus, 6*(1), 3–14.

Ohayon MM, & Schatzberg AF. (2003). Using chronic pain to predict depressive morbidity in the general population. *Archives of General Psychiatry, 60*(1), 39–47.

Papakostas GI. (2009). Managing partial response or nonresponse: Switching, augmentation, and combination strategies for major depressive disorder. *Journal of Clinical Psychiatry, 70*(Suppl. 6), 16–25.

Papakostas GI, Mischoulon D, Shyu I, Alpert JE, & Fava M. (2010). S-adenosyl methionine (SAMe) augmentation of serotonin reuptake inhibitors for antidepressant nonresponders with major depressive disorder: A double-blind, randomized clinical trial. *American Journal of Psychiatry, 167,* 942–948.

Rocha DM, Vilarim MM, & Nardi AE. (2010). What is the effectiveness of the use of polyunsaturated fatty acid omega-3 in the treatment of depression? *Expert Review of Neurotherapeutics, 1*(7), 1117–1129.

Rohan KJ, Roecklein KA, Tierney LK, Lindsey KT, Johnson LG, Lippy RD, et al. (2007). A randomized controlled trial of cognitive-behavioral therapy, light therapy, and their combination for seasonal affective disorder. *Journal of Consulting and Clinical Psychology, 75*(3), 489–500.

Rose N, Koperski S, & Golomb BA. (2010). Mood food: Chocolate and depressive symptoms in a cross-sectional analysis. *Archives of Internal Medicine, 170*(8), 699–703.

Ryff CD, & Singer B. (1996). Psychological well-being: meaning, measurement, and implications for psychotherapy research. *Psychotherapy and Psychosomatics, 65*(1), 14–23.

Saeed SA, Bloch RM, Antonacci MD, Davis CE, & Manuel C. (2009). CAM for your depressed patient: Six recommended options. *Current Psychiatry, 8*(10), 39–47.

Sanchez-Villegas A, Delgado-Rodriguez M, Alonso A, Schlatter J, Lahortiga F, Majem LS, et al. (2009). Association of the Mediterranean dietary pattern with the incidence of depression in primary care. *Archives of General Psychiatry, 66*(10), 1090–1098.

Sarris J, Schoendorfer N, & Kavanagh DJ. (2009). Major depressive disorder and nutritional medicine: A review of monotherapies and adjuvant treatments. *Nutrition Reviews, 67*(3), 125–131.

Schatzberg AF, & Nemeroff CB. (2006). *Essentials of Clinical Psychopharmacology* (2nd ed.). Arlington, VA: American Psychiatric Publishing.

Schwartz DJ, Kohler WC, & Karatinos G. (2005). Symptoms of depression in individuals with obstructive sleep apnea may be amenable to treatment with continuous positive airway pressure. *Chest, 128*(3), 1304–1309.

Segal ZV, Bieling P, Young T, MacQueen G, Cooke R, Martin L, et al. (2010). Antidepressant monotherapy vs. sequential pharmacotherapy and mindfulness-based cognitive therapy, or placebo, for relapse prophylaxis in recurrent depression. *Archives of General Psychiatry, 67*(12), 1256–1264.

Shelton, RC. (2009). Long-term management of depression: Tips for adjusting the treatment plan as the patient's needs change. *Journal of Clinical Psychiatry, 70*(Suppl. 6), 32–37.

Shipowick CD, Moore CB, Corbett C, & Bindler R. (2009). Vitamin D and depressive symptoms in women during the winter: A pilot study. *Applied Nursing Research, 22*(3), 221–225.

Siegel, RD. (2010). *The Mindfulness Solution.* New York: Guilford Press.

Spurgeon JA, & Wright JH. (2010). Computer-assisted cognitive-behavioral therapy. *Current Psychiatry Reports, 12,* 547–552.

Teasdale JD, Segal ZV, Williams JMG, Ridgeway VA, Soulsby JM, & Lau MA. (2000). Prevention of relapse/recurrence in major depression by mindfulness-based cognitive therapy. *Journal of Consulting and Clinical Psychology, 68*(4), 615–623.

Viscott D. (1983). *How to Live with Another Person.* New York: Pocket Publishing.

Walsh R. (2000). *Essential Spirituality: The Seven Central Practices to Awaken Heart and Mind.* New York: Wiley.

Weissman MM, Markowitz JC, & Klerman GL. (2000). *Comprehensive Guide to Interpersonal Psychotherapy.* New York: Basic Books.

Westrin A, & Lam RW. (2007). Seasonal affective disorder: A clinical update. *Annals of Clinical Psychiatry, 19*(4), 239–246.

Williams M, Teasdale JD, Segal ZV, & Kabat-Zinn J. (2007). *The Mindful Way through Depression.* New York: Guilford Press.

Wright JH, & Basco MR. (2002). *Getting Your Life Back: The Complete Guide to Recovery from Depression.* New York: Touchstone.

Index

Bold indicates an exercise.

367

About the Authors

Jesse H. Wright, MD, PhD, is Professor of Psychiatry and Director of the Depression Center at the University of Louisville. A well-known authority on depression and cognitive-behavior therapy, he is the author of award-winning books for both the general public and professionals. Dr. Wright was Founding President of the Academy of Cognitive Therapy, is a Fellow of the American College of Psychiatrists, and received the Distinguished Educator of the Year Award from the University of Louisville.

Laura W. McCray, MD, practices family medicine in Burlington, Vermont, with a focus on mental health in primary care. She is Clinical Assistant Professor of Family Medicine and Associate Director of the Family Medicine Residency Program at the University of Vermont. A recipient of four Family Medicine Teaching Awards from the University of Pennsylvania and the University of Vermont, Dr. McCray lives in rural Vermont with her husband and young son. She is very pleased to be collaborating with her father on this book.

THE GUILFORD SELF-HELP WORKBOOK SERIES
Martin M. Antony, Series Editor

Workbooks in this series are crafted by respected scientists who are also seasoned therapists. Each volume addresses a specific psychological or emotional problem, putting powerful change strategies directly into the reader's hands. Special features include self-assessment tools, worksheets, skills-building exercises, and examples—plus the support and motivation readers need to achieve their goals.

The Anti-Anxiety Workbook: Proven Strategies to Overcome Worry,
Phobias, Panic, and Obsessions
Martin M. Antony and Peter J. Norton

Getting Over OCD: A 10-Step Workbook for Taking Back Your Life
Jonathan S. Abramowitz

Breaking Free from Depression: Pathways to Wellness
Jesse H. Wright and Laura W. McCray

Breaking Free from Depression